The Road to a Healthy Heart

Runs Through the Kitchen

The Road to a Healthy Heart

Runs Through the Kitchen

by Joseph C. Piscatella

Recipes by Bernie Piscatella

Workman Publishing • New York

Library of Congress Cataloging-in-Publication Data

Piscatella, Joseph C.
The road to a healthy heart runs through the kitchen / by Joseph C. Piscatella ; recipes by Bernie Piscatella.
  p. cm.
Includes index.
ISBN-13: 978-0-7611-3518-0; ISBN-10: 0-7611-3518-9 (alk. paper)
ISBN-10: 0-7611-4092-1; ISBN-13: 978-0-7611-4092-4 (HC)
1. Heart—Diseases—Diet therapy. 2. Heart—Diseases—Diet therapy—Recipes.
3. Heart—Diseases—Nutritional aspects. I. Piscatella, Bernie. II. Title

RC684.D5P58 2005
616.1'20654—dc22   2005056966

Cover design by Paul Gamarello
Cover photos by Rich Frishman (front) and Scott Leen (back)

Workman books are available at special discounts when purchased in bulk for premiums and sales promotions as well as for fund-raising or educational use. Special editions or book excerpts can also be created to specification. For details, contact the Special Sales Director at the address below.

Workman Publishing Company, Inc.
708 Broadway
New York, NY 10003-9555
www.workman.com

First printing November 2005
10 9 8 7 6 5 4 3 2 1

The material in this book is provided for information only and should not be construed as medical advice or instruction. Always consult with your physician or other appropriate health professionals before making any changes in diet, physical activity and/or drug therapy.

*As always,
this book is for Bernie.
Thank you for a lifetime of
answered prayers.*

Foreword

Joe Piscatella is not a physician or a Ph.D., but he knows more about healthy eating and the health impact of our dietary choices than any doctor out there. After his coronary bypass operation in 1977, he began a crash course in heart-healthy eating and wrote his first book just five years later. That best-selling book, the *Don't Eat Your Heart Out Cookbook,* was the product of his efforts to keep alive and yet eat food that his wife and two kids would also enjoy. Six more successful books followed, including *Fat-Proof Your Child* and *Take a Load off Your Heart,* and now comes *The Road to a Healthy Heart Runs Through the Kitchen.* This new one discusses the most up-to-date scientific evidence, in a very understandable way, and shows you how to apply that science to everyday eating. By following his Mediterranean-style diet, you not only take care of your heart but enjoy meals and snacks that satisfy your taste buds.

His book is packed full of facts and sound advice. For instance, we learn that the daily requirement for fat can be fully satisfied by consuming the equivalent of one teaspoon of vegetable oil, but the average American eats eight times that amount—the equivalent of one full stick of butter each day—and gains one to two pounds each year from age 20 to 50. Yet Mr. Piscatella does not advocate avoiding fat, since an extremely low-fat diet is too hard to follow. His Mediterranean-style diet includes moderate amounts of the good fats, which he identifies in the text portion of the book.

He also emphasizes the proper role of carbohydrates in a healthy diet: more complex carbohydrates and fewer refined carbs, such as white bread, cookies and cakes. He points out that complex carbohydrates are about the most nutritious foods on the planet and aid in weight control because they contain bulk, mass and fiber but are not calorically dense. As he says, "They will fill you up, not out."

And finally, he shows that extreme eating is never a solution. Rather than banning this food or eating nothing but that food, the smartest approach is a program of balanced eating. This can include "discretionary calories," such as the occasional hamburger or piece of cake, but mainly promotes the fruits, vegetables and whole grains that are central to the Mediterranean-style diet. He is also not against eating out; instead, he is for eating properly whether you're out or at home. And he doesn't forget the importance of exercise.

In summary, this is a splendid book. When I was in medical school from 1954 to 1958, my class did not receive a single lecture on nutrition or foods or calories. When I graduated from medical school, I did not know the caloric content of any food. Since then, I've collected about 150 books on nutrition and healthy eating, and the Piscatella ones are my favorites. If we all followed his advice, the health of this nation would skyrocket.

William C. Roberts, M.D.
Director, Baylor Heart & Vascular Institute,
Baylor University Medical Center,
Dallas, Texas
Editor in Chief, *The American Journal*
of Cardiology

Contents

Part One
Starting Out

Part Two
On the Cutting Edge

Part Three
Getting Practical

Cookbook

A NOTE TO THE READER

It will be very hard (and maybe impossible) for some of you to resist going directly to the recipe section of the book. I understand. When I first learned I had heart disease, I wanted to do something right away and had little patience for learning why. If that describes you, go ahead . . . jump right to the back and start cooking. But then, after you've enjoyed a week or two of heart-healthy eating, I urge you to come back to the beginning and read up on what the right sort of foods can do for your heart. Over the long haul, you'll need to engage your head—along with your stomach—in the quest for a lifestyle that will really make a difference.

Introduction

L OOKING BACK, I WISH I COULD SAY my commitment to healthy eating was the result of native intelligence. But that wouldn't be true. It was born purely out of need. For the first 32 years of my life, healthy eating had taken a backseat to other, seemingly more important issues. Besides, I'd always been in good health. Sure, there were things that could be improved. At around 250, my cholesterol was certainly high, but in the mid-1970s many doctors considered that level to be "average" and not a cause for alarm. And I could stand to lose a few pounds. There would be plenty of time, I thought, to improve my diet and my health in the future.

Then, in July 1977, I found out how wrong I had been. For the second time in a week, I was sitting in the office of Dr. John Nagle, a prominent cardiologist in Tacoma, Washington. I'd gone to see my family physician, Dr. James Early, five days earlier because I'd been experiencing shortness of breath and a low-grade but nagging chest pain as I warmed up to play tennis. The pain was dull, more like a feeling of fullness, and it would usually disappear by the end of the warm-up. But one day it stayed with me through two hours of play, so I called Dr. Early. "I've got a problem in my lungs, probably a touch of bronchitis," I told him. He asked me to come in right away. I had seen him just four months earlier for my annual physical, and the results were excellent, so I wasn't expecting anything more than a quick visit and perhaps a prescription.

This time, however, my electrocardiogram indicated an obstruction of a coronary artery.

Dr. Early said there was no evidence of a heart attack, but he wanted me to see a cardiologist that same afternoon. Three hours later, I found myself undergoing a thorough cardiac examination with

Dr. Nagle. I was given an exercise stress test, which indicated that the cardiac muscle wasn't getting enough blood, but it would take an X-ray to determine the extent of the problem. A thin plastic tube was inserted into an artery in my leg and threaded into my heart. Then a dye was injected into the tube, and Dr. Nagle traced its progress through my coronary arteries.

Now we were ready to review the results. Dr. Nagle began speaking. He told me that my chest pain was caused by three arterial blockages, ranging from 50% to 95%. "This is called coronary heart disease," he said. "Buildups of fat and cholesterol are interfering with blood flow to your heart. The largest blockage is badly located. A blood clot could seal off the opening and trigger a fatal heart attack. I recommend immediate coronary bypass surgery . . ." There was more, but those words hit me like a hard slap in the face. *Just get up and leave,* I told myself. *You're not supposed to be here.*

Like most people, I knew something about the workings of the heart and the coronary arteries, but the information was chiefly of the Biology 101 variety. Some decent information was out there, but what did it have to do with me, a young guy in the prime of his life? Unknowingly, I had succumbed to the "what I don't know won't hurt me" syndrome. In reality, however, what I didn't know could not only hurt me, it could kill me.

Facing Reality

As the diagnosis sank in on that July afternoon, my own age of innocence and ignorance came to an end. My initial reaction was the typical "Why me?" response. Bernie and I had not yet celebrated our 10th wedding anniversary. Our daughter was six; our son was just four. I was in the midst of building a career and contributing to my community. Then I remembered reading a comment by President John F. Kennedy reflecting the fact that life was basically unfair—that unfairness was part of its nature. The randomness of death existed for everyone. All at once, I understood. Why *not* me?

I was gripped by pure, stomach-churning fear. Old age was something I had always looked forward to sharing with Bernie and my kids. Now I had to face the fact that death not only *could* happen in the near future, but probably *would* happen as a result of the time bomb inside my chest. As we talked that day, Dr. Nagle calmly and deliberately explained the many facets of my situation. Soon the late afternoon shadows began to turn into evening twilight, and I was suddenly aware of the importance of time.

Less than a week later, Dr. Kari Vitikainen, a gifted cardiac surgeon, performed a five-hour operation in which a piece of vein was taken from my left leg and used to create a new arterial channel. The new channel literally bypassed the blocked area, allowing blood to again flow freely to my heart.

Ten days after surgery, I went home to recover, happy to be alive but very concerned about my future. Bypass had not "cured" me. Dr. Early put it in perspective: "You had heart disease the day before surgery, you had heart disease the day after surgery, and you have it today as well. The surgery took away the pain and the threat of an imminent heart attack. But it did not remove the disease. Only a change in your lifestyle can reduce your future heart attack risk."

This knowledge was complicated by the prediction of another doctor, a well-known lipids specialist at a national university. I saw him after the surgery for advice on how to manage my cholesterol.

"Shouldn't I change my diet?" I asked.

"Don't bother," he said. "You have an aggressive form of coronary heart disease at a very early age. I'm not sure what you can do to help yourself. Frankly, I'd be surprised if you live to be forty."

Now, for the first time, I was mad! *He's wrong,* I thought. *I'm going to find a way to beat this disease.* My anger and determination became the twin foundations of a resolve to eat a better diet and live a healthier life. Finally, I had reached a point in time when I was ready to listen and learn. Once again, I turned to Dr. Nagle. "My advice is for you to focus on making healthy lifestyle changes," he said. "You need to find a new diet pattern that meets your physical and emotional needs, fits your way of life and can be sustained for the long term. And you have to make it work in the real world. Only you and Bernie can do that."

And so, in the midst of much confusion, we began.

The Mediterranean-Style Diet

When I started to collect information, to simply figure out what to do, the connection between diet and heart health was still controversial. One cardiologist who saw the importance of diet was Dr. John Farquhar of Stanford University Medical School.

I met Dr. Farquhar at a cardiac conference where he delivered a lecture called "The American Diet May Be Hazardous to Your Health." I had listened to a number of speakers at this conference and had yet to learn anything that helped with daily living—that answered the basic question *What can I eat today?* That question was addressed in Dr. Farquhar's discussion of the late Dr. Ancel Keys, a pioneer in cardiac research. In the early 1950s, Dr. Keys went to Italy to observe a curious dichotomy. Italians ate much more fat in their diet than Americans did, yet heart disease was virtually unheard of in their country. While Americans were feasting on steak and potatoes, white bread and butter, and whole milk, Italians ate very few animal foods and favored fruits, vegetables, whole grains, olive oil and wine. Could there be a link between diet and health?

Compelled to learn the answer, Dr. Keys instituted the Seven Countries Study, in which diet, blood cholesterol and frequency of heart attack were measured in communities in Finland, Greece, Italy, Japan, the Netherlands, the United States and Yugoslavia. In all, some 12,000 men in the 40-to-49 age range were tested and observed. The study illustrated that cultures in which saturated fat made up a significant percentage of total caloric intake demonstrated elevated cholesterol levels and a higher incidence of coronary heart disease than cultures with a lower percentage. Thus the Finns, who ate 20% of their calories as saturated fat, had cholesterol levels that averaged 265. The Japanese ate only 5% of their calories as saturated fat and had correspondingly lower cholesterol levels, averaging just 165. A most important point was that the heart attack rate for middle-aged Finnish men was six times greater than for Japanese men of the same age. American men in the study had a heart disease rate twice that of Italian men and four times that of Greek men. Dr. Keys' conclusion: "Saturated fat in the diet leads to high blood cholesterol and then to heart attacks."

As Dr. Farquhar clearly connected the dots between diet, cholesterol and heart disease, he provided a realistic vision of how to eat. His recommendation was the same as that of Dr. Keys: a *Mediterranean diet* emulating the traditional eating habits of southern Europe (Italy, Spain, Portugal and southern France), parts of North Africa (especially Morocco and Tunisia), parts of Turkey and parts of the Middle East (especially Lebanon and Syria). This diet emphasizes food from plant sources, such as whole grains, fruit, vegetables, nuts and olive oil. It also includes moderate amounts of poultry and fish while restricting meat, processed foods and refined grains.

The Mediterranean approach made great sense to me on a scientific level, since heart health is not based on either eating or eliminating a single food group. Instead, the Mediterranean diet looked to a combination of healthy factors. It wasn't just about what you *didn't* eat; it was also about what you *did* eat. But while the Mediterranean diet appealed to both my brain and my taste buds, significant obstacles were in the way of its implementation. For one thing, I didn't live in a country that would support this dietary lifestyle. Consider the contrast between a hypothetical "Mediterranean man" and an "American man":

■ The Mediterranean man eats whole-grain bread for breakfast, then walks to work in the fresh air. The American man grabs a doughnut (rich in added sugar, trans fat and calories) to fortify a stressful freeway commute.

■ The Mediterranean man eats his main meal at midday and centers it on vegetables, whole-grain bread, cheese, yogurt, fruit and perhaps a glass of wine. After a sedentary morning in front of a computer screen, the American man makes quick work of a cheeseburger or a deli sandwich and washes it down with a soft drink.

■ Both men work until six o'clock. The Mediterranean man comes home to a light meal of salad, a small bowl of pasta and fruit. Dinner with family and friends lasts 90 minutes, followed by a stroll in the piazza. The American man brings home Chinese takeout for dinner. The kids have soccer practice and his wife is working late, so he eats his dinner in 15 minutes of solitude in front of the TV set.

Bernie and I were well aware of these differences. We had lived as students in Italy, where lunch was the main meal, supper was light, fresh fruits and vegetables were in abundance, people walked everywhere and the lifestyle was neither hurried nor harried. But now we lived in the United States, where, like everyone else, we were pressed for time. On more days than not, lunch was a quick sandwich and the main meal was steak and potatoes.

Another obstacle. The Mediterranean diet included meat about once a month, fish and chicken once a week or so, and milk virtually never. But I *liked* meat and milk! If I had to restrict meat to once a month and give up milk altogether, the diet was doomed to fail. So, instead of adopting the Mediterranean diet as it was traditionally eaten, we adapted it to our way of life and food preferences. It became a *Mediterranean-style* diet that took the principles of healthy Mediterranean eating and applied them to the American lifestyle. For example, I ate meat, fish and poultry more often than Mediterranean people do, but a lot less frequently than the typical American. Fat-free milk was included in my new diet, as were soy foods.

The Mediterranean-style diet was a great compromise in favor of balance, familiarity, taste and practicality. Bernie cooked meal after meal, trying new recipes and adapting old ones. She took our family favorites and began to make them healthier without sacrificing taste.

This was neither an easy nor a quick effort. Progress was slow and measured in small increments. Trial-and-error ruled. Some meals were disasters; others were great. Some new cooking techniques worked well; others did not and had to be abandoned. But Bernie's focus never strayed. From each bit of experience, she gleaned new information, insight and techniques. We were building the proverbial bicycle as it was being ridden, but we kept at it, knowing that the alternative—returning to our old diet—was not the answer.

Finally, progress started to take root, and a new, healthier way of eating began to take shape. Bernie's techniques and recipes had made it possible.

The Road Back

After six months, my biometric measurements—weight, cholesterol, triglycerides, blood pressure—had improved dramatically. Dr. Nagle remarked that all his cardiac patients and their families should follow what we were doing. He asked if we would put our dietary experience into a book, and that's how the *Don't Eat Your Heart Out Cookbook* came to be.

I never planned to write books on diet and heart health. That first book and the books that followed were the product of our work to beat the odds and keep me alive. But for more than 20 years, they've been dietary bibles for other heart patients and for people interested in preventing heart disease. Endorsed by health professionals and used by thousands of hospitals in cardiac rehabilitation programs, they offer a blend of current science, commonsense advice, meal plans and delicious recipes that have helped millions of people eat better, lose weight, lower cholesterol and improve heart health. Two of the books, the *Don't Eat Your Heart Out Cookbook* and *Take a Load off Your Heart*, have been presented by PBS as television specials.

So, why this new book? First, we know far more today about what constitutes a heart-healthy diet than we knew in the past. This is reflected in the current USDA Dietary Guidelines, which call for more fiber-rich fruit, colorful vegetables and whole grains every day, while limiting foods with saturated fat, trans fat, salt (sodium) and added sweeteners. In addition, a number of foods have now been identified as providing health benefits beyond basic nutrition, such as playing a role in reducing the risk of heart disease. These "functional foods" are central to the balanced dietary program presented here.

Next, the American dietary lifestyle has changed over the last decade—and not necessarily for the better. Home cooking and eating together as a family have virtually disappeared. Instead, we take out, order in, open cans and microwave prepackaged meals, or just head for a restaurant to gobble down supersized servings. Life may be more stressful and move at a faster pace than in the past, but the plain fact is that we have to get back to whole foods, unprocessed and easily prepared. This book has information, tips, menus, a realistic "pick-and-choose" meal plan and over 300 recipes to help you do this efficiently and effectively.

And finally, I'm still here, almost 30 years after bypass surgery, which should say something about the effectiveness of my balanced-eating program. I haven't been seduced by fad diets that ban entire food groups, and I don't subscribe to one-dimensional eating: one week spareribs, the next week grapefruit. Unlike those diets, which are strong on theory but fail to produce long-term results, my program has staying power. And it works in the real world. I recently celebrated the 28th anniversary of my bypass surgery by hiking on Mount Rainier with Bernie. I've experienced the joy of seeing our daughter and son graduate from high school, college and graduate school; of walking our daughter down the aisle and making a toast at our son's wedding; of celebrating 38 years of marriage; and of holding our first grandchild. None of this would have happened without the principles of healthy eating set forth in this book.

Joe Piscatella

Part One

Starting
Out

Chapter One

Understanding Your Heart

F ROM THE EARLIEST TIMES, we've used the heart as a symbol of courage, kindness, generosity and love—all the highest ideals of the human spirit. But what about the heart itself? When poets were writing about sweethearts and hearts of gold, how much did they know about the real thing? Beating more than 4,000 times each hour, this amazing organ pumps blood through 60,000 miles of vessels throughout our bodies. And it does this day after day, year after year, with little or no help from us. Yet even in today's atmosphere of scientific inquiry, knowledge about the heart is still building among the experts as well as the general public.

Given the awesome amount of work it does, people tend to think of the heart as one of our largest organs. In fact, it's quite small, about the size of a man's clenched fist, and usually weighs between 7 and 12 ounces depending on the size of the individual. Another misconception is that the heart is located on the left side of the chest cavity; in fact, it sits in the center, nestled between the lungs. And finally, the heart is not "heart-shaped." It might come as a shock to romantics and candy manufacturers, but the heart looks a lot like an eggplant. Can you imagine eggplant-shaped lockets, valentine cards and boxes of chocolate? For most of us, this might take "truth in advertising" a step too far!

The Heart at Work

Picture a freeway system connected to a city with a line of food trucks on the incoming roads and a caravan of refuse trucks on the outgoing roads. The life of the city depends on the constant movement of these vehicles; any slowing or stopping could result in famine or disease. It's the same for our vascular system. Blood must circulate nonstop to nourish and cleanse the 300 trillion cells that make up the human body. Each of these cells needs to receive oxygen and nutrients and expel waste products, and this process of "in with the good, out with the bad" must occur continuously if the cells are to remain healthy. Of critical importance is an uninterrupted supply of oxygen, since no cell can live for more than about 30 minutes without it. Some cells, notably those in the brain and heart, survive for a much shorter time when deprived of oxygen.

TWO PUMPS IN ONE

While the heart is considered a single organ, for all practical purposes it's two distinct pumps working together. Separated by a wall of muscle, each pump has an atrium, or holding chamber, and a ventricle, or pumping chamber.

A CROSS SECTION OF THE HUMAN HEART

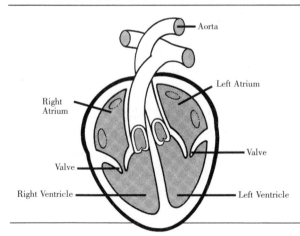

Aorta

Left Atrium

Right Atrium

Valve

Valve

Right Ventricle

Left Ventricle

The right side of the heart (at left in the illustration) collects blood from the body and pumps it into the lungs. The left side receives oxygenated blood from the lungs and pumps it back out to the body through the aorta.

Blood from the veins fills the right atrium and passes into the right ventricle, which pumps it to the lungs. The lungs cleanse this blood of carbon dioxide, supply it with oxygen and send it to the left atrium, from which it passes to the left ventricle below. The left ventricle is the powerhouse, the chamber

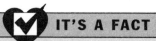

IT'S A FACT

The heart pumps with such force that it takes only about 24 seconds for a drop of blood to make a round trip through the body.

that pumps oxygenated blood to distant parts of the body through arteries and into tiny capillaries that may be only 1/2,500th of an inch in diameter. Even when you're sound asleep or just reading or watching television, your heart is beating 50 to 80 times a minute, steadily pumping about five quarts of blood to your brain and every other vital organ.

THE CORONARY ARTERIES

It may be a super organ in terms of energy and efficiency, but the heart needs its own constant supply of blood in order to do its job. Surprisingly, the gallons of blood that pass through its chambers cannot be used for this purpose. Only blood that reaches the heart through the coronary arteries can provide the nourishment it requries. That's why the health of these arteries is essential to proper cardiac functioning.

By establishing the coronary arteries as the supply line for the heart, nature has devised an almost perfect method of delivery. Each time the heart pumps oxygenated blood to the body, a portion of that blood is siphoned through the coronary arteries back to the heart itself, like a commission received for work performed. When everything is working properly, 95% of the oxygenated blood is supplied to the body and 5% goes to the heart.

Unfortunately, the design of this delivery system has a fundamental flaw. The coronary arteries are extremely small, and any narrowing or clotting can easily impede the flow of oxygenated blood to the

THE CORONARY ARTERIES

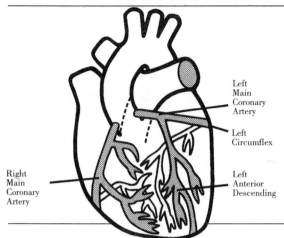

Descending from the aorta, the two principal coronary arteries curl around the surface of the heart and divide into numerous smaller branches that penetrate the muscle, ensuring a continuous blood supply to every region of the heart.

Left Main Coronary Artery

Left Circumflex

Right Main Coronary Artery

Left Anterior Descending

heart. The first sign of damage usually appears in the delicate artery lining called the endothelium. Risk factors such as smoking, high cholesterol levels and high blood pressure can cause injury to this lining so that it roughens in places where cholesterol can collect. Plaque forms at these sites, making the artery itself a weak link in the circulatory chain.

Heart Disease 101

Currently, an estimated 100 million Americans, or about half the adult population, are afflicted with cardiovascular disease, which includes coronary heart disease, high blood pressure and rheumatic heart disease. And, while AIDS and accidents may get the headlines, cardiovascular disease has the deadly distinction of being the number one killer, taking the lives of over a million Americans each year.

The type of cardiovascular disease most responsible for heart attacks is called coronary heart disease. This is the disease I have, along with some 13 million other Americans. Every year, coronary heart disease contributes to more than 1.5 million heart attacks and as many as 800,000 deaths.

SOME HARD FACTS

There is a general feeling that the war against heart disease is being won, but the opposite is true. "The reality," says Dr. Jan L. Breslow, former president of the American Heart Association, "is that the prevalence of the disease is increasing." This discouraging observation is echoed by Dr. Edward Schneider of the University of Southern California, who states, "A hundred years from now, people will look back and realize there was an epidemic of coronary heart disease in the western world that was unique in history. The tragedy is that much of it was—and is—preventable."

A second misconception has to do with *who* gets heart disease. Some people still believe that only men are at risk. (A woman once told me, "I came to your seminar to take notes for my husband. I'm not concerned myself, because women get to circumvent heart disease.") In truth, heart disease is just delayed in women. Men tend to develop signs of the disease about age 40. It usually occurs in women after menopause, when hormonal protection (estrogen) is no longer in effect. Between ages 45 to 64, one out of nine women has heart disease; over age 65, the ratio is one out of three.

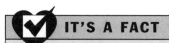 **IT'S A FACT**

Only 8% of American women realize that heart disease is a greater threat than cancer. Yet according to Dr. Nanette Wenger of Emory University Medical School, twice as many females die each year of heart and blood vessel disease as of all forms of cancer combined. Women also tend to have more complications after bypass surgery and heart attack. Whether this is related to their older age when they develop coronary heart disease or to their smaller coronary arteries is unclear.

HOW THE DISEASE DEVELOPS

Coronary heart disease begins when plaque forms on the interior walls of the coronary arteries, compressing the channel and severely obstructing blood flow to the heart. This process is often described as rust accumulating in an old water pipe. One doctor put it this way:

"If rust builds up in the pipe and narrows the opening, pretty soon there is no water at the tap. If plaque narrows the coronary arteries, pretty soon blood flow to the heart is compromised. Insufficient flow can produce chest pain. Stopping blood flow can result in a heart attack."

The buildup of plaque results in atherosclerosis, literally translated from the Greek as "hard mush." Blockages begin as soft, mushy clumps of cholesterol and fat and end up as deposits of hard, encrusted material, producing critical consequences by 1) narrowing the channel opening and gradually pinching off blood supply to the heart; 2) causing arteries to "harden" and impeding blood flow to the heart; 3) generating an inflammatory response in the arteries, which raises heart attack risk; and 4) causing plaque to rupture, producing a blood clot that could trigger a heart attack. The result is that a steady supply of oxygenated blood to the heart may no longer be available, a state that can seriously impair cardiac performance and put the heart—and life itself—at great risk.

A prime characteristic of coronary heart disease is its slow, silent progression over a period of 20 to 40 years, starting as early as childhood. Year after year, plaque continues to accumulate, the arteries harden and lose their elasticity, and the channel openings become more and more obstructed. The insidiousness of the disease lies in the fact that a person with severe blockages may have no symptoms at all until the moment when "sudden" manifestations of the disease appear.

ALL THE SIGNS

How do you know if you have coronary heart disease? As the disease progresses and arteries become compromised, many people experience *angina pectoris,* Latin for "pain in the chest." Angina occurs when the heart muscle receives insufficient oxygen, usually as the result of partial blockages in one or more of the coronary arteries. Symptoms are described as tightness, heaviness, numbness, burning, pressure or crushing pain behind the breastbone (one patient told me it felt like having an elephant sit on his chest) or a sharp pain in the jaw, neck, back or left arm. Frequently, angina is misinterpreted as gas pain or indigestion that will not go away. It's usually experienced more intensely by men than by women.

Doctors recommend seeking immediate medical care if the onset of angina is not relieved by rest and/or medication. New treatments, such as emergency balloon angioplasty and clot-busting drugs, can stop a heart attack and save heart muscle if you can get to a hospital within the first few hours of the onset of symptoms. While angina is not necessarily predictive of an impending heart attack, *it can be*. In fact, the American College of Cardiology recently broadened the definition of a heart attack to include many instances of angina. "This should be a positive thing," says Dr. Sidney Smith, former president of the American Heart Association. "It will get patients' attention and help them to focus on necessary behavior changes, such as stopping smoking and eating a low-fat diet."

A *heart attack,* or *myocardial infarction,* occurs when the heart's own blood supply is severely reduced or stopped completely. Cardiac muscle tissue is replaced by scar tissue, which lacks the ability to contract and expand and is therefore useless in the pumping activity. As a result, the undamaged area of the heart must work harder, creating additional stress on the unaffected muscle.

Heart attack symptoms typically include sharp chest pain, shortness of breath, fainting and nausea. According to the American Heart Association, men usually experience uncomfortable pressure, fullness, squeezing or pain in the center of the chest lasting more than a few minutes; sharp pain may also be felt in the shoulders and arms. Women generally experience pain that radiates through the neck, jaw, shoulders, arms or back; other symptoms include chest discomfort with nausea, sweating, shortness of breath, unexplained anxiety, fatigue or weakness, palpitations and/or lightheadedness. Acting on warning signs quickly can dramatically reduce the risk of coronary fatality. If you think you're having a heart attack, doctors advise chewing and swallowing one regular uncoated adult aspirin (325 mg). In fact, it's estimated that this recommendation, if widely adopted, would save an additional 5,000 to 10,000 lives in the United States each year.

The term *congestive heart failure* refers to a condition in which the heart has become a "weak pump." (Instead of pumping two or three ounces of blood with each beat, it may pump only one to two ounces of blood, putting serious strain on the cardiac engine.) Some three million Americans suffer from congestive heart failure, often as a consequence of muscle being replaced by scar tissue following a heart attack. The loss of pumping ability can have serious consequences, particularly if scarring has occurred only in the left ventricle. The undamaged right ventricle will continue to pump blood normally into the lungs, and the difference in pumping ability of the two chambers may cause blood to back up in the lungs and in the large veins in the legs; this disrupts the normal circulatory flow and causes distention of the tissues and a leaking of fluid into the abdomen and extremities. That's why people with congestive heart failure often have swelling in their ankles and feet, and weight gain due to edema, or the presence of abnormally large amounts of fluid in the tissues. If fluid backs up into the lungs, the result is a condition called pulmonary edema, or extreme shortness of breath.

Almost everyone has heard of someone who suddenly collapsed and died of a heart attack, often without known risks or warning signs. It seems like a mystery, but that's the nature of *sudden cardiac death*, also called *cardiac arrest*. SCD is not the same thing as a heart attack. The most common cause of this event is ventricular fibrillation. Under normal conditions, orderly electrical impulses signal the heart to pump blood throughout the body; however, during ventricular fibrillation, normal electrical impulses in the heart muscle suddenly stop, causing the lower chambers to quiver and cease pumping blood properly. As a result, there is an inadequate blood supply to all the organs, including the heart itself.

STROKE: A "BRAIN ATTACK"

When blockages caused by atherosclerosis interrupt blood flow to the heart, a heart attack occurs. When they cut off blood flow to the brain, a stroke results. The part of the brain that receives insufficient blood suffers damage and death to its cells and can no longer work. Neither can the part of the body it controls.

Because the similarities between a heart attack and a stroke are so great, strokes are often called "brain attacks." Every year, over 500,000 people suffer a stroke. Some of the most common consequences include speech impairment, paralysis, mobility loss, memory loss, mental confusion and visual disorders.

Fast treatment is critical to managing an episode of cardiac arrest. Immediate cardiopulmonary resuscitation (CPR) can be an important lifesaving technique. In addition, a doctor, nurse or trained paramedic can steady any potentially lethal irregular heart rhythms by using defibrillation paddles (the type you might have seen on *ER* and other TV shows). Specially modified, easier-to-operate defibrillators are now found in public places such as major airports, shopping malls and sports stadiums. A survival rate as high as 90% has been reported when defibrillation is achieved within the first minute of collapse.

The best way to reduce the risk of SCD is to modify behaviors that put you at high risk for coronary heart disease: eat a balanced diet, control your weight, exercise regularly and don't smoke. If you experience warning signs and symptoms such as lightheadedness, palpitations or extremely fast or irregular heart rhythms, medical evaluation is required. In some cases, patients with a history of resuscitated SCD, threatening rhythm irregularities or disease of the electrical conduction system of the heart may require a permanent pacemaker or defibrillator.

THE GOOD NEWS

For many years, heart disease and heart attacks were regarded as inevitable consequences of aging and genetics. Now, after more than 50 years of sustained investigation, specific conditions such as elevated cholesterol, high blood pressure and diabetes have been identified as critical risk factors.

Moreover, certain aspects of lifestyle have been shown to have great influence on cardiac functioning. Says Dr. William Roberts, editor in chief of the *American Journal of Cardiology*, "For every one person with heart disease because of family genes, there are 499 people who have it because of lifestyle decisions." And of these decisions, none are more influential than those concerning diet.

Reversal *Is* Possible

It's a well-known fact that coronary heart disease can be prevented. But what if you've already been diagnosed with the disease? What if you've had a heart attack or bypass surgery? Can you take action to reverse the disease and cause plaque to shrink? For many people, the answer appears to be "yes."

Recent studies suggest that lowering cholesterol can cause plaque to shrink at the rate of 1% to 2% per year. At first glance, these percentages may not seem significant. But coronary heart disease can progress at the rate of 2% to 4% a year when cholesterol levels remain high, which means the net gain from lowered cholesterol may be as much as 6% a year. The late Dr. David Blankenhorn at the University of Southern California and Dr. Greg Brown at the University of Washington directed two consequential trials using a combination of low-fat eating and drug therapy to reduce cholesterol. In both trials, the majority of patients with lowered cholesterol showed a slowing of disease progression. But even more noteworthy was the finding that coronary regression, a *reversal* of the disease process, was achieved in up to 30% of patients with significant cholesterol improvement.

Trials involving lifestyle changes alone, without drug therapy, have produced similar results. At the Preventive Medicine Research Institute, Dr. Dean Ornish studied 48 men and women whose coronary arteries were 40% to 100% clogged. The entire group was counseled to follow standard medical recommendations such as quitting smoking, exercising aerobically three times a week for 30 minutes and using stress dissipation techniques. However, about half the group followed the American Heart Association's 30% fat diet. The rest of the group ate a strict vegetarian diet with only about 10% of calories from fat, exercised moderately at least three hours a week, meditated regularly for stress management and met twice weekly in support group sessions. After a year, the first half showed an average drop in cholesterol of only 13 points, with either no improvement or a worsening of their disease. Conversely, the remaining participants showed an average drop in cholesterol of 55 points; more importantly, the vast majority showed less disease and 17 people experienced regression.

Virtually all physicians agree that eating less fat is necessary to improve cholesterol. But how *low* in fat you need to go is a matter of controversy. Dr. Ornish recommended a diet with no more than 10% of calories from fat. Other experts recommend higher fat levels. In Heidelberg, Germany, Dr. Gerhard Schuler conducted a study of 56 men who were suffering from angina due to partially blocked coronary arteries. These men were put on a fairly stringent diet of no more than 20% of calories from fat and a program of regular exercise (at least three hours per week). After a year, 60% of the participants showed no disease progression and 32% had experienced reversal. This study is particularly important because it helps to prove that coronary regression is achievable with a more moderate percentage of calories from fat and therefore a diet much easier to achieve in the real world.

The work of Drs. Ornish and Schuler illustrates the effectiveness of dietary changes along with other modifications of lifestyle. "What

---

DON'T STOP NOW!

Research shows that men who begin and then quit a healthy regimen actually *increase* their risk of heart attack. A study of 1,222 men revealed that the heart condition of those who dieted and exercised improved over time. After treatment stopped, however, they were more at risk than men who never had been treated. "If there is a message here, it's 'Don't stop,' not 'Don't start,'" says Dr. Stuart Rich, chief of cardiology at the University of Illinois at Chicago. And "Don't stop" is often dependent on a low-fat diet that is interesting, tasty and easy to stick to.

---

appears to happen first is that you stabilize the plaque," says Dr. John LaRosa of George Washington University. "So, even though the opening of the artery hasn't changed that much, the plaque is no longer susceptible to clot, spasm and hemorrhaging, which are the things that cause the final closing off of the blood vessel and trigger the heart attack." But while the outcomes of the Ornish and Schuler studies were much the same, the dietary guidelines of each program differed greatly. Dr. Ornish recommended a diet of about 10% fat consisting mostly of vegetables, grains, beans and fruit. No meat, poultry, fish or whole-milk products; in fact, no animal foods at all, except for a daily cup of nonfat milk or yogurt and the occasional egg white. A diet so low in fat doesn't promote long-term compliance, and Dr. Ornish himself admits that the point of his study was to determine what is *possible,* not what is *practicable.* While a very restrictive diet may be a useful goal for some people with significant coronary disease, this kind of extreme curtailment should certainly not be recommended as a lifetime plan for healthy people who simply want to manage their cholesterol levels and lose weight. Such a plan would just set them up for failure in the long run.

In the long run, Dr. Schuler's 20% fat diet is the more reasonable choice because it's easily practiced at home, as well as in restaurants, and offers a balance between taste and health that's critical to long-term compliance. The recommendation of the American Heart Association and the USDA guidelines is a diet with no more than 35% of calories from fat. In my own experience, a diet somewhere between 20% and 35% works best, provided that the fats eaten are healthy ones.

Working with an easy-to-use diet is especially important in light of the popularity of statin drugs. While they can be very effective in managing cholesterol, these drugs are not magic pills. "Don't think you can have prime rib for dinner, then double your statin drug and you're even," says Dr. John Nagle. "Drug therapy must be accompanied by healthy eating in order to get the most benefit from the drug." The point to remember is that stabilizing and reversing coronary heart disease has been established in numerous studies using diet and drugs. While more testing is necessary, using larger groups and improved methods, at this point the data provide much hope for cardiac patients. Findings show that each person with coronary heart disease has an opportunity through realistic lifestyle changes and, if necessary, drug therapy to avoid progression and improve chances for regression.

The findings of the studies discussed in this chapter also provide substantial proof that low-fat eating, by itself, is not a panacea. This fact takes on new meaning today, when we have a more global view of heart disease progression and reversal. Says Dr. Michael Mogadam of Georgetown University Medical School, "It's no longer just about lowering cholesterol. What is responsible for improved cardiovascular health and regression is a whole package of lifestyle changes—giving up cigarettes, stress management, exercise, weight loss, control of blood pressure, improving other lipid abnormalities and altering other risk factors. To give all the credit to a low-fat diet misses the point."

What makes sense, then, is to start by evaluating your own risk factors. As you'll see in the next chapter, not all of these factors have equal importance. Indeed, some of them—your age and gender, for example—will be beyond your control. But your personal lifestyle is in your own hands. If changes are warranted, it's up to you to make them. If you smoke, stop. If your life seems out of control, learn about stress management. And most important of all, if you're eating the wrong foods, change your diet.

We'll show you how.

Chapter Two

Assessing Your Risk

CORONARY HEART DISEASE WOULD BE A LOT EASIER to manage if we could trace it to a virus or some other single source. Instead, we're dealing with a disease that involves more than 250 risk factors. Some of these factors may seem relatively obscure. For instance, research suggests that men who are severely bald on top have up to a 36% greater risk of heart attack than those with full heads of hair. But other factors are out there in plain sight as possible risks that we all have to take into consideration. Elevated cholesterol is one of the best examples. According to data from the Framingham Heart Study, a 1% rise in your total cholesterol level can produce a 3% rise in heart attack risk.

Focus on Diet

Some of the most important cardiac risk factors are influenced by what and how much you eat. These factors include not only total cholesterol, but also LDL and HDL cholesterol, triglycerides, weight, blood pressure, diabetes, coronary inflammation, blood clotting and metabolic syndrome. And that's good news because it means that once you know your risk levels, you can neutralize many factors that can penalize cardiovascular health by taking the right steps to change your diet.

TOTAL CHOLESTEROL

High cholesterol levels have long been viewed as a major cardiac risk factor, and rightly so. Indeed, Dr. Robert Levy, former director of the National Heart, Lung and Blood Institute, points to elevated cholesterol as "the chief factor for heart attack." But just as higher cholesterol levels increase the risk for heart attack, *decreased* levels forecast a reduction in risk.

The amount of cholesterol in the blood is determined by a blood test and is expressed as the number of milligrams (mg) of cholesterol in one deciliter (dl) of blood. (For example, a person with 210 milligrams of cholesterol in a deciliter of blood has a cholesterol level of 210 mg/dl, popularly expressed as a cholesterol "count" of 210.) Initial cholesterol readings should not be etched in stone. Many health professionals now recommend a second test within one to eight weeks of the first. If the readings are within 30 points of each other, use the average of the two values; otherwise, a third test should be performed and the average of all three tests used. You should also be aware that exercise, stress, dieting, body weight change, medications and the phases of a woman's menstrual cycle can affect total cholesterol readings. Morning levels are usually higher than those later in the day. Smoking before a test can cause higher readings, as can failure to fast for 12 hours beforehand. And lying down for a test can cause lower readings, while sitting up tends to produce higher ones.

The National Cholesterol Education Program, in collaboration with the American Heart Association and a number of other medical authorities, has issued the following guidelines for assessing total cholesterol levels:

Total Cholesterol	Risk Classification
Below 200	Desirable
200 to 239	Borderline high
240 and above	High

If your total cholesterol level is somewhere around 200, you're considered "normal" (think "average") by today's standards. But that's not the best level for cardiac health. The optimal, or ideal, level is actually around 150 and below, particularly for heart patients.

There are a number of tried-and true dietary actions that you can take to control cholesterol effectively:

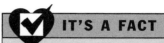

IT'S A FACT

Chronic stress can have a direct impact on cholesterol levels. Researchers found the cholesterol numbers of certified public accountants to be twice as high when they faced tax deadlines in April as when they were on their vacations in August— with no change in diet.

■ Cut down on foods rich in saturated fat (such as red meat and whole-milk dairy products) and trans fat (products made with hydrogenated oils) in favor of foods with fats that promote heart health (olive oil, seafood and walnuts).

■ Increase foods rich in complex carbohydrates (such as fruits and vegetables), soluble fiber (oat bran, oatmeal and beans), bioflavonoids (strawberries and eggplant) and antioxidants (foods rich in vitamins C and E and beta-carotene).

■ Choose cardioprotective foods. Substitute soy protein for animal protein; consider using cholesterol-lowering margarines containing sterol or sterol esters.

■ Use portion control to moderate caloric intake (along with increased physical activity) to lose weight, if necessary.

LDL CHOLESTEROL

Important as it is, total cholesterol seems at best to be a crude indicator of risk. Knowing only that number may leave you dangerously uninformed since the whole is less than the sum of its major parts: LDL ("bad") and HDL ("good") cholesterol. Unable to travel alone through the bloodstream, cholesterol is transported in chemical packages called lipoproteins. Low-density lipoproteins, or LDLs, are predominantly fat. Circulating in the blood for several days after their creation, they drop off cholesterol wherever needed for useful work such as cell building. Unfortunately, if they penetrate an artery wall and "unravel," unused cholesterol is released and deposited in the blood vessel, thus beginning the clogging process.

How low should your LDL cholesterol be? Research published in the *Journal of the American Medical Association* found that LDL levels below 100 could stop the progression of heart disease. Certainly heart patients and people at high risk for heart disease should strive for this level, and it may take diet plus drug therapy to achieve it. The National Cholesterol Education Program has issued the following guidelines:

LDL Cholesterol	Risk Classification
Below 100	Optimal
100 to 129	Near optimal
130 to 159	Borderline high
160 to 189	High
190 and above	Very high

As shown above, the optimal level for LDL cholesterol is below 100. But today, after trials on thousands of people, the National Heart, Lung and Blood Institute says a level below 70 is more beneficial. If you have heart disease or are at high risk, ask your doctor about this new goal.

Dietary habits play an important role in controlling LDL cholesterol. Suggested actions parallel those recommended for managing total cholesterol.

HDL CHOLESTEROL

High-density lipoproteins, or HDLs, contain very little fat. Unlike LDLs, these lipoproteins form stable packages that do not unravel when they come in contact with artery walls, so the cholesterol they carry does not become available for deposit. Furthermore,

HDLs act as scavengers, picking up excessive LDLs from artery walls and transporting them back to the liver for removal from the body.

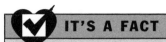

IT'S A FACT

The current estimate is that every increase of one milligram in HDL cholesterol can decrease cardiac risk by 4%.

While HDLs average only about 25% of total cholesterol, they are crucially important in determining heart attack risk. The National Cholesterol Education Program has proposed the following scale for risk from HDL cholesterol:

HDL Cholesterol	Risk Classification
60 and above	Low
40 to 59	Moderate
Below 40	High

Average HDL levels are 45 for men and 55 for women. Female sex hormones tend to raise HDL levels, a difference that in part explains the lower rates of coronary heart disease in women during their childbearing years.

While experts emphasize that HDLs and LDLs are separate and independent factors, the ratio of total cholesterol to HDL cholesterol is often helpful in estimating cardiac risk. To calculate your ratio, divide your total cholesterol number by your HDL number. For example, if you have a total cholesterol of 250 and an HDL of 50, your HDL ratio is 5.0. The scale below illustrates the relationship between ratio and risk:

HDL Ratio	Risk Classification
Below 3.5	Optimal
3.5 to 5.0	Average
5.1 to 6.0	Borderline high
Above 6.0	High

According to the American Heart Association, an HDL ratio should not be above 4.5 for men or 4.0 for women.

Although the first line of defense against low HDL levels is increased physical activity and smoking cessation, diet can make a real difference. Smart actions include:

■ Use portion control to moderate caloric intake (along with increased physical activity) to lose weight, if necessary.

■ Choose healthy unsaturated oils over unhealthy saturated fats and trans fats.

■ Consume alcohol in moderation.

■ Instead of relying on supplements, concentrate on foods that are rich in vitamin E, such as avocados, multigrain cereals, seafood, nuts and seeds.

In addition, a number of new HDL-raising drugs are being developed. Check with your doctor to see if drug therapy is appropriate.

TRIGLYCERIDES

Calories consumed during a meal and not used immediately by tissues are converted into triglycerides and transported to fat cells. (Most of the fat in your body is in the form of triglycerides.) At normal levels, triglycerides play a positive role in good health; however, more than 26 studies suggest that higher levels are a risk for coronary heart disease and heart attack, particularly in women who are overweight, hypertensive and diabetic. In addition, elevated triglycerides are a main component of metabolic syndrome (see page 33).

The National Cholesterol Education Program has issued the following risk classifications:

Triglycerides	Risk Classification
Below 150	Desirable
150 to 199	Borderline high
200 to 499	High
500 and above	Very high

Dietary habits count. The following steps can be taken to lower triglyceride levels:

■ Use portion control to moderate caloric intake (along with increased physical activity) to lose weight, if necessary. A loss of just three to five pounds can lower triglycerides by 30%.

■ Cut down on refined carbohydrates, especially those foods rich in added sugars and other sweeteners.

■ Reduce intake of saturated and trans fats.

■ Increase consumption of healthy oils.

■ Eat foods rich in fiber and complex carbohydrates.

■ Consume alcohol in moderation.

WEIGHT

Carrying too much weight is linked to elevated cholesterol levels and high blood pressure, among other factors that increase the risk of coronary heart disease. An eight-year study of more than 110,000 American women aged 30 to 55, for example, revealed that those who were as little as 5% overweight were 30% more likely than their lean counterparts to develop heart disease. That risk increased to 80% in women who were moderately overweight, while those who were obese were more than 300% more likely to develop heart disease. On the other side of this coin, data show that maintaining an ideal body weight, as compared with being obese, can reduce the risk of coronary disease by 35% to 55%.

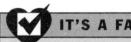

IT'S A FACT

Women who gain 21 to 30 pounds after the age of 18 are about 40% more likely to get breast cancer than women who gain 5 pounds or less. Women who gain more than 70 pounds have twice the risk of breast cancer as women who gain 5 pounds or less.

The National Institutes of Health recommends using the Body Mass Index (BMI) reproduced on pages 24–25. Find your height and weight on the chart and the corresponding BMI. Then assess your BMI in light of the guidelines on page 26.

BODY MASS INDEX TABLE

	HEALTHY WEIGHT						OVERWEIGHT					OBESE					
BMI	**19**	**20**	**21**	**22**	**23**	**24**	**25**	**26**	**27**	**28**	**29**	**30**	**31**	**32**	**33**	**34**	**35**
Height (feet/ inches)	**Body Weight (pounds)**																
4'10"	91	96	100	105	110	115	119	124	129	134	138	143	148	153	158	162	167
4'11"	94	99	104	109	114	119	124	128	133	138	143	148	153	158	163	168	173
5'0"	97	102	107	112	118	123	128	133	138	143	148	153	158	163	168	174	179
5'1"	100	106	111	116	122	127	132	137	143	148	153	158	164	169	174	180	185
5'2"	104	109	115	120	126	131	136	142	147	153	158	164	169	175	180	186	191
5'3"	107	113	118	124	130	135	141	146	152	158	163	169	175	180	186	191	197
5'4"	110	116	122	128	134	140	145	151	157	163	169	174	180	186	192	197	204
5'5"	114	120	126	132	138	144	150	156	162	168	174	180	186	192	198	204	210
5'6"	118	124	130	136	142	148	155	161	167	173	179	186	192	198	204	210	216
5'7"	121	127	134	140	146	153	159	166	172	178	185	191	198	204	211	217	223
5'8"	125	131	138	144	151	158	164	171	177	184	190	197	203	210	216	223	230
5'9"	128	135	142	149	155	162	169	176	182	189	196	203	209	216	223	230	236
5'10"	132	139	146	153	160	167	174	181	188	195	202	209	216	222	229	236	243
5'11"	136	143	150	157	165	172	179	186	193	200	208	215	222	229	236	243	250
6'0"	140	147	154	162	169	177	184	191	199	206	213	221	228	235	242	250	258
6'1"	144	151	159	166	174	182	189	197	204	212	219	227	235	242	250	257	265
6'2"	148	155	163	171	179	186	194	202	210	218	225	233	241	249	256	264	272
6'3"	152	160	168	176	184	192	200	208	216	224	232	240	248	256	264	272	279
6'4"	156	164	172	180	189	197	205	213	221	230	238	246	254	263	271	279	287

VERY OBESE

36	37	38	39	40	41	42	43	44	45	46	47	48	49	50	51	52	53	54
172	177	181	186	191	196	201	205	210	215	220	224	229	234	239	244	248	253	258
178	183	188	193	198	203	208	212	217	222	227	232	237	242	247	252	257	262	267
184	189	194	199	204	209	215	220	225	230	235	240	245	250	255	261	266	271	276
190	195	201	206	211	217	222	227	232	238	243	248	254	259	264	269	275	280	285
196	202	207	213	218	224	229	235	240	246	251	256	262	267	273	278	284	289	295
203	208	214	220	225	231	237	242	248	254	259	265	270	278	282	287	293	299	304
209	215	221	227	232	238	244	250	256	262	267	273	279	285	291	296	302	308	314
216	222	228	234	240	246	252	258	264	270	276	282	288	294	300	306	312	318	324
223	229	235	241	247	253	260	266	272	278	284	291	297	303	309	315	322	328	334
230	236	242	249	255	261	266	274	280	287	293	299	306	312	319	325	331	338	344
236	243	249	256	262	269	276	282	289	295	302	308	315	322	328	335	341	348	354
243	250	257	263	270	277	284	291	297	304	311	318	324	331	338	345	351	358	365
250	257	264	271	278	285	292	299	306	313	320	327	334	341	348	355	362	369	376
257	265	272	279	286	293	301	308	315	322	329	338	343	351	358	365	373	379	386
265	272	279	287	294	302	309	316	324	331	338	346	353	361	368	375	383	390	397
272	280	288	295	302	310	318	325	333	340	348	355	363	371	378	386	393	401	408
280	287	295	303	311	319	326	334	342	350	358	365	373	381	389	396	404	412	420
287	295	303	311	319	327	335	343	351	359	367	375	383	391	399	407	415	423	431
295	304	312	320	328	336	344	353	361	369	377	385	394	402	410	418	426	435	443

BMI	Condition	Risk Classification
19 to 24.9	Healthy weight	Desirable
25 to 29.9	Overweight	Borderline high
30 to 39.9	Obese	High
40 to 54	Very obese	Very high

The link between heart disease and overweight is particularly strong if the excess weight is carried around the middle. Says Dr. William Castelli, former director of the Framingham Heart Study, "People with wide hips and flat bellies may seem overweight, but the extra weight does not seem to increase their cardiac risk as much as that of people with narrow hips and potbellies. Abdominal obesity, which is more a male problem, is predictive of coronary disease." (See also page 34.)

Striking a balance between calories in and calories out is the key to managing weight. It's that simple. If you want to lose weight, take in fewer calories and exercise a little more. Some tested principles for managing caloric intake include:

■ Don't diet! Crash dieting is a game for fools. The only thing lost in the long run is money. Smart dietary decisions are based on the question "How do I want to eat for a lifetime?"

■ Do not skip meals.

■ Do a kitchen makeover. If your refrigerator and cupboard shelves are filled with all kinds of junk food, that's what you'll eat. Clean out the high-calorie snacks and restock your kitchen with healthier choices.

■ Cut your normal portion size by a third and watch out for supersizing in restaurants.

■ Reduce high-calorie foods rich in fat and low-fiber carbohydrates. Eat protein-rich snacks to curb hunger.

■ Drink eight glasses of water daily, or other healthy fluids.

■ Aim for 60 to 90 minutes of exercise on most days to lose weight, and 30 to 60 minutes to maintain weight loss.

BLOOD PRESSURE

Blood pressure is the force needed to move blood through the vascular system against the resistance of artery walls. *High* blood pressure, or hypertension, occurs when blood pressure exceeds an upper limit for an extended period of time. This condition can take place when arteries become narrow and hardened, often the result of atherosclerosis. Then additional resistance is created, increasing the pressure needed to move blood through the system and making the heart work harder than normal. Over time, this added strain can cause injury to coronary artery walls and result in inflammation. According to the Framingham Heart Study, people with high blood pressure have five times the risk of a heart attack as those with normal blood pressure. Unfortunately, the percentage of people with high blood pressure has been steadily increasing in recent years, particularly in females, African Americans and Mexican Americans.

"The view of blood pressure is changing," says Dr. Paul Wheaton of Tulane University Health Sciences Center. "Doctors used to consider high blood pressure a disease people either had or did not have. But today we understand that the risk of dying from heart complications caused by high blood pressure is a graded risk. The higher the blood pressure, the higher the risk. The more you can take that pressure down, the more you can get the risk back down."

Blood pressure is measured when the heart beats (systolic pressure) and then rests (diastolic pressure) and is expressed as two numbers representing millimeters of mercury (mm Hg). A systolic pressure of 120 and a diastolic pressure of 80 are typically expressed as 120/80, or "120 over 80." "Normal" systolic pressure is below 120; "normal" diastolic pressure is below 80. High blood pressure is defined as any reading above 140/90. In recent years, however, readings between 120/80 and

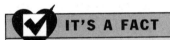

IT'S A FACT

Every one-point drop in diastolic pressure produces a 2% to 3% reduction in the risk of heart attack.

139/89 have been labeled indications of a condition called prehypertension. The standards below, established by the National Heart, Lung and Blood Institute, reflect the debilitating effect of blood pressure even at lower levels. New science suggests that the risk of heart disease starts to rise with readings as low as 115/75 and doubles for each increase of 20/10.

BLOOD PRESSURE READING

Systolic	Diastolic	Risk Classification
Below 120	Below 80	Optimal
120 to 139	80 to 89	Prehypertension
140 to 159	90 to 99	Stage 1 hypertension
Above 160	Above 100	Stage 2 hypertension

As Americans get older and fatter, the number of adults with high blood pressure has climbed to almost one in three. Fortunately, healthy eating can have a very positive impact on blood pressure. One study found that overweight people lowered their blood pressure by one point for every kilogram (2.2 pounds) of body weight they were able to lose.

Suggested dietary actions include:

■ Use portion control to moderate caloric intake (along with increased physical activity) to shed excess pounds, if necessary.

■ Eat less salt and sodium.

■ Emphasize potassium-rich foods (such as white beans, tomato paste, yogurt, bananas, apricots, avocados, sweet potatoes, lima beans, tuna, cantaloupe, winter squash and spinach). Cut down on foods low in potassium (such as white bread, doughnuts, soft drinks and junk food).

■ Limit alcohol and caffeine.

■ Eat foods rich in antioxidants (fruits, vegetables and nuts).

Regular exercise, along with not smoking and stress management, can also help.

THE SODIUM-POTASSIUM RATIO

While high sodium grabs the headlines, current studies suggest that high blood pressure is aggravated by an excess of sodium *in relation to potassium.* Experts counsel that we should get five times as much potassium as sodium in our diet. (The National Academy of Sciences recommends 4,700 milligrams of potassium daily for people over age 14.) Unfortunately, the American diet has it backwards, providing twice as much sodium as potassium. The best way to get sufficient potassium is to eat three servings a day of potassium-rich foods. (See Chapter Fourteen for more detailed information.)

DIABETES

Glucose, or blood sugar, is used by the body for energy. Insulin, a hormone produced by the pancreas, is necessary for the body to absorb glucose. But in the 16 million Americans with diabetes, the pancreas does not produce insulin (or produces too little of it) or the body does not properly use the insulin that *is* produced. Type 2 diabetes, the form most commonly linked to cardiovascular disease, usually strikes people in their forties or older and accounts for 90% to 95% of all diabetic cases. *Experts estimate that a third of the people who have it don't know they have it.* Although African American, Hispanic/Latino and Native American populations seem to be more genetically predisposed than Caucasians, most type 2 diabetes is triggered by obesity; indeed, more than 85% of type 2 diabetics are overweight. But the opposite is also true. You can lower your risk of getting diabetes by at least 80% if you lose as little as 5% of your body weight and exercise just 30 minutes a day.

It's important to know your estimated risk for diabetes, particularly if you have a family history. Experts recommend that all adults over age 45 be tested for diabetes every three years with a fasting blood glucose test. The American Diabetes Association suggests using the following scale to estimate risk:

Glucose	Risk Classification
Below 110	Desirable
110 to 125	Borderline high
Above 125	Confirmed diabetes

IT'S A FACT

According to the Centers for Disease Control and Prevention, one in three children born in the United States in the year 2000 will become diabetic unless our emphasis changes to eating less and exercising more.

Diet can play an important role in reducing risk for diabetes:

■ Use portion control to moderate caloric intake (along with increased physical activity) to reduce weight, if necessary.

■ Eat a balanced diet that provides adequate protein, complex carbohydrates and fiber. Reduce foods rich in fat (especially saturated and trans fats) and refined carbohydrates.

Type 2 diabetics should also talk with their physician about the appropriateness of taking cholesterol-lowering statin drugs.

CORONARY INFLAMMATION

Injury to the coronary arteries can occur easily as they twist and turn in response to the beating of the heart 100,000 times a day. It can also result from smoking and chronic stress. Whenever it occurs, however, injury is quickly followed by inflammation, a natural part of the repair process that can do more harm than good if it becomes chronic. Ongoing inflammation can destabilize plaque, causing the protective cap to rupture and release cholesterol into the bloodstream. Then a clot is formed, which can staunch blood flow to the heart. An estimated 25 to 35 million middle-aged Americans have normal cholesterol but above-average inflammation, putting them at increased risk of heart attack.

Research has now identified homocysteine and C-reactive protein (CRP) as two markers for coronary inflammation. A study of nearly 15,000 male physicians aged 40 to 84 revealed that high homocysteine tripled their heart attack risk. In the Nurses' Health Study, those with the highest levels of CRP had more than four times the risk of heart attack even if they were nonsmokers with normal cholesterol and no family history. Lower levels of CRP are linked to a slower progression of atherosclerosis and fewer heart attacks and deaths.

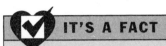 **IT'S A FACT**

Researchers have discovered that gum disease, a chronic bacterial infection of the gums, can trigger coronary inflammation.

Homocysteine and CRP levels can be established by blood tests. The traditional CRP test, used for arthritis and other inflammatory diseases, cannot accurately assess coronary inflammation, so be sure your doctor uses the *highly sensitive CRP test*, or *hs CRP*. The following scales have been established to indicate relative risk:

Homocysteine Level	Risk Classification
Below 5	Desirable
5 to 9	Normal
10 to 30	Moderate
31 to 100	High
Above 100	Severe

CRP Level	Risk Classification
Below 0.7	Lowest
0.7 to 1.1	Low
1.2 to 1.9	Average
2.0 to 3.8	Higher
3.9 to 15.0	Highest

The science of managing inflammation is still evolving. At this point, it's not clear whether CRP and/or homocysteine *reflect* coronary inflammation or actually *cause* it. Also, there is no evidence yet that lowering CRP and/or homocysteine reduces the risk of heart attack. However, CRP, homocysteine and coronary inflammation do appear to be linked, so if your numbers are elevated, it makes sense to take action. Talk with your doctor about aspirin therapy and statin drugs, which have been shown to reduce the inflammatory effect. And take these dietary steps:

■ Use portion control to moderate caloric intake (along with increased physical activity) to lose weight, if necessary.

■ Eat foods rich in folic acid (such as whole grains, oranges, fortified breakfast cereals and leafy green vegetables), vitamin B_6 (such as whole grains, fish and bananas) and vitamin B_{12} (meat, poultry, eggs and fortified cereals).

■ Choose oils rich in omega-3 fatty acids (found in seafood, walnuts and flaxseed) and omega-9 fatty acids (olive oil and canola oil), and moderate intake of omega-6 fatty acids (corn and safflower oils).

BLOOD CLOTTING

Many people believe that cholesterol triggers a heart attack. It does not. True, cholesterol forms blockages and can be released into the bloodstream, but it's the resulting clot that seals off the artery, chokes off the blood supply and causes the attack.

Clotting occurs when fragments of white blood cells group together. The more these cells aggregate, the greater the number of clots and the larger they become. Therefore, a tendency for blood to clot easily is an important cardiac marker. Many experts recommend assessing your risk by screening for fibrinogen, a protein in the blood that promotes clotting. One study of 2,600 people found that the participants with the highest levels of fibrinogen had more than twice the risk of coronary heart disease and heart attack as those with the lowest levels.

EMERGING RISK FACTORS

Recent evidence has illustrated less obvious effects of stress on cardiac health. Depression caused by chronic stress is now being viewed as a risk factor. So is stress-caused sleep deprivation, which has been shown to increase risk for heart disease, diabetes and overweight. Nearly two-thirds of adults do not get the eight hours of nightly sleep recommended by the National Sleep Foundation.

To test fibrinogen levels, blood is drawn and evaluated as milligrams per deciliter (mg/dl). Levels between 200 and 400 are considered normal. The following scale is an overall guide to risk:

Fibrinogen	Risk Classification
Below 200	Desirable
200 to 400	Borderline high
Above 400	High

Currently, there are no established medical treatments for lowering fibrinogen, but if your blood tends to clot too easily, cover the basics in heart-healthy living by not smoking, exercising regularly, eating right and managing stress. Talk to your doctor about aspirin therapy and niacin. From a dietary standpoint, moderate alcohol consumption and eating more fish seem to reduce the clotting mechanism.

METABOLIC SYNDROME

Also known as Syndrome X, metabolic syndrome is actually a cluster of symptoms: abdominal obesity, high triglyceride levels, low HDL cholesterol levels, high blood sugar levels and high blood pressure. Each of these symptoms is a cardiac risk in its own right; however, in combination, the sum of the parts is greater. People with metabolic syndrome are twice as likely to have a heart attack and three times as likely to develop diabetes.

Because people with this condition typically have a moderate level of total cholesterol (often under the national goal of 200), metabolic syndrome is sometimes missed. Consider the following profile of a 51-year-old male in the Framingham study:

Total cholesterol	195 mg/dl
LDL cholesterol	108 mg/dl
HDL cholesterol	32 mg/dl
Triglycerides	264 mg/dl

Given his low total cholesterol level and his "near optimal" LDL level, an assumption might be that this man has a low cardiac risk. But, according to Dr. William Castelli, such an assumption would be in error. In fact, this man has progressive coronary heart disease caused primarily by elevated triglycerides and low HDL cholesterol. Says Dr. Castelli, "Metabolic syndrome is a new cardiac risk factor, and the people who have it form a new group. In our Framingham study, we found that when triglycerides are over 250 and HDL is below 40, the risk of heart attack doubles—even when total cholesterol is in line."

WHAT ABOUT LIPOSUCTION?

Abdominal fat carried in a "potbelly" is linked to metabolic syndrome, but using liposuction to get rid of this fat will not make anyone healthier. A study of women who had 20 pounds of surface fat removed through liposuction indicated that risks associated with obesity (high cholesterol, high blood pressure, inflammation, elevated insulin and blood glucose) showed no improvement; however, women who lost 20 pounds of fat through diet and exercise exhibited improvement in all these metabolic abnormalities.

The National Cholesterol Education Panel has published the following risk profile for metabolic syndrome:

- Is your HDL number below 40 (men) or below 50 (women)?
- Is your fasting triglycerides number over 150?
- Is your waist size 35 inches or above (women) or 40 inches or above (men)?
- Is your blood pressure consistently 130/85 or greater?
- Are you diabetic (a fasting glucose of 110 or greater)?

If you answered "yes" to two of the five questions above, you probably have metabolic syndrome. If you answered "yes" to three or more, you definitely have a metabolic syndrome profile. See your doctor about monitoring your profile and possible drug therapy. Then get to work losing excess weight, increasing physical activity and adding fiber-rich and healthful high-fat foods to your diet, along with foods low in refined carbohydrates and sodium. A recent study found that maintaining such a diet cut the prevalence of metabolic syndrome in participants by 50%. A very low-fat diet, with 20% or fewer calories from fat, is *not* recommended. Eating so little fat inhibits satiety and invariably bumps up carbohydrate consumption, which can cause both triglycerides and blood glucose to rise. In any case, people with metabolic syndrome should concentrate on complex carbohydrates, found in vegetables, fruits, whole grains and beans.

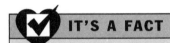 IT'S A FACT

The Internet can help you estimate your risk of a heart attack. Log onto the Web site of the National Heart, Lung and Blood Institute, *www.nhlbi.nih.gov,* and use its 10-year heart attack risk calculator.

The Importance of Lifestyle

It's imperative to ask this basic question: *Why do so many Americans have heart disease?* An examination of risk factors suggests that while noncontrollable risks like age and family history must be taken into account, controllable factors related to lifestyle play a much bigger role.

Studies show that about 85% of Americans with heart disease have it because of the choices they make every day. As Dr. JoAnn Manson of Harvard University says, "When it comes to heart attacks, most of us control our own destiny." Dr. Manson and her colleagues reviewed nearly 200 studies on coronary heart disease to evaluate the role of known preventive measures. The results, published in the *New England Journal of Medicine*, suggest taking the following steps:

Behavior Change	Estimated Reduction in Heart Attack Risk
Stop smoking	50–70% lower risk within 5 years of quitting
Reduce cholesterol	1% reduction = 2–3% decline in risk
Manage blood pressure	1 mm Hg reduction in diastolic pressure = 2–3% decline in risk
Exercise regularly	Active lifestyle = 45% decline in risk
Maintain ideal weight	35–55% lower risk, as compared with obesity

Whether your interest is prevention, stabilization or reversal of heart disease, these findings show how much you can do just by shaping healthy lifestyle habits. "To prevent heart disease, risk factor modification and lifestyle changes are absolutely critical," said cardiologist Dr. John Canto in an editorial in the *Journal of the American Medical Association.* "You can't smoke, gain weight, not exercise and just take a statin drug and expect to have a great outcome."

A cardiologist friend, Dr. Steve Yarnall, put it more succinctly: "You don't have to be a scientist to understand that the grease you sandblast from your oven and soak off your dishes isn't something you want in your arteries. You don't have to be a physiologist to understand that regular, moderate exercise is preferable to no exercise. And you don't have to be a genius to figure out that setting fire to tobacco leaves and inhaling the smoke doesn't make a whole lot of sense."

Chapter Three

What's Wrong with Our Diet?

A MERICAN DIETARY HABITS may never have been as unhealthy as they are today, reflecting not only what we eat but also what we *don't* eat. As a result of dining higher on the food chain, we consume fewer whole foods and more refined, low-fiber, highly processed foods. Marbled red meat, sugary desserts and other foods that were eaten occasionally in the past have gradually replaced fruits, whole grains, beans and vegetables as regular fare. According to the Department of Agriculture, on any given day:

- 3% of Americans will eat a hot dog, ham or luncheon meat.
- 25% will consume a hamburger, cheeseburger or meat loaf.
- 41% will eat a doughnut, cookies or a piece of cake.
- 23% will consume at least one serving of steak or roast beef.
- 41% will down two glasses of whole milk.

This modern eating pattern is the result of daily decisions based on impulse, availability, advertising, stress, convenience, economics, status, taste and cravings—on influences other than positive nutrition. Says Dr. Mark Hegsted, former director of the federal government's Human Nutrition Center, "The menu we happen to eat today—high in fat, sugar, salt and calories, and low in fiber and complex carbo-hydrates—was never planned on the basis of health. The fact that we consume it is no indication that it is balanced or desirable."

To give it its due, our modern diet has banished rickets, scurvy and other diseases of malnutrition. But still, as the surgeon general has warned, we are "gobbling our way to the grave." Indeed, 5 of the 10 leading causes of death are directly linked to our national diet: heart disease, cancer, high blood pressure, stroke and cirrhosis. Many experts believe that diet actually contributes to *six* of the leading causes of death, thanks to obesity's critical role in the development of type 2 diabetes.

In his critically acclaimed book *The Perfect Storm*, Sebastian Junger describes three ferocious weather fronts off Nova Scotia's fishing banks that combine to produce the most disastrous storm in weather bureau history. In a way, the three key elements of the modern American diet match that scenario. Poor food choices, too much food and a toxic environment have come together in a "perfect storm" to threaten cardiac health on a nationwide scale.

Poor Food Choices

Nutritional experts often rail against the "typical American diet," but in reality no such diet exists. There is no single way of eating in the United States. Anyone who has enjoyed cheesecake in New York, huevos rancheros in Los Angeles or prime rib in Kansas City knows that favorite foods differ across the country, reflecting regional preferences and ethnic heritage.

But there is a commonality. From Massachusetts to California, Oregon to Florida, our national diet can be described as made up of "sweet and salty fat." In fact, a comparison of foods consumed today with those consumed a century ago, when the USDA first started to keep figures on the food supply, shows a dramatic shift in the source of calories. A century ago, dietary fat made up just 27% of calories. Today, we eat some 37% of calories as fat. This means that the average person takes in over 100 pounds of fat a year. Not only has this level contributed to our epidemic weight problem, but much of the fat eaten is the kind that raises LDL cholesterol.

Another serious problem is our consumption of added sweeteners, which has more than doubled to 156 pounds per year. "America's sweet tooth is out of control," says dietitian Bonnie Liebman of the Center for Science in the Public Interest. "Added sweeteners now account for about 24% of calories eaten, mostly in the form of soft drinks, candy and commercially baked goods." This is well beyond the World Health Organization's recommendation of no more than 10% of calories from added sugar. The high level of sugar intake bears much responsibility for a steady rise in the number of Americans who are overweight and have elevated triglycerides and metabolic syndrome.

The average person currently consumes about 15 pounds of salt a year, or some 2 to 4 teaspoons each day. (The USDA recommends no more than 2,300 milligrams of sodium, or about a teaspoon of salt daily.) The intake of salt and other sodium products has risen with the increased popularity of convenience foods, snack foods and restaurant eating. Excess sodium plays a role in the development of high blood pressure, a condition afflicting over 60 million Americans.

And finally, a century ago carbohydrates came in the form of whole foods such as fruits, vegetables and whole grains. These foods have such a positive effect on our health that the new guidelines call for eating nine servings of fruit and vegetables (about 2 cups of fruit and 2½ cups of vegetables) and at least six one-ounce servings of grains daily, three from whole grains (a slice of bread is one serving). But instead of these complex carbohydrates, we are filling up on low-fiber, flour-based foods such as cakes, cookies, tortillas and hamburger buns. In the early 1970s, we ate 136 pounds of flour and cereal products per person; today, that figure is a dangerous 200 pounds.

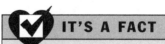

IT'S A FACT

Only about one-fifth of Americans eat even five servings of fruits and vegetables a day, much less the current recommendation of nine servings. In fact, it's estimated that on any given day 40% of adults eat *no* fruit or vegetables.

Too Much Food

Poor food choices aren't the only problem. We also eat too much, period! And the excess pounds aren't just on our bodies—they're on our plates. Cookies are the size of pancakes, bagels look like life rafts, muffins are bigger than baseballs, and soft drinks are practically large enough to swim in.

This trend has translated into a dramatic increase in calories consumed. Women are eating about 1,900 calories a day, while men are averaging more than 2,600 calories. Compare these daily intakes with those recommended by the government—1,600 calories for women and 2,200 calories for men—and it's easy to see why obesity rates have jumped. To put this in more concrete terms, consider that in 1990 only four states had more than half of their population classified as obese. Today, you can't find a single state that does *not* have half its population in that category.

Restaurant foods garner much of the blame by offering high-calorie foods in large amounts. "Portions are getting much larger," says Dr. Denise Bruner, past president of the American Society of Bariatric Physicians. "Dinner plates used to be 10.5 inches in diameter at sit-down restaurants; now they're closer to 12.5 inches. As a result, an 8-ounce serving of pasta has evolved into a 16-ounce serving to fill the larger plate." And fast-food restaurants have kept pace. Five years ago, the standard was a 3.5-ounce hamburger, 2 ounces of French fries and an 8-ounce soft drink. "Supersizing" has expanded the average meal to a 5-ounce hamburger, 4 ounces of French fries and a 20-ounce soft drink. Typical of many chains, Ruby Tuesday offers a giant burger consisting of almost a pound of meat with cheese.

For the record, the champion appears to be a roadhouse in western Pennsylvania that not only offers a 6-pound cheeseburger with 12 pieces of cheese for $23.95 (presumably for sharing) but recently challenged any customer to eat a colossal 11-pound burger. The winner was a petite, 115-pound college coed.)

AVERAGE PORTIONS THEN AND NOW

Food	20 Years Ago	Today	Difference
Bagel	140 calories (3" diameter)	350 calories (6" diameter)	250 calories
Cheeseburger	333 calories	590 calories	257 calories
Spaghetti and meatballs	500 calories (1 cup pasta, 3 small meatballs)	1,025 calories (2 cups pasta, 3 large meatballs)	525 calories
French fries	210 calories (2.4 oz.)	610 calories (6.9 oz.)	400 calories
Soda	85 calories (6.5 oz.)	250 calories (20 oz.)	165 calories
Turkey sandwich	320 calories	820 calories	500 calories
Chicken stir-fry	425 calories (2 cups)	865 calories (4.5 cups)	430 calories
Coffee	45 calories (8 oz. with whole milk and sugar)	350 calories (16 oz. with whole milk and mocha syrup)	305 calories
Muffin	210 calories (1.5 oz.)	500 calories (4 oz.)	290 calories
Pepperoni pizza	500 calories (2 slices)	850 calories (2 slices)	350 calories
Chicken Caesar salad	390 calories (1.5 cups)	790 calories (3.5 cups)	400 calories
Popcorn	270 calories (5 cups)	630 calories (11 cups)	360 calories
Cheesecake	260 calories (3 oz.)	640 calories (7 oz.)	380 calories
Chocolate-chip cookie	55 calories (1.5" diameter)	275 calories (3.5" diameter)	220 calories

SUPER PORTIONS

The impact of serving size was demonstrated in the 2004 award-winning documentary *Super Size Me: A Film of Epic Portions.* For one month, filmmaker Morgan Spurlock ate all his meals at McDonald's. Whenever supersizing was offered, he accepted, which usually meant his meals included a 7-ounce carton of French fries and a 42-ounce soft drink. From a weight of 185 pounds at the start of the experiment, he ballooned to 210 pounds by month's end. His cholesterol rose by 60 points.

Portion distortion is also going on at home. Even popular cookbooks have given in to the trend. Recipes that used to feed six now feed only four. The Nestlé Toll House Chocolate Chip Cookie recipe from 1949 yielded 100 cookies; that same recipe today is 60 cookies. What is particularly disturbing is that studies show two-thirds of Americans eat everything on their plates, no matter what the size. Indeed, new research suggests that when people are given larger portions, they eat 30% more food before feeling full. In one study, participants were served lunch on four separate occasions, each time with a bigger entrée; despite their stable hunger levels, the participants ate increasingly larger amounts as portions increased. These results confirmed suspicions that human hunger can be expanded merely by offering more and bigger options. The fact is, we pay little attention to the actual need for food.

The root of the problem, according to many experts, is that many people don't know what a normal portion is. The USDA Handbook #8, published in 1963, was the first to list "standard portion sizes" for a variety of foods. For the next 12 years, food products pretty much came in those sizes. Then, after some marketing genius decided to increase portion size, a dietary culture of giant bagels and monster muffins began to evolve. "People are currently taking in more calories because of big portions that no longer reflect a single serving," says

Robyn Flipse, a registered dietitian. "It isn't that we want to eat multiple servings. It's just that people no longer know what one serving looks like, and this has played a critical role in the ever-expanding American waistline."

For example, the USDA defines one portion of bread as "one ounce." But a large bagel today can weigh in at about 4 ounces—the equivalent of four pieces of toast. The single portion size for a muffin is 1.5 ounces, but often one muffin will contain three or four portions. And when is the last time you saw a 4-ounce glass of juice, 3.5 ounces of meat or fish, or a 3-ounce baked potato—all single-portion sizes? We even overeat the good stuff. One 4.5-inch banana constitutes a single portion of fruit, but today bananas are grown a foot long, representing approximately three portions. Dr. Marion Nestle sums it up: "There's no end in sight to the supersizing of portions and the supersizing of us."

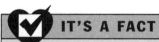

IT'S A FACT

Okinawa claims the longevity trophy for the planet, with an average life expectancy of 81.8 years. (The average in the U.S. is only 77.1 years.) While the Okinawan diet (rich in vegetables, fish and soy) gets much credit, a critical factor is that Okinawans do not overeat. They leave the table when they're *hara hara bu,* roughly translated as "8 parts out of 10 full."

A Toxic Environment

Food supply has been inconsistent for more than 99% of human history, and this hard fact of evolutionary life may have caused us to be hardwired when it comes to food choices. In other words, we may have an instinctive desire for basic tastes—sweet, fat, salt—that evolved during times of scarcity. "As a result," says Rutgers University anthropologist Lionel Tiger, "we don't have a cutoff mechanism when it comes to eating. Our bodies tell us, 'Fat is good to eat but hard to get.'" Even though the second half of that equation is no longer true, evolutionary development has made overeating a powerful drive.

While our physiology may set us up for dietary excesses, according to most experts it's not the principal source of our difficulties today. Our ancestors had the same preferences, but they didn't have high cholesterol or obesity problems. One reason is that they didn't live in an environment that allowed basic food preferences to run amok. Early man was pleased to eat meat, but that meat was wild game, not a double cheeseburger. And early woman may have gorged on fruit, but she couldn't eat anywhere near the amount of added sweeteners that comes in a couple of doughnuts.

As reported in a 2002 cover story in *Time* magazine, "Hunting and gathering food took virtually nonstop physical activity. Just 100 years ago, if you wanted butter, you had to churn it. If you wanted meat, you had to hunt it or butcher the cow. If you had a craving for a pie, you had to pick the fruit, roll out the dough, fire up the stove and bake the pie. But today technology has removed physical exercise from the day-to-day lives of most Americans, including how we get food. Forget hunting and gathering. Instead, we just jump in the car and head to the nearest supermarket, which is filled with cheap, mass-produced, good-tasting food packed with calories. Or go to the convenience store for a bag of chips and a 32-ounce soft drink. And if that's too much effort, just dial up the Internet or make a phone call and the food—probably pizza!—will be delivered to your door."

IT'S A FACT

According to a study published in the *Journal of Nutritional Education*, in one year the average child in the United States watches nearly 10,000 commercials touting food or beverages. Hamburgers, candy and soft drinks lead the list. Fruits and vegetables are near the bottom.

The result, according to obesity expert Dr. Kelly Brownell of Yale University, is that we live today in an atmosphere that makes it all too easy to make unhealthy food choices and to overeat. "Everywhere you turn, there is an opportunity to eat poorly," says Dr. Brownell, "backed up by an advertising industry that encourages overeating. Such a toxic environment has shaped a modern-day eating pattern that practically guarantees obesity. It's like trying to treat an alcoholic in a town where there's a bar every 10 feet. Bad food is cheap, heavily promoted and engineered to taste good."

Dr. Brownell points to the experience of immigrants from low-obesity countries such as India and Japan. "When people move to countries where there is more obesity, they tend to gain weight," he says. "Did they suddenly become less responsible when they moved? More likely, they are responding to their new environment's cues to eat more calories." Mark Krikorian, executive director of the Center for Immigration Studies, puts it this way: "Assimilation often means assimilation into eating too much Cheez Whiz."

A second aspect of this toxic environment is a stressful, pressure-packed lifestyle that can override even the best of intentions. People are hurried and harried, working longer hours, commuting farther, trying to balance work and home life. The result is that many people constantly feel like they're out of time, which results in chronic stress. A woman in one of my seminars told me, "I'm answering e-mails at nine in the evening, doing laundry at midnight and grocery shopping at six in the morning. I don't have enough time to shop, cook or make food choices based on good nutrition. I barely have time to eat! I feel lucky just to get something on the table." Too often that "something" is a frozen, packaged or takeout meal. In addition, restaurant eating has soared, leading one observer to remark that "restaurants have become the ultimate kitchen appliance." Data show that at 4:00 P.M. on any given day, 70% of Americans do not know what they'll be hav-ing for dinner that night, so it's easy to choose foods that someone else has already made.

Another result of our stressed-out society is the demise of official mealtimes. For many families trying to balance long work hours, soc-cer practice and school activities, dinnertime lasts from 4:00 P.M. to 8:00 P.M. as parents and children drift in and out on their own. "By the time children go to middle school," says Dr. Marquisa LaVelle of the University of Rhode Island, "many families have basically stopped eating together. Solitary eating can be uncontrolled eating—snacks, sweets and meals in the car. Everyone in the family can feed themselves whatever they want—and they do."

According to Dr. Nancy Wellman, former president of the American Dietetic Association, "Many of us would like to eat healthier, but demographic changes, the number of meals eaten away from home, the convenience pull, nutritional naïveté and plain confusion confound our attempt." The bottom line is that we've traded nutrition for convenience. And as a nation we're paying the price in rising rates of heart disease and obesity.

But it doesn't have to be that way. The information and recipes in this book can help you choose healthier foods and smarter portion sizes. Your taste buds, your waist and your heart will thank you.

Part Two

On the Cutting Edge

Chapter Four

The New Guidelines

H EART-HEALTHY EATING HAS TO BE ANCHORED in sound nutritional science; otherwise, you might find yourself trying to survive exclusively on high-protein cabbage soup or some other fad of the moment. Fortunately, today there's a wide body of knowledge on which to base a balanced lifetime eating pattern. Recent information from the American Heart Association, the American Dietary Association, the surgeon general and other accepted sources has contributed to changes in recommended food choices. In particular, the Dietary Guidelines for Americans issued by the Department of Human and Health Services and the Department of Agriculture are essential in creating the principles for a program that promotes healthy eating habits.

How Much, How Often?

M any of the foods recommended in the new guidelines are central to our Mediterranean-style dietary plan, so our recipes and menus reflect the latest science. But keep in mind that guidelines are not mathematical formulas. They're intended to help you make wise food choices. Says Gail Frank, R.D., Ph.D., a spokesperson for the American Dietetic Association, "The guidelines give families a daily intake to strive for. For example, if we meet our fruit and vegetable requirements, that's the first step toward healthy eating."

MINIMUM DAILY SERVINGS
OF MAJOR FOOD GROUPS

The recommendations below are premised on a 2,000-calorie-a-day diet. (If you eat fewer or more calories per day, see the section beginning on page 53.)

■ *Five servings or two and a half cups of vegetables,* including fresh, frozen, canned and dried vegetables and vegetable juices. In general, one cup of raw or cooked vegetables or vegetable juice, or two cups of raw leafy greens can be considered one serving.

■ *Four servings or two cups of fruit,* including fresh, frozen, canned and dried fruits and fruit juices. In general, one-half cup of dried fruit can be considered one cup.

■ *Six servings of grains,* including three servings of whole grains. This group includes all foods made from wheat, rice, oats, cornmeal or barley, such as bread, pasta, oatmeal, breakfast cereals, tortillas and grits. A serving is generally one ounce, the equivalent of one slice of bread, half an English muffin or one cup of ready-to-eat cereal. For cooked grains (oatmeal, pasta, rice, polenta), one serving is equal to one-half cup.

■ *Three servings of fat-free or low-fat milk* or fluid milk products and foods made from milk that retain their calcium content, such as yogurt and cheese. A serving is one cup of milk or yogurt, or one and a half ounces of cheese. (Foods made from milk that have little or no calcium, such as cream cheese, cream and butter, are not part of the recommended milk group.) This recommendation is a major change from past guidelines. Once mere supporting players, fat-free and low-fat dairy products now rank with fruits, vegetables and whole grains as a "food group to encourage."

■ *Five and a half one-ounce equivalents of fish, meat, beans and nuts.* In general, one ounce of cooked lean fish, poultry or meat, one egg, one tablespoon of peanut butter, one-quarter cup of cooked beans, peas or lentils, or one quarter-cup of nuts and seeds can be considered one-ounce equivalents.

THE RIGHT FATS

Choose liquid oils. The guidelines keep the minimum fat intake at 20% of total calories but allow for a more liberal cap of 35%. However, they strongly recommend eating monounsaturated oils (such as olive or canola oils) and polyunsaturated oils (corn, safflower and soybean, for example). For every 2,000 calories, the guidelines suggest 6 teaspoons of heart-healthy oils daily.

The recommendation is to get no more than 10% of your calories as saturated fat (found in beef fat, chicken fat and butter) and to keep trans fat (hydrogenated stick margarine and shortening) as low as possible. Many experts believe trans fat should be limited to no more than 1% of calories since it clearly penalizes heart health.

LESS SODIUM, MORE POTASSIUM

The guidelines call for no more than 2,300 milligrams of sodium (about a teaspoon of salt) per day. People with hypertension, middle-aged and older adults, and African Americans should consume no more than 1,500 milligrams daily. At the same time, experts recommend increasing foods rich in potassium, such as fruits and vegetables.

LESS SUGAR

Watch out for added sugar and other sweeteners like high-fructose corn syrup, which can increase weight and triglycerides. While the guidelines urge us to eat fewer sugary foods, they stop short of specific limits on how much sugar should be consumed. The World Health Organization's recommendation is less than 10% of calories from sugar.

WEIGHT MANAGEMENT

If you consume more calories than you use, you'll gain weight. And it's hard not to overconsume with fast-food places on every corner, snack machines within easy reach and dinner plates as large as hubcaps. If weight is a problem, you have to pay more attention to "calories in." That means eating lower-fat, lower-sugar foods and just plain eating less.

TOO LITTLE DIETARY FAT?

If you need to lose weight, keep your consumption of dietary fat under control. Says Dr. Marion Nestle, chairman of New York University's Department of Nutrition and Food Studies, "Since fat has more than twice the calories of an equal amount of carbohydrates or protein, managing fat intake will help you to take in fewer calories and maintain a healthy weight." *But don't cut out too much fat!* When fat falls below about 20% of calories, people tend to increase their carbohydrate consumption. The net effect can be weight gain.

And exercise regularly. Yes, this is a dietary principle! While the guidelines' goals (30 to 90 minutes daily) are certainly ambitious, they do emphasize that accumulating activity over time—taking the stairs, doing gardening, washing your car—can help you meet your activity quota.

THE RIGHT CARBOHYDRATES

Choose high-fiber carbohydrates such as fruits, vegetables and whole grains. Limit low-fiber carbohydrates like desserts, cookies, white bread, crackers, many cereals and doughnuts. Too many of these foods, typically rich in saturated fat and trans fat, added sugars and calories, can penalize your heart and your waistline.

LIMITS ON ALCOHOL

If you drink alcohol, do so in moderation. This means no more than one drink a day for women, two for men.

ADDITIONAL CONSIDERATIONS

While not part of the guidelines per se, five additional principles should be included in designing a healthy eating plan:

■ *Treat food as good medicine.* Eat a variety of foods, particularly those that are whole (not processed) and plant-based. *But no food should be forbidden.* Everything from red wine to red meat has its place within the context of healthy eating.

■ *Don't diet.* If any of the quick fad diets had been effective over the past 50 years, we'd be a nation of skinny folks. Don't fall into that trap.

■ *Stay hydrated.* Trade in your soft drinks for water and other healthy fluids such as sparkling water, flavored seltzer and decaffeinated green and black teas. They'll help to curb your daily snacking habits.

■ *Choose cardioprotective foods.* Look for "functional foods" with properties that give an edge to cardiac health. (See Chapter Seven.)

■ *Make palatability a priority.* No one will eat nutritious food if it doesn't taste good. Take the time to prepare delicious meals that also boost well-being.

One Size Does *Not* Fit All

Unlike the one-size-fits-all guidelines that premised healthy-eating advice on a 2,000-calorie-a-day diet, the new recommendations take into consideration the fact that people of different heights, weights and activity levels have different nutritional needs. Says Eric Hentges, director of the Department of Agriculture's Center for Nutritional Policy and Promotion, "From previous consumer research, we knew we had to personalize the guidance." That's why the USDA has provided 12 new pyramid versions under the heading MyPyramid Plan, based on calorie levels that best match individual needs.

Follow these three simple steps to construct a personalized plan:

Step 1: Estimate the number of calories you need based on your level of activity. You can do this by logging onto the Internet and visiting *www.mypyramid.gov.* Just fill in your age, gender and activity level, and MyPyramid will take you to one of 12 pyramid versions that will fit your needs.

The USDA chart on pages 54–55 also shows the differences in suggested caloric intake based on age, gender and level of physical

CALORIES NEEDED

ACTIVITY LEVELS—MALES

AGE	Sedentary*	Moderately Active*	Active*
2	1,000	1,000	1,000
3	1,000	1,400	1,400
4	1,200	1,400	1,600
5	1,200	1,400	1,600
6	1,400	1,600	1,800
7	1,400	1,600	1,800
8	1,400	1,600	2,000
9	1,600	1,800	2,000
10	1,600	1,800	2,200
11	1,800	2,000	2,200
12	1,800	2,200	2,400
13	2,000	2,200	2,600
14	2,000	2,400	2,800
15	2,200	2,600	3,000
16	2,400	2,800	3,200
17	2,400	2,800	3,200
18	2,400	2,800	3,200
19–20	2,600	2,800	3,000
21–25	2,400	2,800	3,000
26–30	2,400	2,600	3,000
31–35	2,400	2,600	3,000
36–40	2,400	2,600	2,800
41–45	2,200	2,600	2,800
46–50	2,200	2,400	2,800
51–55	2,200	2,400	2,800
56–60	2,200	2,400	2,600
61–65	2,000	2,400	2,600
66–70	2,000	2,200	2,600
71–75	2,000	2,200	2,600
76 and up	2,000	2,200	2,400

Sedentary = less than 30 minutes a day of moderate physical activity in addition to

Moderately active = at least 30 minutes up to 60 minutes a day of moderate physical

Active = 60 or more minutes a day of moderate physical activity in addition to daily

PER DAY

AGE	ACTIVITY LEVELS—FEMALES		
	Sedentary*	Moderately Active*	Active*
2	1,000	1,000	1,000
3	1,000	1,200	1,400
4	1,200	1,400	1,400
5	1,200	1,400	1,600
6	1,200	1,400	1,600
7	1,200	1,600	1,800
8	1,400	1,600	1,800
9	1,400	1,600	1,800
10	1,400	1,800	2,000
11	1,600	1,800	2,000
12	1,600	2,000	2,200
13	1,600	2,000	2,200
14	1,800	2,000	2,400
15	1,800	2,000	2,400
16	1,800	2,000	2,400
17	1,800	2,000	2,400
18	1,800	2,000	2,400
19–20	2,000	2,200	2,400
21–25	2,000	2,200	2,400
26–30	1,800	2,000	2,400
31–35	1,800	2,000	2,200
36–40	1,800	2,000	2,200
41–45	1,800	2,000	2,200
46–50	1800	2,000	2,200
51–55	1,600	1,800	2,200
56–60	1,600	1,800	2,200
61–65	1,600	1,800	2,000
66–70	1,600	1,800	2,000
71–75	1,600	1,800	2,000
76 and up	1,600	1,800	2,000

daily activities.

activity in addition to daily activities.

activities.

Food	1,000	1,200	1,400	1,600	1,800
Fruits	1 cup	1 cup	1.5 cups	1.5 cups	1.5 cups
Vegetables	1 cup	1.5 cups	1.5 cups	2 cups	2.5 cups
Grains	3 oz.	4 oz.	5 oz.	5 oz.	6 oz.
Meat and beans	2 oz.	3 oz.	4 oz.	5 oz.	5 oz.
Milk	2 cups	2 cups	2 cups	3 cups	3 cups
Oils	3 tsp.	4 tsp.	4 tsp.	5 tsp.	5 tsp.
Discretionary calorie allowance	165	171	171	182	195

DAILY AMOUNT OF FOOD

CALORIES NEEDED PER DAY

activity. A construction worker who pours concrete all day, for instance, needs more calories than an office worker of the same age and gender who spends eight hours a day sitting quietly in front of a computer screen. (When I went to the site and put in my information, I learned that I could eat 2,600 calories because I exercise more than 60 minutes daily.) And here's a nice bonus. After you've filled up on essential calories from foods that meet the basic requirements for vitamins, minerals and other necessities for good health, you can indulge in some "discretionary calories." The new USDA guidelines define these calories as those from occasional treats like sugary snacks, solid fats, refined foods or alcoholic beverages. The more physically active you are, the more discretionary calories you're allowed. (See Chapter Sixteen.)

Step 2: Estimate the daily amount of each food group you should consume for good nutrition. Again, *www.mypyramid.gov* will calculate this for you, or you can use the chart above to estimate your needs.

Step 3: Track your progress. Since you'll need to know what foods to include each day in order to meet your daily quota, the USDA has

FROM EACH GROUP

CALORIES NEEDED PER DAY						
2,000	**2,200**	**2,400**	**2,600**	**2,800**	**3,000**	**3,200**
2 cups	2 cups	2 cups	2 cups	2.5 cups	2.5 cups	2.5 cups
2.5 cups	3 cups	3 cups	3.5 cups	3.5 cups	4 cups	4 cups
6 oz.	7 oz.	8 oz.	9 oz.	10 oz.	10 oz.	10 oz.
5.5 oz.	6 oz.	6.5 oz.	6.5 oz.	7 oz.	7 oz.	7 oz.
3 cups	3 cups	3 cups	3 cups	3 cups	3 cups	3 cups
6 tsp.	6 tsp.	7 tsp.	8 tsp.	8 tsp.	10 tsp.	11 tsp.
267	290	362	410	426	512	648

provided a tracking tool called MyPyramid Tracker, which can be found at *www.mypyramid.gov.*

You can also keep track of your progress by using the checklist reproduced on page 58. With your caloric intake as a guide, decide the number of servings (boxes) daily that apply to you in each food group. Then check off a box when you've eaten a serving of the food. (We've added water consumption as a line item because it's so important.) You'll soon know how you're doing and can make adjustments if necessary. For example, at 2,000 calories a day, you should eat six one-ounce servings of grains daily. If you need more than 2,000 calories, use the extra boxes to record additional servings. A person who consumes 2,200 calories a day, for instance, should eat seven servings of grains and check off that many boxes. For less (say, a 1,600-calorie diet), fewer boxes would be checked off, in this case five.

Using a checklist does not have to be a lifelong activity. It's simply a way to get used to dietary change. If you miss some of the servings or food groups one day or overdo on another, don't let it upset you. Heart-healthy eating is all about balance. Just choose wisely the next day.

HAVE YOU FILLED YOUR DAILY QUOTA?

The number of servings for each group below is based on a diet of 2,000 calories per day. Serving equivalents are listed on page 50.

✓ **water** ☐ = one 8-ounce glass

☐ ☐ ☐ ☐ ☐ ☐ ☐ ☐

✓ **dairy** ☐ = one cup

☐ ☐ ☐ ☐ ☐ ☐ ☐ ☐

✓ **vegetables** ☐ = one cup

☐ ☐ ◺ ☐ ☐ ☐ ☐ ☐

✓ **fruit** ☐ = one cup

☐ ☐ ☐ ☐ ☐ ☐ ☐ ☐

✓ **oils** ☐ = one teaspoon

☐ ☐ ☐ ☐ ☐ ☐ ☐ ☐

✓ **grains** ☐ = one ounce

☐ ☐ ☐ ☐ ☐ ☐ ☐ ☐

✓ **fish, poultry, meat, beans and nuts** ☐ = one ounce

☐ ☐ ☐ ☐ ☐ ◺ ☐ ☐

Chapter Five

The Truth About Fats

FOR MANY YEARS, fat was considered the supreme dietary villain. Cardiac experts railed at the American "high-fat" way of eating and called for a cut in fat consumption; some even counseled a diet close to "no fat." But science marches on, and today we have a different take on the proper role of fat. The extremes of "high fat" and "no fat" have given way to "moderation and balance."

The fact is that dietary fat plays a legitimate and important role in maintaining good health. Polyunsaturated fats supply us with essential linoleic (omega-6) and linolenic (omega-3) fatty acids. Monounsaturated fats arm us against heart disease by reducing LDL cholesterol and decreasing blood clots. Dietary fat is also used in the transportation of important fat-soluble vitamins in the body; without it, we wouldn't be able to absorb vitamins A, D, E and K. And with double the amount of calories as protein and carbohydrate, dietary fat provides us with a concentrated source of energy; our bodies store fat as an energy reserve and draw upon it when extra fuel is needed. Fat also provides satiety, an important element in appetite control.

The key issue is how to consume fat in a way that maximizes health and reduces the risk of heart disease. The current consensus suggests that balance revolves around the *amount* and *type* of fat consumed.

THE CHOLESTEROL CONNECTION

There is plenty of evidence to show that a high-fat diet can increase cholesterol and cardiac risk. But simply eating a diet lower in fat is not the answer. In a study published in *Annals of Internal Medicine,* 120 adults were divided into two groups. One group ate a low-fat diet that included packaged foods such as reduced-fat cheeses, lunch meats, frozen dinners, diet sodas and fat-free cookies. After a month, their LDL cholesterol levels had dropped by 4.6%. The second group followed a low-fat diet with large quantities of plant-based foods—vegetables, fruits, beans, legumes, whole grains and soy—and limited amounts of meat and dairy. Their LDL levels were lowered by 9.4%, double the reduction shown in the first group. Says Dr. Christopher Gardner, director of nutrition studies at Stanford University's Prevention Research Center, "The effect of diet on lowering cholesterol has really been minimized because we simply focused on the negative—what foods to avoid. This study confirms that reducing LDL cholesterol is not just about what you don't eat. It's about what you *do* eat as well."

■ *Amount.* The new guidelines recommend getting 20% to 35% of our calories from fat. More than 35% generally increases saturated fat intake and makes it more difficult to avoid consuming excess calories. Southern Europeans, who are seldom overweight and enjoy good heart health, eat far more fat—sometimes over 40% of calories. But most Americans don't follow the Mediterranean lifestyle, which involves more physical activity, eating more fruits and vegetables, and consuming smaller portions. So, for reasons of weight management, we need to moderate fat content.

■ *Type.* Most of the fat in our diet should come from monounsaturated and polyunsaturated oils. The efficacy of monounsaturated oils is reflected in the decision by the USDA to allow labels on olive oil to contain this message: *Two tablespoons daily may benefit cardiac health.* According to the guidelines, no more than 10% of calories should come from saturated fat (the American Heart Association calls for a 7% limit) and trans fats should be kept to the barest minimum (some experts say no more than 1% of calories). From the standpoint of cardiac risk, there's a huge difference between olive oil and fish oil on one hand and butterfat and lard on the other.

Consuming a moderate amount of fat and choosing heart-healthy oils are two fundamental principles of Mediterranean-style eating, emphasized in the advice and recipes throughout this book.

Fat and Weight

It's old news that Americans weigh too much. Our weight is the subject of numerous books, articles, TV specials and warnings from health groups and the government. It's also immediately evident if you look around you at the beach, the mall or a baseball game.

It's not that dietary fat makes us overweight all by itself. It's that we eat too much of it. From a nutritional standpoint, the daily requirement for fat can be fully satisfied by consuming the equivalent of one tablespoon of vegetable oil, but the average American eats eight times that amount—between 800 and 1,000 calories, or about the equivalent of one full stick of butter a day! Not surprisingly, two-thirds of Americans are officially overweight; even worse, 50% of this group are obese and about 5% are morbidly obese. Much more than an aesthetic problem, this profile is connected to heart disease, high blood pressure, type 2 diabetes and a host of other debilitating ailments.

While it's tempting to blame the overweight epidemic on bad genes or sluggish metabolism, many studies suggest that high-fat food choices are the leading cause. "Most people really cannot invoke some genetic cause as the only explanation for obesity," says

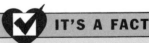 **IT'S A FACT**

Studies show that Americans gain an average of one to two pounds each year between the ages of 20 and 50. That may not seem like much, but at the rate of one and a half pounds yearly, by the time you're 50 you've put on an extra 45 pounds!

Dr. Steven Heymsfield, medical director of the weight-control unit at St. Luke's–Roosevelt Hospital Center in New York City. "The main reason they're overweight is that they consume too many calories. And it's hard not to do this when your diet is too high in fat."

FAT IS CALORICALLY DENSE

Food supplies us with energy in the form of calories. As long as energy input (calories consumed) is in balance with energy expenditure (calories burned in physical activity and basic bodily functions), all is well. But when caloric input is greater than caloric output, the extra calories are stored as body fat. If 3,500 extra calories have been accumulated, one pound of body fat has been created. It will take an energy expenditure of 3,500 calories to burn this pound of fuel. Unfortunately, the ability of the body to store fat is virtually limitless.

It's not easy to put on a pound of body fat in a single day. In order to increase your input by 3,500 calories, you'd have to down eight McDonald's Quarter Pounders, or binge on 16 pieces of pepperoni pizza, or drink a case of beer. The point is that, for most of us, gaining a few pounds of body fat doesn't happen overnight. As few as 50 extra calories a day, a single chocolate-chip cookie, can add 350 calories a week, or 18,200 in a year. That doesn't sound like much, but it equates to a gain of 5 pounds in a year or 52 pounds in a decade.

Of course, it's possible to gain weight by overeating any type of food. Gobble down enough carrots or shrimp and, at least in theory, you're on your way to becoming overweight. But fats aren't the same as carbohydrates or proteins, either in the number of calories they contain or in the way we metabolize them. At 9 calories per gram, dietary fat has more than twice as many calories as

IT'S A FACT

Between the ages of 19 and 50, the average American consumes 230 calories more on weekends than on weekdays. Most of these extra calories, which come from fat and alcohol, translate into a five-pound weight gain every year.

A LOW-FAT FIASCO

As the connection between fatty foods and overweight became clearer, Americans answered the call to slash dietary fat, but all the new low-fat and fat-free products failed to produce a healthier population. In my opinion, we did two things wrong. First, we thought a diet with 37% of calories from fat was real progress (after all, just a few decades before, fat made up over 40% of calories). What we overlooked was the fact that we were still consuming the same number of fat-grams per day—they just made up a smaller percentage of total calories. Second, many of us paid a price in terms of constant hunger, which we tried to satisfy with more low-fiber carbohydrates such as pasta, white rice, potatoes and commercially baked goods, the last often appealingly labeled "low-fat" or "fat-free." The addition of these foods created an excess of calories that contributed in a major way to today's overweight epidemic.

carbohydrates and proteins at 4 calories per gram. A small package of M&M peanut candies, for example, contains 250 calories, 47% of them from fat. This isn't a lot of food (only 1.74 ounces), but it's calorically dense because it's so rich in fat. Just the opposite is true of low-fat foods. An entire pound of apples contains only 240 calories.

Research proves that people who eat high-fat diets actually take in less food but a lot more calories. One study measured food intake by two different groups. The first group ate a diet low in fat and rich in complex carbohydrates and fiber; the second group ate a diet rich in fat. The first group ate more than the second group but lost weight. The second group ate a 13% lower volume of food but, because of the prominence of dietary fat, took in 56% more calories and gained weight. Study after study has reached the same conclusion: People who eat a diet moderate in fat but rich in complex carbohydrates and fiber eat a greater volume of food but lose weight because of fewer calories consumed.

DIETARY FAT TURNS INTO BODY FAT

For many years, scientists held to the belief that "a calorie is a calorie is a calorie." A growing body of evidence now suggests that once a calorie is eaten, this simple rule of dieting dogma doesn't always hold true. Says Dr. Eric Jequier of the University of Lausanne in Switzerland, "There is a marked difference in the body's metabolic response to dietary fat. Calorie for calorie, fat is more fattening."

Some of the calories we consume are immediately utilized as fuel. Those not used right away are converted to body fat for future use. This process takes energy, which is produced by some of the calories being converted, but not all foods call for the same *amount* of energy. A hundred calories of butter needs only 3 calories for processing, which means 97 calories can be converted to body fat. A hundred calories of a baked potato, on the other hand, needs 23 calories for processing, so just 77 calories are converted to body fat. (In reality, only about 1% of calories from complex carbohydrate and protein end up as body fat because the body would rather use them up right away than waste energy to store them.) Therefore, by eating a diet moderate in fat and higher in complex carbohydrates, the calories you consume are less likely to be converted into body fat.

Fat and Heart Health

The type of fat consumed can either bolster or undermine cardiac health. For example, of the four types of dietary fat, monounsaturated oils should be part of your daily diet, while trans fats top the list in the high-risk category. The distinction lies in the profound effect each type exerts on blood cholesterol levels.

THE GOOD

The best choice for heart health is *monounsaturated oils* rich in omega-9 fatty acids. Good examples include olive oil, canola oil, green and black olives, avocados, peanuts, peanut butter, hazelnuts, cashews, almonds and almond oils. Studies indicate that omega-9s reduce total and LDL cholesterol, lower triglycerides, reduce the risk of blood clots and minimize decreases in protective HDL cholesterol. This may partially explain the low incidence of heart disease among Mediterranean populations that use olive oil and Asian populations that use canola oil.

At the time of this writing, *polyunsaturated oils* have become a subject of scientific inquiry. Some of these oils, such as those found in seafood, walnuts and flaxseed, are rich in omega-3 fatty acids that protect cardiac health by reducing blood clotting, regulating contraction and relaxation of artery walls and modulating inflammation. On the other hand, polyunsaturated oils with omega-6 fatty acids may be unsafe. Some studies suggest that consuming *excessive* quantities of omega-6s, as in safflower oil, soybean oil, sunflower oil, corn oil, cottonseed oil and sesame oil, may work against cardiac health by increasing coronary inflammation, promoting constriction of blood vessels and raising the risk of blood clots.

This was not a concern in the past. Back when our diet included wild plants, seeds, fish and game, the ratio of omega-6s to omega-3s was four to one, considered a healthy balance. But when medical research in the 1960s strongly suggested that the epidemic of heart disease in America was caused by our intake of saturated fat, vegetable oil products boomed. Margarine took the place of butter, vegetable shortenings replaced lard and over time the ratio of omega-6s to omega-3s has widened to 15 to one. It's too early to determine an exact connection to coronary risks such as inflammation, but in the meantime there's good reason to cut back on omega-6s in favor of omega-3s.

THE BAD

One of the most harmful dietary fats is *saturated fat,* found in animal foods, dairy products and three vegetable oils: palm oil, palm kernel oil and coconut oil. Saturated fat works to increase both total and LDL cholesterol. The chart on the next page breaks down the sources.

MAJOR SOURCES OF SATURATED FAT

Food	% of Total Saturated Fat Consumed
Cheese	13.1%
Beef	11.7
Milk (including whole, low-fat and fat-free)	7.8
Oils	4.9
Ice cream/sherbet/frozen yogurt	4.7
Cakes/cookies/doughnuts	4.7
Butter	4.6
Shortening and animal fats	4.4
Salad dressings/mayonnaise	3.7
Poultry	3.6
Margarine	3.2
Sausage	3.1
Potato chips/corn chips/popcorn	2.9
Yeast bread	2.6

For the average American, saturated fat makes up 13% to 18% of calories; however, for some it makes up as much as 33%. Because of its impact on cholesterol, experts advise that saturated fat should make up no more than 10% of calories. "But," says Dr. Virgil Brown, past president of the American Heart Association, "the guideline of 10% is an upper limit, not a target. A better goal is 7%—and less than that if you have heart disease." The table below shows how much saturated fat you can eat to keep below 10% of total calories:

Calories	Grams of Saturated Fat
1,600	18 or less
2,000	20
2,200	24
2,500	25
2,800	31

Sometimes it takes just a small adjustment in food choices or cooking methods to reduce saturated fat:

Food	Grams of Saturated Fat
Cheese	
Regular cheddar, 1 oz.	6.0
Low-fat cheddar, 1 oz.	1.2
Ground beef	
Regular (25% fat), 3 oz. cooked	6.1
Extra-lean (5% fat), 3 oz. cooked	2.6
Milk	
Whole milk, 1 cup	4.6
1% milk, 1 cup	1.5
Breads	
Croissant, 1 medium	6.6
Bagel, oat bran, 1 medium	0.2
Table spreads	
Butter, 1 tsp.	2.4
Soft margarine with zero trans fat, 1 tsp.	0.7
Chicken	
Fried, leg with skin, 3 oz. cooked	3.3
Roasted, skinless breast, 3 oz. cooked	0.9

THE UGLY

Trans fats, or trans fatty acids, are even more harmful than saturated fats. Appearing on food labels as "partially hydrogenated" or "hydrogenated" oils, these fats deliver a cardiovascular double whammy. The more trans fats you consume, the higher your LDL cholesterol level will climb. And worse, they can produce smaller LDL particles in your bloodstream, raising heart attack risk. That's why the new guidelines recommend limiting trans fat to less than 1% of total calories on a 2,000-calorie diet, or about 2 grams per day. Americans, however, consume closer to 5% of calories, or 11 grams per day.

IT'S A FACT

In the Nurses' Health Study, women who consumed lots of trans fat on a regular basis had a 66% higher risk of heart disease than those who did not.

Trans fats do not occur naturally; they're created in food processing when vegetable oils are changed to solid or semisolid fats in order to extend the shelf life of products or to improve their taste and texture. For example, it takes oil to make cookies, but cookies don't turn out right if liquid oil is used, so the manufacturer chemically hardens or stiffens the oil by adding hydrogen to it. This process, called hydrogenation, may make the cookies turn out well, but it also produces trans fat that acts like saturated fat.

Margarine is another good example of how hydrogenation can alter the health properties of a food product. Spray and squeeze-type margarines, soft tub margarines and "diet" margarines are seen as healthful alternatives to butter because their oils (usually canola, corn or safflower) remain in a liquid form. But when the oils are hardened into stick form, cholesterol-raising trans fat is created. So, if you're concerned enough about your cholesterol to avoid butter and other saturated fats, it makes sense to also avoid stick margarine and other hydrogenated food products.

Almost half the supermarket foods in North America contain trans fats. Here are some examples:

Food	% of Total Trans Fats Consumed
Cakes, cookies, crackers, bread, etc.	40%
Animal products	21
Margarine	17
Fried potatoes	8
Potato chips, corn chips, popcorn	5
Other (including candy and breakfast cereal)	5

Trans fat is also used in restaurant foods such as salad dressings, chicken nuggets, fried foods and many desserts. Fast foods supply an inordinate amount of trans fat, particularly since many companies moved from deep frying in beef fat to frying in heavily hydrogenated oils. The impact of processed and fast foods can be significant. Remember, if you eat 2,000 calories a day, you should aim for no more than about 2 grams of trans fat daily. Then consider this:

■ You can eat *twice* that amount with a Burger King Big Fish Sandwich, two Little Debbie Swiss Cake Rolls or a KFC Biscuit.

■ You can eat *four* times that amount with 10 pieces of McDonald's Chicken Select chicken strips.

Because they now have to disclose trans fats on labels, food manufacturers are scrambling to reduce them or eliminate them altogether. After all, the words "trans fat free" on a label can boost sales. But it's not easy to remove hydrogenated oils without compromising taste, texture and shelf life, so many manufacturers are substituting palm oil, which is about 50% saturated fat. They're being a little cagey about it, using the name "palm fruit oil" to promote a healthier image, but that doesn't keep the oil from being heavily saturated. So, buyer beware. Foods like margarine spreads, cereals, energy bars and cookies are losing trans fats but gaining palm oil. This is not a good a trade-off.

Fat and Palatability

All the science in the world won't keep you eating right if the food doesn't taste good. That's where a moderate amount of dietary fat can help. Fat provides texture, makes food "melt in your mouth" and is digested slowly, so it provides an enjoyable feeling of satisfaction. My friend Graham Kerr, the Galloping Gourmet, once told me that when he trained as a chef, commercial kitchens kept butter in nut-size chunks. "The rule was, *When in doubt about the recipe, throw in a nut of butter.* The extra fat made everything taste better."

I've found this to be true with our Mediterranean-style recipes. Bernie uses judicious amounts of olive oil, cheese, meat, poultry and

---

WHAT ABOUT DIETARY CHOLESTEROL?

Cholesterol in food is no longer the lone villain it once was. Says Dr. Margaret Denke of the University of Texas Southwestern, "The main problem with cholesterol-rich foods is that they also tend to be high in dietary fat, particularly saturated fat." Dr. Ernst J. Schaefer of Tufts University puts it this way: "Reducing saturated fat consumption by 50% may lower blood cholesterol twice as much as a similar drop in dietary cholesterol."

---

seafood to create delicious, satisfying meals. But there's another benefit to cooking this way. Anyone offering advice on healthy eating pushes fruits and vegetables. And frankly, eating more fruit is easy. But, as one dietitian observed, "You know you're *really* hungry when you're hungry enough to eat vegetables." After all, how many people get excited over a pile of Brussels sprouts or okra? With this in mind, we often follow the Mediterranean tradition of dressing or sautéing vegetables in a small amount of olive oil. You might not like raw carrots, but toss them with a little olive oil and stir-fry or roast them, and your family will make them disappear.

Moderation and Balance

Heart-healthy eating is not the "all-the-fat-you-can-eat" high-protein diet, allowing up to 20% of total calories from saturated fat. Nor is it the severely restrictive plan that provides a far from palatable 10% or fewer calories from fat. Rather, a truly balanced diet is reasonable in total fat, provides for a healthy range of unsaturated fats and balances carbohydrate, fiber and protein. It allows for tasty, satisfying foods that you can eat for a lifetime. Indeed, Dr. Walter Willett of the Harvard School of Public Health suggests that healthy fats should join complex carbohydrates as foods to eat on a regular basis.

Chapter Six

The Truth About Carbohydrates

MERICA SEEMS TO HAVE A SERIOUS CASE of anxiety about food. Or, to be more accurate, about certain components in food. We tend to isolate them, categorize them as dangerous and exert superhuman efforts to avoid them. A decade ago, we were caught up in a low-fat mania. Today, we're aware that our zeal was misguided. But when it comes to carbohydrates, it appears that we haven't learned our lesson.

There's a lot of contradictory information around these days about carbohydrates. High-carb, low-carb. Which diet is better? The fact is, it depends on which kinds of carbohydrates you're talking about. Refined carbohydrates carry few nutrients, are usually high in sweeteners and calories, and break down quickly in your body. Complex carbohydrates, on the other hand, are just about the healthiest foods on the planet. They're full of great nutrients—fiber, vitamins, phytochemicals and antioxidants—and they're easy to recognize because they look much like they did in their original form.

If, like me, you're worn out from advice to cut down on one food and eliminate another altogether, you need to put together a dietary plan centered on foods you *can* eat. Complex carbohydrates fill the bill. They're the secret to an eating pattern that promotes good health and delicious food.

Low-Carbohydrate Diets

The appeal is obvious. You don't have to measure portion sizes or count calories. Even better, you can load up on favorite foods: hamburgers, steaks, bacon and cheese. And there's a so-called "nutritional theory" to back it up. Cut carbohydrates, says the theory, and you can't help but lose weight. Too many carbohydrates can cause blood sugar to surge, which spurs insulin production, which in turn causes blood sugar to dive abruptly, which leads to an increase in appetite . . . and so on.

But short-term weight loss is not the best measure of a diet's ultimate value, particularly for cardiac health. Besides, once you get past the anecdotal success stories, the data reveal mixed results. On one hand, at least five clinical trials indicated that low-carbohydrate diets were as effective as low-fat diets—and in most cases better—in helping very overweight people shed pounds quickly. On the other hand, there is little evidence that low-carbohydrate diets are as effective as low-fat diets over the long term. In fact, research shows just the opposite. While both low-fat and low-carbohydrate diets help people shed pounds initially, low-fat plans work better at keeping weight off.

In addition, low-carbohydrate diets turned out to be as difficult to stick with as any others and may actually be harder to maintain since the choice of foods is more restricted. Says Harvard's Dr. Frank M. Sacks, "Unless larger studies show that low-carbohydrate eating helps people keep weight off for a long time, and that this weight loss brings the expected health benefits, studies showing short-term weight loss don't mean very much."

 IT'S A FACT

Low-carb claims on food labels have no legal status, says the U.S. Food and Drug Administration. In fact, its Canadian counterpart, Health Canada, has banned all "low-carb" labeling. That government agency concluded there's no solid evidence to support carb-related health claims.

Low-carbohydrate diets also have several negative side effects:

■ Since carbohydrates provide the body's only source of glucose (blood sugar), limiting their intake means that our organs, including the brain, are deprived of fuel. Experts recommend eating no fewer than 130 grams of carbohydrates each day as the minimum amount needed for brain function. This is in striking contrast to most low-carbohydrate diets, particularly in the initial phase, which calls for a 20-gram maximum. Some people follow this guideline for their entire time on the diet.

■ An MIT study found that low-carbohydrate diets reduce levels of serotonin, which can regulate mood. Low serotonin levels often result in chronic fatigue.

■ Low-carbohydrate eating can produce ketosis, a toxic condition in which the body breaks down fats due to carbohydrate deficiency. Ketosis can cause the excretion of calcium and potassium in the urine and may harm the bones and kidneys.

■ Low-carbohydrate diets are low in fiber, vitamin C, B-complex vitamins, potassium and magnesium. At the same time, these diets are traditionally high in fat and cholesterol.

■ Some studies found that LDL cholesterol levels rose by at least 10% in about one-third of people on low-carbohydrate diets.

■ A study at Duke University suggests that low-carb diets can produce headaches, bad breath, constipation and hair loss.

The Glycemic Index

Hand in hand with the low-carbohydrate theorists are those who recommend using a scale called the Glycemic Index (GI) as a final arbiter of food selection. It's a given that not all carbohydrates act the same in the body. A key variable is how rapidly a food breaks down into glucose, or blood sugar. Over the past few years, there has been a movement to categorize carbohydrate foods according to the speed with which they break down in the body and how much and how fast they increase blood sugar. The Glycemic Index ranks foods that break down very rapidly as "high" and those that break down more slowly as "low." The index sets glucose at 100 and scores foods against that number.

■ Foods that are digested and absorbed slowly have a low GI value of less than 55.

■ Foods with a GI of 55 to 70 have an intermediate value.

■ Foods with a GI above 70 have a high value.

As shown in the table on page 75, most foods with a high GI tend to be refined carbohydrates. These foods, including junk food, instant rice, French fries, cakes, muffins and jelly beans, are considered to have a faster rate of absorption, resulting in rapid swings in insulin levels. Foods with a GI substantially below 70 are absorbed more slowly.

Most complex carbohydrates, such as fruits, vegetables, beans and whole grains, break down and enter the bloodstream gradually, triggering only a moderate rise in insulin. But when converted into refined carbohydrates (think of grains being pulverized into fine flour), these foods break down quickly and can make blood sugar levels rise rapidly. This action causes the body to crank out more insulin, which in turn makes blood sugar plummet by converting it to triglycerides and body fat. Have you ever eaten a meal of Chinese food and been hungry less than an hour later? According to GI proponents, this happens because the rice and noodles, both high on the index, are converted rapidly to sugar and disappear quickly from the bloodstream. The result is that you're left feeling lethargic, so you eat again—a bag of chips or a couple of cookies—to cause another rush of glucose and restore your energy. Of course, this effect doesn't last very long, so you eat another snack and the destructive cycle continues.

While the science behind the GI may be sound, many experts question its use as a valid mechanism for shaping dietary patterns. To begin with, there are some anomalies. White bread, for instance, has almost the same rating as whole wheat bread. And some healthy

Food	GI Score
Table sugar	100
Carrots	92
Cornflakes	80
Gatorade	78
Potato, mashed	74
Bagel, white	72
White bread	71
Instant white rice, long-grain	68
Whole wheat bread	64
Cereal, muesli	66
Potato, baked	60
Sweet corn	60
White rice, long-grain	60
Bread, rye, whole-meal	58
Apple	55
Coca-Cola	53
All-bran cereal	50
Sweet potato	48
Banana	46
Cake, sponge	46
Pumpernickel bread, whole-grain	46
Grapes	43
Kidney beans	42
Oatmeal	42
Spaghetti, white	42
Apple juice, unsweetened	41
Yogurt	36
Chickpeas	33
Milk, fat-free	32
Barley, pearled	25
Lentils	22

foods, such as baked potatoes, have a high GI. Also, the GI applies to individual foods, but we eat foods in groups. And the effects of foods eaten as part of a meal differ from those of foods consumed alone. Even the inventor of the index, Dr. David Jenkins at the University of Toronto, says it's "only one way of looking at carbohydrate foods—perhaps not even in some cases the most important way. My interest has been to look at the total physiological impact of a meal. The Glycemic Index was only the beginning of that kind of classification, not the end."

So, until the science is farther along, you probably don't need a list of GI numbers to tell you what you already know. For weight loss and good health, eat your carrots and skip the carrot cake.

A Different View

There are some marked differences between our Mediterranean-style dietary plan and that of the extreme low-carbohydrate advocates. But, with a bit of tweaking, there's also some common ground.

The principal area of disagreement is the amount of red meat, cheese and other sources of saturated fat found on many low-carbohydrate plans. (As a heart patient, it makes no sense to me to eat a plateful of bacon as a weight-loss technique.) The common ground is the recommendation to reduce carbohydrates. But low-carb proponents need to better define their terms. The only carbohydrates that cause weight gain are *refined* or *low-fiber* carbohydrates. Says Dr. P.K. Newby of the Jean Mayer USDA Human Nutrition Center at Tufts University, "It's not the carbohydrates you eat that expand your waist, it's the *kind* of carbohydrates you eat. In other words, follow the fiber and skip the processed foods when you're picking carbs with an eye on your weight."

The carbohydrates that benefit heart health and promote weight control are *complex* carbohydrates. Therefore, a carbohydrate-restricted diet should minimize only refined or low-fiber carbohydrates. However, a good number of low-carbohydrate proponents treat both as an enemy of weight loss. This is a major mistake.

Low-carbohydrate eating became popular because the old recommendation to scale back on fat caused some people to gain weight. Aggressive food processors reduced fat to meet the recommendation, but their products were now bursting with added sweeteners and low-fiber carbohydrates, not to mention calories. "We said nothing about calories, and neither did the food industry," says Nancy Ernst, nutrition coordinator of the National Cholesterol Education Program. "As a result, what was promoted was high-sugar, no-fat products that translated into weight gain."

Indeed, sometimes the lower-fat version of a food had more calories than its full-fat counterpart. But because such foods were advertised as heart-healthy (and also because eating too little fat kept some people constantly hungry), a lot of us ate an excess of refined carbohydrates in the form of high-calorie bagels, cookies and potato chips. To make matters worse, people tend to overeat fat-free foods. According to Dr. Chris Rosenbloom of Georgia State University, "Research shows that if people are told a food is fat-free or lower in fat, they tend to eat three to five times as much as they normally would if the food contained fat."

Now fast-forward to current times and note that carbohydrates have replaced fat as the nutritional scapegoat. But here's the critical point: *Carbohydrates are not the enemy.* People did not gain weight on low-fat diets because they ate too many carbohydrates. They ate too many calories, period. The best approach is to balance both carbohydrates and fat, and choose the healthiest sources of each. Many people learned the hard way that eating boxes of low-fat cookies adds calories. Well, eating boxes of low-carbohydrate cookies does the same. Says Dr. Gary D. Foster of the University of Pennsylvania School of Medicine, "There are no data to support the idea that carbohydrates make you hungry or that they're addictive. What puts weight on is eating too many calories—from whatever source."

The Benefits of Carbohydrates

Throughout history, complex carbohydrates have been the chief source of calories for humans: corn for American Indians, bread for Europeans, rice for Asians, grains and beans for Africans and South Americans. Unfortunately, the lack of an adequate intake of complex carbohydrates in the modern American diet, coupled with an excessive intake of low-fiber carbohydrates, ranks right up there with too much dietary fat as a major negative influence. Instead of analyzing the effects of regular versus low-fat or low-carb cookies for dessert, we should have been promoting fruit.

 IT'S A FACT

A high-fiber diet, particularly one rich in green, orange and yellow vegetables and citrus fruits, has been shown to decrease susceptibility to colon cancer.

"There are two things that make a carbohydrate healthy," says registered dietitian Janis Jibrin. "It's nutrient- and fiber-rich. And it doesn't send your blood sugar soaring. The complex carbohydrates found on the Mediterranean diet—fruits, vegetables, legumes and whole grains—fit the bill." Many foods rich in complex carbohydrates also contain cardioprotective compounds called phytochemicals, including:

- Flavonoids (in apples, citrus fruits, onions and grapes)
- Anthocyanidins (in blueberries, red grapes, cherries and plums)
- Indoles (in cabbage, bok choy, cauliflower, cabbage, Brussels sprouts, broccoli and other cruciferous vegetables)
- Carotenoids (in orange, red and yellow vegetables)
- Isoflavones (in soy foods)
- Lycopene (in tomatoes and tomato products)

HEART HEALTH

Studies throughout the world have concluded that people who habitually consume a diet rich in plant food have a low risk of coronary heart disease. In the 1950s, researchers studied three groups of Japanese subjects, each residing in a different environment and eating a different diet. Differences in heredity and physiology were set aside in this study, allowing the researchers to concentrate on diet patterns and blood cholesterol levels. This is how it worked out:

■ The first group lived in Japan and ate a traditional low-fat Asian diet: lots of vegetables, fruit, legumes, soy products, rice, fish and little meat. Members of this group had low cholesterol levels and a low incidence of heart attacks.

■ The second group lived in Hawaii and ate a mixture of Asian and American meals, which meant less fruits, vegetables and grains, and more meat and butter. This group had higher levels of cholesterol and a greater incidence of heart attacks.

■ The third group lived in Los Angeles and consumed a totally American diet . . . from steaks to ice cream. Their intake of fruits, vegetables and grains was decreased substantially, and this group had the highest levels of cholesterol and greatest incidence of heart attacks.

More recent studies have reaffirmed the benefits of plant foods. The Harvard Nurses' Study, with some 95,000 participants, found that those who ate whole grains and five servings a day of fruits and vegetables lowered their risk of heart attack by 35%. The Harvard Physicians' Study also concluded that unrefined foods rich in complex carbohydrates and fiber are cardioprotective and can help to control blood pressure and weight.

And finally, as reported in Chapter Five, a Stanford University study showed that people who eat a low-fat diet packed with complex carbohydrates reduce their LDL cholesterol levels by twice as much as people who eat a low-fat diet heavy on processed foods.

WEIGHT CONTROL

Unlike their refined counterparts, complex carbohydrates aid weight control because they fill you up, not out. You can eat a whole pound of apples and (although their bulk would cause some discomfort) take in less than 250 calories. Compare that with eating a pound of chocolate-covered peanuts (which almost anyone would find easy to do) and taking in more than 2,200 calories.

In addition, certain complex carbohydrates—especially whole fruits, raw vegetables, beans, whole grains and nuts—are rich in fiber. Says carbohydrate researcher Joan Slavin, R.D., "There's very strong evidence that people who eat high-fiber diets are less likely to be obese." Fiber passes through the digestive system intact, so not all calories consumed stay with the body. Also, high-fiber foods produce satiety, which means you're more likely to feel full for a longer period of time. Unfortunately, the average American consumes only 15 grams of dietary fiber each day, falling far short of the Surgeon General's recommendation of 25 to 35 grams. Luckily, there are many simple ways to boost fiber in your diet:

■ Eat a high-fiber cereal for breakfast.

■ Choose whole-grain foods such as whole wheat bread, brown rice and whole wheat pasta.

■ When baking, add bran cereal, ground flaxseed or wheat bran to your batter.

■ Replace white flour with whole wheat flour or use one-half of each when baking bread.

■ Add beans, peas and lentils to soups and salads.

■ Make fruits and vegetables your premier snack.

Another point to be made is that foods like apples and carrots need a lot of chewing, take a long time to eat and therefore provide sufficient time (about 20 minutes) for satiety to be attained. These foods also absorb water in the digestive system, thereby helping to create a feeling of fullness and satisfaction that keeps you from overeating. The fact is that most overweight people cannot eat enough complex carbohydrates to maintain their weight. They lose pounds automatically when they replace fatty and sugary foods with fruits, grains and vegetables.

And finally, there's no question that complex carbohydrates promote dietary compliance, particularly among men. Let's take a 60-

year-old man who's used to eating a small salad and a giant steak for dinner. Now he has a heart problem, so his diet changes to a small salad, a half-cup of rice and half a chicken breast. Needlesss to say, he's starving! And when men get too hungry, they cheat. One woman in a seminar audience told me that she had really cranked down on the fat in her husband's diet after he had undergone bypass surgery. "He's a new man," she said. "He's always going off by himself for a drive in the country." I didn't have the heart to tell her that his outings probably included a stop at the Golden Arches. Instead, I advised her to offer her husband a large salad, a full cup of wild rice, two other vegetables and half a chicken breast. With enough complex carbohydrates to keep him satisfied, he probably wouldn't revert to his old high-fat diet.

Moderation and Balance

Amid all the hype and contradictory and confusing advice about carbohydrates, one thing is crystal-clear: *Extreme eating is never a solution.* Banning carbohydrates, or eating nothing but carbs, has very little to do with science. "The fact is," says Dr. Judith Wurtman at the MIT Clinical Research Center, "it's completely natural to eat carbohydrates. If nature didn't mean for us to eat carbohydrates, we wouldn't have this elaborate system in place that makes them so important to our brains."

While Dr. Wurtman is certainly correct about carbohydrates in general, the devil is in the details. Low-fiber carbohydrates, such as presweetened cereals, sugary drinks and snack cakes, should be eaten in minimal amounts. Much of the nutritional value has been removed in such products by the refining process, and because of added sweeteners their calorie content is usually high. But we also have to take into consideration what they replace when we make them a regular part of our diet: the cardioprotective nutrients in neglected foods such as fruits, vegetables, whole grains, nuts, fish and soy products.

So, what's the bottom line? The experts tell us that complex carbohydrates should make up at least 55% of our total calories. (For those with metabolic syndrome, the appropriate amount is more on the order of 45% of calories.) And according to the new guidelines, all Americans should eat two cups of fruit, two and a half cups of vegetables and at least six one-ounce servings of grains (three from whole grains) every day.

In Chapter Eight, we'll show you how to adjust your dietary program so that meeting these requirements becomes an easy, satisfying part of your day-to-day plan.

Chapter Seven

Beyond the Basics

THE SCIENTIFIC COMMUNITY has only just begun to understand the complex interactions between nutritional components and the human body. However, it's becoming more evident every day that some foods provide extra health benefits when eaten on a regular basis. These foods, now incorporated into the dietary guidelines, have been dubbed "functional foods." According to the Institute of Medicine's Food and Nutrition Board, the term "functional" describes any food or food ingredient that may provide a health benefit beyond the traditional nutrients it contains.

Tomatoes, for instance, are high in vitamin C, but they also contain lycopene, which has been found to decrease the risk for developing certain cancers. Other foods found to fight cancer include broccoli and other cruciferous vegetables, citrus fruits and green tea. Many functional foods positively impact heart health. Foods rich in monounsaturated fats and omega-3 fatty acids reduce LDL cholesterol and triglycerides, lower the risk of blood clots and minimize decreases in protective HDL cholesterol.

In this chapter, we'll discuss some of the most important functional foods for your heart. Please note they're not ranked in order of importance. *All* of them are important, and you should be eating them on most days—if not every day.

Oats and Other Foods Rich in Soluble Fiber

The fiber in plant foods can contribute to lower risks of heart disease, diabetes and cancer. Fiber falls into two broad categories: insoluble and soluble. Insoluble fiber passes through the digestive track largely unchanged; found in wild rice, whole wheat bread, the skins of fruits, and vegetables such as carrots and broccoli, this kind of fiber may protect against certain types of cancer. In contrast, soluble fiber forms a gel that not only interferes with cholesterol absorption, but also binds with cholesterol and causes it to be excreted naturally. Both actions help to reduce total and LDL cholesterol levels.

It's important to understand that foods rich in soluble fiber help only when they become part of a healthful, low-fat eating plan accompanied by exercise. Foods rich in soluble fiber are listed below:

 IT'S A FACT

Studies conducted at the University of Kentucky by Dr. James Anderson showed that people with blood cholesterol levels above 200 could reduce their numbers by 13% to 19% simply by eating one cup of oat bran cereal per day.

SOLUBLE FIBER IN COMMON FOODS

Food	Grams of Soluble Fiber	Grams of Total Fiber
Fruits		
Apple, 1 medium	1	4
Banana, 1 medium	1	3
Blackberries, ½ cup	1	4
Grapefruit, 1 medium	2	2–3
Orange, 1 medium	2	2–3
Peach, 1 medium	1	2
Pear, 1 medium	2	4
Plum, 1 medium	1	1.5
Prunes, ¼ cup	1.5	3
Tangerine, 1 medium	1	2

Vegetables

Broccoli, cooked, ½ cup	1	1.5
Brussels sprouts, cooked, ½ cup	3	4.5
Carrots, cooked, ½ cup	1	2.5

Beans and Other Legumes

Black beans, cooked, ½ cup	2	5.5
Chickpeas, cooked, ½ cup	1	6
Kidney beans, cooked, ½ cup	3	6
Lentils, cooked, ½ cup	1	8
Lima beans, cooked, ½ cup	3.5	6.5
Navy beans, cooked, ½ cup	2	6
Northern beans, cooked, ½ cup	1.5	5.5
Pinto beans, cooked, ½ cup	2	7
White beans, cooked, ½ cup	0.4	4.2

Cereal Grains

Barley, cooked, ½ cup	1	4
Oatmeal, cooked, ½ cup	1	2
Oat bran, cooked ½ cup	1	3

A good suggestion: For breakfast, have oatmeal or oat bran with your orange juice at least three times a week. Topped with fresh or frozen berries, raisins, dried cranberries, chopped nuts, a sprinkle of bran or ground flaxseed and a dash of cinnamon, it makes a healthful *and* tasty start to your day.

Fruits, Vegetables and Other Foods Rich in Antioxidants

When I first heard about the effectiveness of antioxidants in protecting coronary artery cells, I assumed that this would mean popping a vitamin pill or two. Not necessarily so. Study after study has confirmed the disease-fighting role of beta-carotene and vitamins C

IT'S A FACT

A review of clinical trials conducted by the American Heart Association concluded that antioxidant supplements cannot match the heart-protective effects of a diet rich in whole grains, fruits, vegetables and beans. Says Dr. Alice Lichtenstein of Tufts University, "There are no quick fixes. We need to focus on making better choices while shopping for food, preparing food and eating out."

and E *when they come from whole foods.* A study at the University of Texas, for example, showed a 30% reduction in the risk of heart disease in men whose daily intake of vitamin C equaled that found in one or two oranges and who consumed an amount of beta-carotene equal to that found in one or two carrots. The Harvard Nurses' Study showed that those who ate at least five servings a day of fruits and vegetables lowered their risk of heart attack by 33%. Such research provides a strong incentive for everyone, and particularly heart patients like me, to eat at least 2 cups of fruits and 3 cups of vegetables per day.

My recommendation is to get your antioxidants from food. Then, if you wish, use supplements as . . . well, supplements. If you want to use vitamin pills, it's important to first check with your physician or a registered dietitian.

BETA-CAROTENE

Eating bright orange fruits and vegetables ensures a diet high in mixed carotenoids (alpha, beta, delta and gamma) known to favorably impact cardiac health and reduce cancer risk. Beta-carotene, the best-known carotenoid, is concentrated in carrots, sweet potatoes and pumpkin; tomatoes and tomato products; sweet red pepper; leafy greens like spinach, collards, turnip greens, kale, beet and mustard greens, green leaf lettuce and romaine; orange fruits like mango, cantaloupe and apricots; and red or pink grapefruit. While there is no USRDA for beta-carotene, many experts recommend 5 to 30 milligrams a day for optimal antioxidant effect. This can be achieved with a little menu planning.

FOODS HIGH IN BETA-CAROTENE

Food	Milligrams of Beta-Carotene
Carrot juice, 1 cup	38
Sweet potato, cooked, ½ cup	17
Pumpkin (canned), cooked, ½ cup	16
Carrots, cooked, ½ cup	11
Cantaloupe, ½ medium	8
Carrots, raw, ½ cup	5
Mango, 1 medium	5
Collard greens, cooked, 1 cup	4
Spinach, cooked, ½ cup	4
Dried apricots, ½ cup	3
Spinach, raw, 1 cup	3
Winter squash, ½ cup	3
Red pepper, raw, ½ cup	2

Although carrot juice, sweet potato and pumpkin are high in beta-carotene, most people are probably not going to eat them every day. Pick three or four foods you *will* eat regularly and work them into meals. It's as simple as a snack of dried apricots, a bowl of spinach or carrots dipped in salsa.

VITAMIN C
The USRDA for vitamin C is 60 milligrams daily; however, the latest research suggests that the optimal level for cardiovascular protection is 500 to 1,000 milligrams per day. Fortunately, getting an adequate amount from food is relatively easy on a Mediterranean-style diet that emphasizes fruits and vegetables, many of which are excellent sources of vitamin C. For example, just a half-cup of strawberries and three-quarters of a cup of orange juice at breakfast and a half-cup of red bell pepper in a stir-fry at dinner will put you in the range of 250 milligrams.

FOODS HIGH IN VITAMIN C

Food	Milligrams of Vitamin C
Guava, raw, ½ cup	188
Red bell pepper, raw, ½ cup	142
Red bell pepper, cooked, ½ cup	116
Kiwi fruit, 1 medium	70
Orange, raw, 1 medium	70
Orange juice, ¾ cup	61–93
Green bell pepper, raw, ½ cup	60
Green bell pepper, cooked, ½ cup	51
Grapefruit juice, ¾ cup	50–70
Vegetable juice cocktail, ¾ cup	50
Strawberries, raw, ½ cup	49
Brussels sprouts, cooked, ½ cup	48
Cantaloupe, ¼ medium	47
Papaya, raw, ¼ medium	47
Kohlrabi, cooked, ½ cup	45
Broccoli, raw, ½ cup	39
Edible pod peas, cooked, ½ cup	38
Broccoli, cooked, ½ cup	37
Sweet potato, canned, ½ cup	34
Tomato juice, ¾ cup	33
Cauliflower, cooked, ½ cup	28
Pineapple, raw, ½ cup	28
Kale, cooked, ½ cup	27
Mango, ½ cup	23

Several foods are excellent sources of both beta-carotene and vitamin C. Here are some easy ways to boost beta-carotene and vitamin C at the same time:

- Use spinach instead of iceberg lettuce for salads.
- Add chopped bell peppers to omelets, salads, stir-fries and casseroles.
- Add chopped or grated carrots or squash to salads, soups, muffins, casseroles and meat loaf.
- Substitute sweet potatoes for regular potatoes.
- Add tomatoes to salads and sandwiches.
- Reach for dried apricots, peaches or prunes when it's time for a quick snack.
- When baking bread and muffins, think about using pumpkin— but watch out for fat and calories.
- Include mangoes in your menus.

VITAMIN E

The optimal level for vitamin E is 100 to 800 international units (IU), or about 133 to 533 milligrams. Some foods, such as 100% fortified, ready-to-eat breakfast cereals, wheat germ, cooked spinach, turnip greens, tomato sauce, avocado and mangoes, are low-fat sources of vitamin E. However, many sources are higher in fat, including sunflower seeds; sunflower, safflower, canola, corn, olive, peanut and soybean oils; salmon; mayonnaise; Brazil nuts, almonds and hazelnuts; peanuts and peanut butter.

Use these fattier sources to replace less healthy fat in your diet. It takes some planning to get at least 100 IU of vitamin E daily. In fact, I'm not at all sure I reach that level on most days. As with beta-carotene, I've identified a handful of foods that I do eat regularly and that provide a steady source of vitamin E for me. These include fortified cereals, salmon, peanut butter, olive oil and almonds. Since I do a lot of traveling by air, I pack some almonds in my briefcase for snacking on the plane.

FOODS HIGH IN VITAMIN E

Food	International Units of Vitamin E
Wheat germ, 1 tbsp.	26.2
Almonds, dry roasted, 1 oz.	7.5
Safflower oil, 1 tbsp.	4.7
Corn oil, 1 tbsp.	2.9
Turnip greens, cooked, ½ cup	2.4
Mango, 1	2.3
Peanuts, dry roasted, 1 oz.	2.1
Mayonnaise made with soybean oil, 1 tbsp.	1.6
Broccoli, cooked, ½ cup	1.5

Beans, Nuts and Other Foods Rich in B Vitamins

Emerging research shows that one of the best ways to control homocysteine and coronary inflammation is to consume an adequate amount of three B vitamins: folate (called folic acid when used in a supplement or to fortify foods), B_6 and B_{12}. This is a very important finding in view of new science implicating coronary inflammation as a major marker for heart disease and heart attack. In an editorial in the *Journal of the American Medical Association,* Dr. Kilmer S. McCully observed that "consuming an adequate amount of folate, B_6 and B_{12} is as important to reducing coronary risk as quitting smoking, lowering high cholesterol levels and controlling blood pressure."

The current USRDA for adults is 400 micrograms of folate, 1.3 milligrams (women) and 1.7 milligrams (men) of B_6, and 2.4 micrograms of B_{12} daily.

IT'S A FACT

In a study of over 80,000 female subjects, those who consumed more than twice the USRDA of folate, B_6 and B_{12} reduced their risk of a heart attack by more than 45%.

However, these levels may be inadequate to provide maximum protection against heart disease. "Everyone should be at two to three times the current USRDA for folate, B_6 and B_{12} to achieve the maximum reduction in risk," says Dr. Eric B. Rimm of the Harvard School of Public Health.

Fortunately, as shown in the table below, B vitamins are readily found in common foods such as cereal; peas and beans; oranges and orange juice; and deep green leafy vegetables like spinach and mustard greens.

FOODS HIGH IN FOLATE

Food	Micrograms of Folate
100% fortified ready-to-eat cereal, ¾ cup	400
Chickpeas, cooked, 1 cup	280
Cranberry beans, 1 cup	350
Asparagus, cooked, 1 cup	260
Lentils, cooked, 1 cup	260
Spinach, cooked, 1 cup	260
Black-eyed peas, cooked, 1 cup	210
Broccoli, cooked, 1 cup	200
Oatmeal, 1 cup	200
Beef liver, cooked, 3 oz.	185
Avocado, 1 cup	160
Artichoke, cooked, 1 cup	155
Orange juice, 1 cup	110
25% fortified ready-to-eat cereal, ¾ cup	100
Vegetarian baked beans, canned	60
Sunflower seeds, 1 oz.	55

FOODS HIGH IN VITAMIN B₆

Food	Milligrams of Vitamin B₆
100% fortified ready-to-eat cereal, ¾ cup	2.00
Potato, baked with skin, 1 medium	.70
Banana, 1 medium	.68
Garbanzo beans, canned, ½ cup	.57
Chicken breast, cooked, 3 oz.	.52
25% fortified ready-to-eat cereal, ¾ cup	.50
Banana, 1 medium	.48
Avocado, ½ medium	.42
Hamburger, 3 oz.	.39
Pork loin (lean only), cooked, 3 oz.	.32
Fish, 3 oz.	.29
Tuna, canned in water, 3 oz.	.18
Spinach, cooked, ½ cup	.16
Rice, brown, ½ cup	.16
Walnuts, 1 oz.	.15

FOODS HIGH IN VITAMIN B₁₂

Food	Micrograms of Vitamin B₁₂
Beef liver, 3 oz.	68
Clams, canned, ½ cup	19
Oysters, canned, 3.5 oz.	18
100% fortified ready-to-eat cereal, ¾ cup	6
Salmon, cooked, 3 oz.	5
Tuna, 3 oz.	2
Yogurt, 1 cup	1
Milk, fat-free, 1 cup	.9
Halibut, 3 oz.	.8
Egg, 1 large	.8
Chicken, 3 oz.	.4
Cheese, cheddar, 1 oz.	.4

Soy Foods Rich in Protein

Though not part of the traditional Mediterranean diet, soy offers benefits that are hard to ignore. Rich in protein and isoflavones, soy products such as soybeans, soy milk and tofu have a positive impact on cardiac health. In early studies of Asian populations that exhibited lower cholesterol levels and far less heart disease than western populations, it was initially thought that the fat content of their respective diets—low among Asians, high for westerners—was the key factor. Upon further investigation, however, researchers found that the Asian diet of rice, vegetables, whole grains and particularly soy was just as important as the low intake of fat.

Subsequent studies confirmed soy's effectiveness. An analysis of 38 clinical studies showed that substituting soy products for animal foods can lower LDL cholesterol by as much as 8%. In addition, it has been found that soy protein can lower triglyceride levels, raise

FOODS HIGH IN SOY PROTEIN

Food	Grams of Soy Protein
Soybeans, cooked, ½ cup	14
Edamame (green soybeans, cooked/canned, ½ cup	13
Soy nuts, ¼ cup	12
Texurized soy protein, cooked, ½ cup	11
Soybean burgers, 3.5 oz.	10
Soy crumbles, ground, ½ cup	9
Tofu, firm, 3 oz.	8
Soy flour, ¼ cup	8
Tofu yogurt, 8 oz.	8
Soy milk, 8 oz.	6
Tofu, silken, 3 oz.	6
Soybean sprouts, 1 oz.	4
Miso, 1 tbsp.	2

IT'S A FACT

The benefits of soy protein are so compelling that the FDA now permits food manufacturers to post a health claim on the labels of products with at least 6.25 grams per serving.

HDL levels, inhibit inflammation and reduce the risk of blood clots. Indeed, its link to protection against heart disease is so strong that the Food and Drug Administration has suggested an intake of 25 grams of soy protein every day as part of a diet low in saturated fat and cholesterol.

Varieties of soy foods are becoming more plentiful every day. These include soybeans, soy milk, tofu, sports bars, tempeh (a chewy, soft soybean cake), soy nuts, soy burgers, textured vegetable protein (TVP, a good substitute for ground beef), breakfast cereals fortified with soy, and soy flour.

A good suggestion: Copy the Japanese by eating edamame (green soybeans) as a snack. They're delicious cold or hot, and they're right near the top of the list of foods high in soy protein.

Beverages Rich in Flavonoids

While red wine has received most of the publicity concerning alcohol and cardiac health, studies show that moderate and regular consumption of any form of alcohol—including beer and whiskey—is associated with a reduced risk of heart attack and stroke. Says Dr. R. Curtis Ellison of the Boston University School of Medicine, "It's now commonly accepted in the medical community that alcohol can reduce the risk of atherosclerosis, the gradual 'silting up' of arteries that can lead to a heart attack or stroke." Even the American Heart Association acknowledges that moderate alcohol consumption may be cardioprotective.

Alcohol works to improve cardiovascular health by boosting HDL and lowering LDL. Anytime you can get that movement—HDL going up, LDL coming down—your arteries benefit. In addition, many alcoholic beverages, including red wine and beer, contain powerful antioxidants called flavonoids. Recent studies suggest that people who drink moderately show signs of less arterial inflammation when compared with nondrinkers and heavy drinkers; in particular, moderate drinkers have significantly lower levels of C-reactive protein, a marker of inflammation. Flavonoids also have an anticoagulant property similar to that of aspirin.

Says Dr. Arthur Klatsky, a cardiologist with Kaiser Permanente in Oakland, California, "Our studies found that moderate drinkers, those who consume from one to three drinks per day, have a lower risk of dying from heart disease than either those who abstain all together or those who drink heavily. In fact, nondrinkers and heavy drinkers seem to have heart attacks at the same rate. Light drinkers, on the other hand, have a decreased rate."

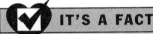
IT'S A FACT

Commercial grape juice and alcohol-free wine have also been shown to confer cardiovascular benefits.

As a heart patient and as a proponent of Mediterranean-style eating, I enjoy a glass of wine with dinner three or four times a week. But despite its cardioprotective nature, alcohol is not for everyone. Heavy drinking can cause elevated blood pressure and coronary inflammation and can contribute to overweight, obesity and metabolic syndrome. For many people, alcohol can slow metabolism. So check with your doctor, particularly if you have high blood pressure, elevated triglycerides, obesity, cardiomyopathy (a weakened heart) or atrial fibrillation, or if you're taking prescription or over-the-counter medications. Then, if you do drink, be smart about it:

■ *Drink in moderation.* This means no more than one to two drinks a day for men, one for women. It *doesn't* mean averaging a drink a day by abstaining on weekdays and binge drinking on weekends. That pattern is clearly harmful to health.

■ *Understand what constitutes a drink.* Twelve grams (a half-ounce) of pure alcohol: this is the amount in 12 ounces of beer, 1.5 ounces of 80-proof liquor or 5 ounces of wine.

■ *Pair your drink with food.* Studies show that moderate drinkers who generally imbibe outside of mealtimes have a 45% higher risk of hypertension than folks who drink with food.

■ *Determine if you can afford the extra calories,* particularly if you're trying to lose weight. Ounce for ounce, alcohol has almost as many calories (7) as fat has (9).

CALORIES IN ALCOHOLIC BEVERAGES

Beverage	Calories
Beer, regular, 12 fl. oz.	144
Beer, light, 12 fl. oz.	108
White wine, 5 fl. oz.	100
Red wine, 5 fl. oz.	105
Sweet dessert wine, 3 fl. oz.	141
80-proof distilled spirits, 1.5 fl. oz. (gin, vodka, whiskey)	96

BLACK TEA

Green tea has long had a reputation for stimulating good health. Now studies suggest that drinking at least one cup of black tea daily could cut your risk of heart attack significantly due to the beneficial action of flavonoids. A 1999 study headed by Dr. Michael Graziano, a heart specialist at Brigham and Women's Hospital, selected 340 men and women who had suffered heart attacks and matched them by age, gender and neighborhood with people who had never had heart attacks. The study then investigated their coffee- and tea-drinking habits for one year. Dr. Graziano found that those who drank one or more cups of black tea every day slashed their heart attack risk by a staggering 44% compared with those who did not drink tea.

Such positive research results translate into a strong lifestyle recommendation to drink more black tea. But don't imagine that drinking tea will offset an unhealthy lifestyle. If you really want to maximize the effect of black tea, add it to healthy habits. It won't work if you're smoking, sitting on a coach and eating junk foods. And keep a sense of perspective. The amount of tea needed to provide a cardioprotective effect is still under debate. Until we know the "threshold" dosage (whether it's one or six cups a day), employ the advice of "moderation in all things."

A good suggestion: Have a cup of tea as your morning drink or as an afternoon pick-me-up. Or, better yet, drink decaf tea to obtain the flavonoids without the caffeine.

Margarine with Plant Sterol Esters

A new type of margarine, made from plant sterol esters, has a cholesterol-lowering effect similar to that of oat bran. Clinical trials have shown that this margarine lowers total cholesterol by 10% and LDL cholesterol by 14%. Some brands can be used only as a spread, while others can also be used in cooking.

While plant sterol margarine may be beneficial for cholesterol control, making it part of your diet raises two concerns. The first relates to weight gain. A single pat of this type of margarine can have 45 or 50 calories, yet two or three pats a day are needed for cholesterol-lowering efficacy. That can add up to a lot of extra calories. If you're replacing other fat calories with plant sterol margarine, your net caloric intake should not change and you should not gain extra weight. But if the margarine is adding calories to your diet to the tune of between 100 and 135 calories a day, weight gain is a distinct possibility.

The second concern is that people might treat this margarine as a cure-all, eating the wrong food and then trying to "correct" their diet with cholesterol-lowering margarine. Obviously, this doesn't work when the margarine is spread on a croissant.

If, like me, you prefer not to eat *any* margarine, cholesterol-lowering or otherwise, be aware that you can get plant sterol esthers in your diet from soy products, nuts and seeds.

Putting It All Together

While it's encouraging to learn that certain foods provide cardiac benefit because of their functional components, in truth most of us can hardly pronounce "phytochemical" or "flavonoid," much less remember to include these components in our diet day after day. Too much emphasis on the scientific elements can sometimes make us feel as if our kitchens have been turned into chemistry labs instead of places for preparing fun, satisfying meals and snacks. That's why we've put a great deal of effort into making certain that functional foods from every food group are contained in our recipes. It's an easy way to eat what you need to eat for your heart but still enjoy your food as food rather than medicine.

SELECTED FUNCTIONAL FOODS

Food	Key Component(s)	Potential Benefit(s)
Oats	Beta-glucan (soluble fiber)	Reduces heart disease risk (lowers total and LDL cholesterol)
Soy foods	Soy protein	Reduces heart disease risk (lowers total and LDL cholesterol)
	Isoflavones	Promote bone health; reduce breast cancer risk
Whole grains	Cereal grains	Reduce heart disease risk (lower total and LDL cholesterol); reduce risk of type 2 diabetes
Fish	Omega-3 fatty acids	Reduce heart disease risk (lower triglyceride levels and risk of blood clotting; increase HDL cholesterol)
Walnuts and almonds	Omega-3 fatty acids; vitamin E	Reduce heart disease risk (lower LDL cholesterol)
Fruits and vegetables	Phytochemicals	Reduce risk of heart disease and cancer

Garlic, onions, leeks and scallions	Sulfur compounds	Reduce risk of heart disease (lower total cholesterol) and cancer
Olive oil	Monounsaturated fatty acids	Reduce heart disease risk (lower total and LDL cholesterol; reduce blood clotting)
Wine	Alcohol flavonoids	Reduce heart disease risk (lower risk of blood clotting; increase HDL cholesterol)
Broccoli, cauliflower and other cruciferous vegetables	Phytochemicals; vitamins A and C	Reduce cancer risk
Legumes/dried beans	Folate; soluble fiber	Reduce heart disease risk (lower cholesterol and homocysteines)
Citrus fruits	Vitamin C; pectin; folate	Reduce heart disease risk (lower cholesterol and homocysteines)
Flaxseed	Omega-3 fatty acids	Reduce heart disease risk (lower total and LDL cholesterol; reduce blood clotting)
Fat-free dairy products	Calcium; vitamin D	Reduce risk of high blood pressure and obesity
Tea, black	Flavonoids	Reduce heart disease risk (protect blood vessel lining from inflammation; reduce blood clotting)
Tea, green	Flavonoids	Reduce cancer risk
Tomatoes	Lycopene	Reduces heart disease risk
Cholesterol-lowering margarine (corn, soy, wheat)	Plant stanols; plant sterols	Reduce heart disease risk (lower LDL cholesterol)
Berries, cherries and red grapes	Antioxidants	Reduce heart disease risk (improve cellular health)
Carrots	Beta-carotene	Reduces heart disease risk (improves cellular health)

A PERFECT DINNER

Dutch researchers have identified the "ideal meal"—one that can help to prevent disease and still taste good. In a review of 44 studies, they found that men and women who ate six key foods daily cut their risk of heart disease by 76%. If they stuck with it, men could increase their life expectancy by 6.5 years and women by about 5 years. Here's how it breaks down:

- ½ teaspoon fresh garlic
- 2 cups of fruits and vegetables (especially citrus fruits and leafy greens)
- 3½ ounces of dark chocolate
- a 5-ounce glass of red wine
- a handful (2.3 ounces) of almonds
- 4 ounces salmon or another fish containing omega-3 fatty acids (2 to 4 times a week)

A number of additional foods are currently being studied for their cardioprotective potential. While it would be premature to label them "functional," the initial research results on dark chocolate, cinnamon and pomegranate juice appear to be positive.

Part Three

Getting
Practical

Chapter Eight

First Steps

THE GOAL OF THIS BOOK IS TO HELP YOU make dietary changes that will last a lifetime. But before you get started, it makes sense to prepare for success. Without a plan, your first thought might be to just jump in and start doing something. That's what I did . . . and it didn't work. In the heat of the decision to change everything overnight, my family and I scurried to find ways to "eat healthy for Dad's heart." Kitchen cupboards were cleaned out. New cookbooks were purchased. And yet we had no plan, no focus, no clear goals at all.

We learned the hard way that significant behavior modification is not the result of a single quantum leap. Rather, it comes with the accumulation of little changes that add up to a major accomplishment. It's about discovering how to eat for a lifetime, not how to diet for a week. Researchers estimate that it takes from six weeks all the way up to six months to establish a lifestyle habit. So, before you start, step back for a moment to consider what you want to achieve. Think in terms of manageable building blocks. For example, having a daily goal of "eating more vegetables" is too nebulous. Instead, set a concrete goal such as eating two cups of veggies at dinner each night. Accomplish that and you've created a solid building block. After a period of time, such building blocks can add up to substantial change.

Set Your Goals

Not all Americans need to lose weight. Those at a healthy weight should strive to maintain it, since research shows that it's far easier to keep from putting on more pounds than to take them off. But if you do need to lose weight, you should have some idea of the outcome you expect and how much time it will take to make it happen. A goal of "losing weight over the next year" is too imprecise for you to make a real commitment to change. Instead, it's better to say, *I'm 10 pounds above my ideal weight. My goal is to lose those 10 pounds in the next three months.* Since eating smart and exercising effectively can produce a weight loss of up to one and a half pounds a week, this is a reasonable and realistic goal.

Do you know what weight is appropriate for your good health? The Body Mass Index (BMI) in Chapter Two can provide you with a range of classifications for weight from "normal" to "extreme obesity." Find where you are and where you'd like to be. Or go to the Web site for the National Heart, Lung and Blood Institute, *www.nhlbi.nih.gov,* and use its BMI assessment tool.

ESTABLISH A FAT GUIDELINE

The new guidelines counsel managing fat intake (and therefore calories) in order to manage weight effectively. But how much fat should you be eating? That question can be answered by calculating your personal fat budget with three simple steps.

Step #1 Start by estimating your ideal weight. This should not be some fantasy weight based on wishful thinking. A reasonable estimate is provided by the following formula, developed by Dr. Richard Freeman of the University of Wisconsin Medical School. First, measure your height in feet and inches:

■ Men get 105 pounds for the first 5 feet of height. Every additional inch is plus 6 pounds. *Example:* A man 5'10" tall has an ideal weight of 166 pounds.

■ Women get 100 pounds for the first 5 feet of height. Every additional inch is plus 5 pounds. *Example*: A woman 5'5" tall has an ideal weight of 125 pounds.

Don't panic if your ideal weight seems unrealistically low. This is less about being a target weight for you and more about providing a scientifically sound basis for creating a personal fat budget.

I like the Freeman Formula because it's based on healthy body-fat levels. Too often, we look to the bathroom scale as our be-all and end-all. Up two pounds and it's the end of the world; down two pounds and it's better than Lotto. The scale records your body *weight*, not its *composition*. How much of your scale weight is lean muscle and bone, and how much is body fat? There can be huge differences in terms of health impact. Let's take two people who each weigh 150 pounds. One has a body-fat level of 30% (i.e., 45 pounds of body fat); the other has a level of 12% (18 pounds of body fat). Their scale weights are the same, but there's a great dissimilarity in body composition. If your "ideal weight" and "scale weight" match up, you probably have a healthy body-fat level. If your scale weight exceeds your ideal weight, it's usually because you're carrying too much body fat.

The Freeman Formula applies to people with a "medium"-size frame. To find out whether your frame is "medium," "large" or "small," measure your wristbone (toward your hand) with a cloth measuring tape. Then use the table below to estimate your frame size:

Men	Frame Size	Women
Under 7 inches	Small	Under 6 inches
7 inches	Medium	6 inches
Over 7 inches	Large	Over 6 inches

If you have a medium frame, the Freeman Formula predicts your ideal weight. For a small frame, subtract 10%; for a large frame, add 10%.

A WORD OF CAUTION

While it's critical to establish ideal weight as a means to a goal, don't become so obsessed with what you weigh that you step on a scale every morning. Your body won't drop weight in a predictable, orderly way. (Indeed, a woman's weight can fluctuate as much as 10 pounds in a month as a result of fluid retention during the menstrual cycle.) As nutritionist Dr. Sandra Haber says, "The scale becomes a judge of how well you've done that day. You may know that you haven't overeaten, but if the scale needle hasn't moved, or worse, it's inched upward, you believe the scale, not your own actions." Discouragement can cause stress, anxiety and overeating. Experts advise weighing yourself no more than twice a week—first thing in the morning, naked, and on an empty stomach.

Step #2 Estimate how many calories you need each day to maintain your ideal weight. To a great extent, caloric intake depends on your level of activity. The more physically active you are, the more calories you can consume. According to the American College of Sports Medicine and the American Dietetic Association, the following levels of activity provide a reliable guideline for estimating daily caloric need:

Level of Activity	Calories Needed per Pound per Day
Extremely inactive or sedentary (*Example:* No aerobic exercise in the course of a week)	11
Moderately active (light activity) (*Example:* Aerobic exercise 2–3 times a week)	13
Active (moderate exercise and/or work) (*Example:* Aerobic exercise 4–5 times a week)	15
Extremely active (heavy exercise and/or work) (*Example:* Aerobic exercise 6–7 times a week)	18

Next, multiply your ideal weight by your level of activity to determine the number of calories needed daily. *Example:* A 190-pound man who is "extremely active" needs about 3,420 calories each day to sustain his ideal weight. The following chart is an easy way to determine daily need:

CALORIES NEEDED DAILY TO SUSTAIN IDEAL WEIGHT

MEN

Ideal Weight	Extremely Inactive	Moderately Active	Active	Extremely Active
118	1,298	1,534	1,770	2,124
124	1,364	1,612	1,860	2,232
130	1,430	1,690	1,950	2,340
136	1,496	1,768	2,040	2,448
142	1,562	1,846	2,130	2,556
148	1,628	1,924	2,220	2,664
154	1,694	2,002	2,310	2,772
160	1,760	2,080	2,400	2,880
166	1,826	2,158	2,490	2,988
172	1,892	2,236	2,580	3,096
178	1,958	2,314	2,670	3,204
184	2,024	2,392	2,760	3,312
190	2,090	2,470	2,850	3,420
196	2,156	2,548	2,940	3,528
202	2,222	2,626	3,030	3,636

Using the chart on page 108, a "moderately active" 125-pound woman would learn that she needs 1,625 calories daily to sustain her ideal weight.

CALORIES NEEDED DAILY TO SUSTAIN IDEAL WEIGHT

WOMEN

Ideal Weight	Extremely Inactive	Moderately Active	Active	Extremely Active
100	1,100	1,300	1,500	1,800
105	1,155	1,365	1,575	1,890
110	1,210	1,430	1,650	1,980
115	1,265	1,495	1,725	2,070
120	1,320	1,560	1,800	2,160
125	1,375	1,625	1,875	2,250
130	1,430	1,690	1,950	2,340
135	1,485	1,755	2,025	2,430
140	1,540	1,820	2,100	2,520
145	1,595	1,885	2,175	2,610
150	1,650	1,950	2,250	2,700
155	1,705	2,015	2,325	2,790
160	1,760	2,080	2,400	2,880

Step #3 Because fat percentages are often misleading, it makes more sense to establish your fat budget in grams. For most people, 20% to 35% of calories from fat is recommended; for people who need to lose weight, 20% to 25% of calories from fat may be more appropriate. Use the chart on the facing page to estimate the maximum grams of total fat you can consume in a day and still maintain a lean diet.

Remember, the figures in the chart are the recommended maximum grams of fat in a day. Unless you're extremely active, i.e., you run 10 miles a day or work in a very cold climate, there is no reason to budget for more than 60 grams of fat per day. Anything above that figure is for reference only. On the other hand, experts warn against falling below 15 grams of fat per day.

MAXIMUM GRAMS OF TOTAL FAT PER DAY

Daily Calories	Percentage of Calories from Fat			
	20%	25%	30%	35%
1,200	27	33	40	46
1,300	29	36	43	50
1,400	31	39	47	54
1,500	33	42	50	58
1,600	36	44	53	62
1,700	38	47	57	66
1,800	40	50	60	70
1,900	42	53	63	73
2,000	44	56	67	77
2,100	47	58	70	81
2,200	49	61	73	85
2,300	51	64	77	89
2,400	53	67	80	93
2,500	56	69	83	97
2,600	58	72	87	101
2,700	60	75	90	105
2,800	62	77	93	108
2,900	64	80	96	112
3,000	67	83	100	116

ESTABLISH A CARBOHYRATE GUIDELINE

There is good cause today to establish a carbohydrate guideline, but not for the reason you might think. *It isn't that we eat too many carbohydrates; it's that we might not be getting enough.* The recommendation is to get at least 55% of calories from carbohydrates for optimum nutrients and fiber and for brain functioning. So, if you eat about 1,800 calories per day, you need about 250 grams of carbohydrates.

The chart on page 110, developed by Jo Ann Hattner, M.P.H., R.D., of the American Dietetic Association, provides a general estimate of how many grams of carbohydrates you need each day.

Height	Grams of Carbohydrates Needed
5'	165
5'1"	170
5'2"	180
5'3"	190
5'4"	195
5'5"	200
5'6"	210
5'7"	220
5'8"	225
5'9"	235
5'10"	245
5'11"	255
6'	260

Write It Down

Most people assume that they eat (and overeat) because of physical hunger, but that's not usually the reason. A great many of us are moved to eat and to select certain foods by external cues. For example, you might eat because of the time of day. A morning coffee break might automatically call for a helping of Danish pastry. Then, when the clock strikes noon, it's time to eat again, whether you're hungry or not. Internal cues can be just as motivating. These include anger, happiness, anxiety, boredom, depression and loneliness. Too often, food becomes a reward, a consolation prize, a pacifier, a stimulant or a security blanket. We all know that emotions do not provide good reasons for us to eat, yet many health professionals believe them to be the single most important cause of overeating in America.

A good way to begin to change the way you eat is to keep a food journal for a week or two. Don't try to be "good." Just record everything you eat. And that means *everything*: the half slice of toast one

SAMPLE FOOD JOURNAL

Day of Week: Wednesday

When/ Where	Why?	With Whom?	Food Eaten	Calories
7:00 A.M. Kitchen	Very hungry	Family	1 cup orange juice	110
			Jelly doughnut	225
			Coffee w/ 2 tsp. sugar	30
10:00 A.M. Conference room	Not very hungry; ate for social reasons	Coworkers	Large mocha coffee	390
			Large bran muffin	350
Noon Cafeteria	Moderately hungry; worried about presentation	Alone	Cheeseburger	425
			French fries, regular	230
			Diet cola, 8 fl. oz.	0
2:00 P.M. Meeting room	Not hungry; feeling anxious	Managers	2 handfuls of jelly beans	250
6:30 P.M. Dining room	Hungry	Family	Grilled chicken breast w/ skin, 5 oz.	300
			Baked potato	145
			w/ 2 tbsp. sour cream	50
			Green salad	15
			w/ 2 tbsp. blue cheese dressing	166
			Glass of white wine	70
8:30 P.M. TV room	Not hungry; social eating	Kids	1 handful of taco chips	180
9:15 P.M. TV room	Not hungry; feeling lonely`	Alone	French vanilla ice cream, 1 cup	285
Total calories				3,210

IT'S A FACT

A study at Northwestern University Medical School tracked 38 people from two weeks before Thanksgiving through two weeks after New Year's. The participants who recorded everything they ate, every day, lost an average of seven pounds, even over the holidays. Those who didn't gained three pounds.

of the kids left at breakfast, the handful of jelly beans from the office receptionist's desk, the bite of dessert your friend offers you at lunch. And be sure to include salad dressings, coffee creamers and other easily forgotten foods. Use one of the popular calorie counters available at most bookstores as a resource.

Don't forget to write down how you're feeling when you eat, so you can identify those internal cues. Overeating and poor food choices are not isolated events; they're linked to lifestyle influences. Once you understand *why* you eat, changing your dietary habits becomes much easier.

This same methodology can also keep you on track with your new eating program. If you find yourself up a few pounds, write down what you eat as you eat it. This kind of record-keeping can be very effective, particularly in the beginning.

Read Food Labels

Even the most serious pro-health activists among us occasionally eat from boxes, cans and packages. And since processed foods lend themselves to hidden fat, sugar and sodium, knowing how to read food labels is critical to making informed choices.

Fortunately, the Food and Drug Administration and the Department of Agriculture have met the need to supply consumers with reliable information about the foods that line the shelves of our supermarkets and delicatessens. The current format isn't perfect, but it makes understanding the label information easier than ever. A sample label from a box of macaroni and cheese is shown on the facing page.

Nutrition Facts

Serving Size 1 cup (228 g)
Servings Per Container 2

Amount Per Serving

Calories 250	Calories from Fat 110

	% Daily Value
Total Fat 12 g	18%
Saturated Fat 3 g	15%
Trans Fat	1.5 g
Cholesterol 30 mg	10%
Sodium 470 mg	20%
Total Carbohydrate 31 g	10%
Dietary Fiber 0 g	0%
Sugars 5 g	
Protein 5 g	

Vitamin A 4%	*	Vitamin C	*	2%
Calcium	20%	*	Iron	*	4%

*Percent Daily Values are based on a 2,000-calorie diet.
Your daily values may be higher or lower depending on your calorie needs:

	Calories	2,000	2,500
Total Fat	Less than	65 g	80 g
Sat Fat	Less than	20 g	25 g
Cholesterol	Less than	300 mg	300 mg
Sodium	Less than	2,400 mg	2,400 mg
Total Carbohydrate		300 g	375 g
Fiber		25 g	30 g

Calories per gram
Fat 9 · Carbohydrate 4 · Protein 4

First, pay attention to the serving size, number of servings and number of calories per serving. In this case, one serving of macaroni and cheese is 250 calories, but the whole package is two servings, or 500 calories.

Next, zero in on the nutrients you want to limit:

■ *Total fat.* Be sure to keep fat content moderate, particularly if weight control is one of your health objectives. A good rule of thumb is no more than 3 grams of fat per 100 calories of food.

■ *Saturated fat* and *trans fat.* If you want to avoid high total and LDL cholesterol, choose whole plant foods over processed and animal foods. Together, saturated and trans fats should make up no more than 10% of total calories consumed.

■ *Cholesterol.* The guideline is no more than 300 milligrams daily for healthy persons; no more than 200 milligrams for heart patients.

■ *Sodium.* The goal is to consume no more than 2,300 milligrams of sodium a day, or approximately one teaspoon of salt. (Check out the sodium in canned soup if you want a shock!)

And finally, make sure the remaining nutrients are in line:

■ *Total carbohydrate.* This category is broken down into dietary fiber and sugars. The recommended level for fiber is 20 to 35 grams a day, so look for foods with high fiber content (4 to 5 grams per serving should be the minimum target). While there is presently no guideline for sugars, it makes sense to limit refined sweeteners. Remember, 4 grams of sugar equals a teaspoon.

■ *Protein.* Most Americans get more protein than they need. For adults, the USRDA for protein is no more than 0.8 grams per kilogram (2.2 pounds) of body weight. (Athletes in training need about 1.2 grams per kilogram of weight.)

■ *Vitamins and minerals.* Your goal here is 100% of each for the day. Let a combination of foods add up to a winning score.

TRANS FATS

You might not find trans fats listed in the Nutrition Facts for certain products. This makes no sense, since trans fats may actually be more harmful to heart health than saturated fats. Until federal regulations take care of this problem, check the ingredients list for hydrogenated oils. If one or more are included, you know that the product contains trans fats. Then subtract the amount of saturated fat listed from the amount of total fat listed. Most likely, the difference can be attributed to trans fats.

Let's use a pancake mix made with hydrogenated cottonseed oil as an example. If it has 3.5 grams of total fat and one gram of saturated fat per serving, it more than likely also has about 2.5 grams of trans fat per serving.

BUTTER VS. MARGARINE

Despite the many healthier oils available, people are still regularly switching back and forth between butter and margarine. It's a difficult choice to make because both contain cholesterol-raising fats: saturated fat in butter and trans fat in margarine. Experts warn against treating saturated and trans fats independently when making food decisions. Instead, add their grams together and choose the product with the lowest total. Look at this comparison of table spreads:

BUTTER	**STICK MARGARINE**	**TUB MARGARINE**
Nutrition Facts	**Nutrition Facts**	**Nutrition Facts**
Serving Size 1 Tbsp (14 g)	Serving Size 1 Tbsp (14 g)	Serving Size 1 Tbsp (14 g)
Servings Per Container 32	Servings Per Container 32	Servings Per Container 32
Calories 100	Calories 100	Calories 100
Calories from Fat 100	Calories from Fat 100	Calories from Fat 60
Total Fat 11 g	Total Fat 11 g	Total Fat 7 g
Saturated Fat 7 g	Saturated Fat 2 g	Saturated Fat 1 g
Trans Fat 0 g	Trans Fat 3 g	Trans Fat 0.5 g
Combined Amount	**Combined Amount**	**Combined Amount**
Saturated Fat 7 g	Saturated fat 2 g	Saturated Fat 1 g
+ Trans Fat 0 g	+ Trans Fat 3 g	+ Trans Fat 0.5 g
Total 7 g	Total 5 g	Total 1.5 g

In this example, tub margarine is the product to choose since it has the lowest combined total.

Manage Portion Size

Most people have little understanding of portion size. They simply eat what's on their plate . . . and then have seconds! The fact is, it's easy to overeat if you don't know what a cup, an ounce or a teaspoon looks like in practical terms. One way to approach this problem is to use your hand—thumb, palm and fist—as a guide.

■ One teaspoon of butter, peanut butter, mayonnaise or sugar is about the size of the top joint of your thumb. Three such portions make up about one tablespoon.

■ A three-ounce serving of cooked meat, fish or poultry is about the size of your palm.

■ One cup of cereal, spaghetti, potatoes, vegetables or cut fruit is about the size of a woman's closed fist. One and a half cups equals the size of a man's closed fist.

■ One ounce of nuts or small candies is just one handful. For chips or pretzels, it's two handfuls.

PICTURE IT . . .

If you're a visual person, it might be easier to compare serving sizes to everyday items:

■ Three ounces of meat, poultry or fish = the size of a bar of soap, a checkbook or a deck of playing cards.

■ Two tablespoons of peanut butter = a golf ball.

■ One medium bagel = a hockey puck.

■ Three ounces of hamburger = the lid of a medium-size jar of mayonnaise.

■ One-half cup of cooked vegetables or cut fruit, or a half-cup of cooked rice and pasta = a cupcake liner.

■ One small baked potato = a small computer mouse.

■ One cup of raw, leafy vegetables or one cup of dry cereal = a baseball.

■ One ounce of cheese = four dice.

A second way to manage portion size is to divide your plate into halves. Fill one half with vegetables and/or fruits and the other half with roughly equal amounts of potato, rice or pasta and a high-protein food such as meat, poultry or seafood. Says Netty Levine, R.D., a nutritionist at Cedars-Sinai Medical Center, "The beauty of the divided plate concept is built-in portion control. You fill the divided plate once. If you're still hungry, have another plate of vegetables, and then you're done."

Aim for half or more of each meal to be vegetables, something that happens naturally on our Mediterranean-style diet, and finish with fruit as a sweet dessert.

Here are a few other tips:

■ Serve food on smaller plates so your meals don't look skimpy. Most of the salad plates used today are as big as your grandmother's dinner plates.

■ Start some meals with a piece of fruit or a cup of soup to take the edge off your hunger. We try to eat two cups of raw veggies (with salsa, hummus, bean or other flavorful fat-free or low-fat dips) before sitting down to dinner.

■ Eat a variety of fruits and vegetables, but limit your choices of everything else. Studies show that people routinely overeat when a wide choice of foods is offered at a single meal. (Remember your last trip to a buffet?)

■ Know the calories you're eating. Spend just a few days measuring, weighing and writing down what you eat and the calories contained. You don't have to do it for a lifetime, but it will give you a good feel for healthy portion sizes.

■ Put your fork down between bites.

■ Disband the "clean plate club." You don't have to keep eating until nothing is left on your plate. Listen to your internal cues and stop eating when you feel full.

■ Allow 20 minutes for your meal to be digested before considering seconds.

Modify Favorite Recipes

Believe it or not, you don't have to give up your family's favorite recipes as you change over to a heart-healthy diet. Just find some ways to make them healthier . . . without sacrificing taste.

Let's say your family likes to have French toast on Sunday mornings. The traditional recipe calls for dipping white bread in whole milk and eggs, then frying it in bacon fat. How can you make this recipe healthier yet still tasty? Use fat-free milk instead of whole milk, and whole-grain bread instead of white. Rather than bacon grease, use a nonstick pan or griddle with a little cooking spray. Now you can afford to top the French toast with fresh fruit, fruit syrup, fruit compote and, if fat and calories permit, even a small dollop of soft margarine and a little maple syrup.

For a detailed look at successful modification, see the recipes for chicken enchiladas on page 119. First check the substitutions:

- Skinless chicken breasts
- Reduced-fat cheddar cheese
- Whole wheat tortillas
- Fat-free sour cream

Now look at how such small changes improve the nutritional makeup of the original recipe without sacrificing taste:

Original Recipe	**Modified Recipe**
Each serving about:	*Each serving about:*
349 calories	191 calories
17 g total fat	4 g total fat
60 mg cholesterol	31 mg cholesterol
30 g carbohydrates	22 g carbohydrates
1 g dietary fiber	7 g dietary fiber
19 g protein	17 g protein
653 mg sodium	568 mg sodium

Calories saved per serving: 158
Fat saved per serving: 13 grams

AN EASY RECIPE MODIFICATION

CHICKEN ENCHILADAS

Original Recipe (8 servings)

2 tablespoons butter

2 whole chicken breasts, boned

1 small ripe tomato, chopped

1 onion, chopped

1 8-ounce can chopped green chilies

1½ cups grated cheddar cheese

1 cup tomato salsa

8 flour tortillas

1 8-ounce can tomato puree

3 cloves garlic

3 drops Tabasco sauce

½ cup sour cream

Melt butter in a heavy skillet. Add chicken breasts and sauté 10 to 15 minutes, or until chicken is cooked. Let cool; tear into shreds.

Combine chicken, tomato, ¼ cup of the chopped onion, 1 tablespoon of the chilies, 3 tablespoons of the cheese and 1 tablespoon of the salsa. Set aside . . .

Modified Recipe (8 servings)

4 cups reduced-fat chicken broth

2 whole chicken breasts, skinned and boned

1 small ripe tomato, chopped

1 onion, chopped

1 8-ounce can chopped green chilies

¾ cup grated reduced-fat cheddar cheese

1 cup tomato salsa

8 whole wheat tortillas

1 8-ounce can tomato puree

3 cloves garlic

3 drops Tabasco sauce

½ cup fat-free sour cream

In a saucepan, bring chicken broth to a boil. Add chicken breasts and bring to a second boil. Reduce to medium heat. Cook 20 minutes, or until chicken is done. Remove chicken and tear into shreds. Reserve broth for later use.

Combine chicken, tomato, ¼ cup of the chopped onion, 1 tablespoon of the chilies, 1 tablespoon of the cheese and 1 tablespoon of the salsa. Set aside.

Heat tortillas on a nonstick baking sheet in 350°F oven for about 3 minutes on each side to soften.

Put 3 tablespoons chicken filling in center of each tortilla, and roll. Arrange seam side down in a shallow ovenproof baking dish. Set aside.

Place tomato puree, garlic and remaining onion in blender. Puree until smooth. Stir in remaining chilies and Tabasco sauce. Pour over enchiladas. Bake at 375°F for 15 minutes. Sprinkle with remaining cheese. Bake 10 minutes longer. Remove from oven. Top each enchilada with remaining salsa and dollops of sour cream.

USE LOW-FAT SUBSTITUTES

Switching to low-fat versions of the foods in your own recipes is one of the easiest modification strategies. This involves simple "one for one" exchanges of lower-fat foods for those higher in fat. If, for instance, your favorite chili recipe calls for hamburger, substitute extra-lean ground round or shredded chicken breast. There will be very little change in taste, but the fat content will plummet.

A second method involves the use of more low-fat ingredients. For example, if your favorite lunch is a tuna salad sandwich, make it with water-packed white albacore tuna and use "light" mayonnaise instead of the regular full-fat version.

Check the labels for products that are lower in fat and calories, then try them. If one brand of fat-free sour cream or low-fat cheese doesn't meet your taste requirements, try others. Keep looking until you find the one that works for you and your family. There's a whole new world of products available in the grocery store to help in healthy low-fat cooking and eating.

LOW-FAT SUBSTITUTIONS

Instead of:	Use:
Dairy Products	
Milk, whole or 2%	Fat-free or 1% milk
Buttermilk	1% buttermilk
Evaporated milk	Light (1%) evaporated milk
American, cheddar, Colby, Havarti, Edam, Swiss	Cheese with 5 grams of fat or less per ounce
Mozzarella	Part-skim mozzarella; mozzarella with 5 grams of fat or less per ounce
Cottage cheese	Fat-free or 1% cottage cheese
Cream cheese	Fat-free or light cream cheese
Ricotta cheese	Fat-free, light or part-skim ricotta cheese
Sour cream	Low-fat or fat-free sour cream or yogurt

Yogurt	Low-fat or fat-free yogurt
Frozen yogurt	Fat-free or reduced-fat frozen yogurt
Ice cream	Low-fat, light or reduced-fat ice cream; fat-free or low-fat frozen yogurt or sherbet; sorbet; frozen fruit bars
Whipping cream	Pressurized light whipped cream (use sparingly)

Fats and Oils

Butter and/or margarine	Reduced-calorie liquid or tub-type margarine made with canola, safflower or corn oils
Mayonnaise	Fat-free, light or reduced-calorie mayonnaise
Oil	Olive, canola, safflower, soybean, corn or peanut oil in moderate amounts

Meat and Poultry

Bacon	Canadian bacon, lean ham
Beef, veal, lamb, pork	Skinless chicken or turkey breast; lean cuts of meat trimmed of all visible fat
Ground beef	Extra-lean ground round or ground turkey breast
Luncheon meats	Sliced skinless turkey or chicken breast; lean cooked ham; lean roast beef
Poultry	Skinless breast
Tuna packed in oil	Tuna packed in water
Turkey, self-basting	Turkey basted with fat-free broth

Miscellaneous

Creamed soups, canned	Reduced-fat or fat-free condensed creamed soups
Creamy salad dressing	Oil and vinegar, lemon juice, reduced-calorie dressings
Fats or oils for frying	Nonstick cooking spray
Fudge sauce	Fat-free fudge sauce or chocolate syrup
Gravy	Broth thickened with flour or cornstarch
Hard shortening, lard	Olive, canola, safflower, corn, sunflower and soybean oils

---

CLEAN UP YOUR ENVIRONMENT

Not long ago, a female heart patient said to me, "I'm watching calories and trans fats, but it's hard to stay away from chocolate-chip cookies before bed. I eat five or six every night." My first thought was: *What are you doing with chocolate-chip cookies in the house?*

Before taking action, go through your cabinets and remove everything that's counterproductive to heart-healthy eating, such as impulse foods and prepackaged foods high in sugar or fat. You're more likely to eat those cookies at 10:00 P.M. if they're sitting on your counter than if you have to get dressed and drive to the store to buy them. Instead, stock up on foods that will help you when a snack craving hits: almonds, raisins, juice bars, fresh or frozen berries, apples with peanut butter.

COOK WITHOUT EXTRA FAT

How you cook is as important as *what* you cook. A well-made heavy-gauge nonstick skillet is indispensable for stir-frying or sautéing in minimal fat. You can use one tablespoon of olive oil, for example, instead of an inch of oil to fry potatoes. Or cook your pancakes on a nonstick griddle instead of the traditional skillet with added fat.

Grilled fish is more flavorful and healthful than fish fried in deep fat. If you're using ground beef, brown and drain it well on paper towels and pat off excess fat before adding it to your recipe. Learn to use herbs and spices like fresh basil, cilantro, fresh ginger, curry powder and mustard, as well as champagne, raspberry and other flavored vinegars to add flavor without the fat. Fresh herbs and the fine flavors of quality ingredients will help you rely less on extra fat to carry the taste.

Make a Meal Plan

It's one thing to talk about limiting fast food and convenience foods in favor of Mediterranean-style meals, but quite another to make it happen. If it's five o'clock and you're shopping for dinner to be served at six, you may be too pressed to make healthy choices. Under pressure to just get *something* on the table, it's very easy to revert to old, familiar but less healthy favorites. This is why planning is essential for success. By preselecting foods and recipes that appeal to your family and meet your dietary guidelines, you ensure the inclusion of healthy foods and minimize selections left to chance.

Over the years and through many books, we have consistently been asked to prepare a 30-day meal plan, similar to that found with many weight-loss diets. "Just give me a diet, tell me specifically what to eat and when to eat it," said one heart patient, "and I'll do it." This concept was certainly attractive, so we decided to test a 30-day heart-healthy meal plan in our home. The result? *It was virtually impossible to stick with.* Real life is not tidy and controllable. It just *happens* sometimes, and when it does, you can't keep to your plan. Working late on a deadline, driving kids in a hockey carpool, running out of time to shop and cook . . . these are realities that can override the best intentions. So, in place of a fixed 30-day plan, we developed a more realistic and effective alternative: pick-and-choose menus.

Start by creating a weekly plan for dinner based on categories of foods that your family likes. Here's an example:

Day	Type of Food
Monday	Poultry
Tuesday	Pasta, grains, soup, stew
Wednesday	Seafood
Thursday	Main-meal salad
Friday	Pizza, casserole, chili
Saturday	Restaurant, takeout
Sunday	Meat

Then, using the recipes in this book, select specific meals to fit into the daily categories. On Monday, you might have Grilled Lemon Chicken. On Tuesday, it might be Mostaccioli with Fresh Tomatoes and Basil. And so on. The point is that you know what you're going to do for the whole week. Dinner is no longer something that just happens. You are now in control.

This method works well for people who have a fairly steady routine. But what if you and your family are pulled and tugged by last-minute changes? At the end of this book, we've included complete pick-and-choose menus (including entrées, side dishes and salads) that are simple and easy to prepare. Use them as a backup plan when a traffic jam has just destroyed your good intentions. These menus will help you to salvage a healthy dinner. Below is a menu that you can put together in just 20 minutes:

> 20-Minute Marinara with Pasta
> Field Greens with Chickpeas and Tomatoes
> Sautéed Spinach with Pine Nuts
> Fresh Fruit

Stay Positive

In the long run, a positive mental attitude is the key to success. This mind-set centers on what can be done rather than on what *cannot* be done. It creates an outlook in which change is seen as a gain, not an irretrievable loss. It also recognizes the possibility of setbacks but views them as learning experiences rather than failures. Malcom S. Forbes once said, "Failure is success if we learn from it." And Babe Ruth went down in history as "the home run king" because he focused on his successes at the plate rather than the 1,330 times he struck out. In dietary terms, succumbing to a hamburger or a chocolate doughnut doesn't mean you've "blown" your healthy eating program.

A few years ago, I was asked to partner with a hospital on a community health initiative. The hospital was concerned about the overweight problem in its community and the influence it was having on diseases and conditions such as heart disease, blood pressure and

HAPPY BIRTHDAY!

It's simply unrealistic to ban certain foods forever. For instance, fresh fruit is a better dessert choice than pie or cake, but a peach with a candle in it may not do much for a birthday celebration. So enjoy a piece of chocolate cake without guilt, satisfying both your taste buds and emotions. But make sure it's *one small piece only*. Afterwards, it's easy to resume a healthy diet and workout program. (Just be sure not to celebrate your birthday once a week!)

type 2 diabetes. We combined our efforts to design and implement a 12-week program of behavior change involving diet, exercise and stress management, and it worked. Some 640 people lowered cholesterol, reduced blood pressure and lost 4,200 pounds! More importantly, four years after the program ended, about 70% of participants reported that they were still eating healthfully, exercising effectively and managing stress—and that the weight was still off.

While I was pleased with the results, what amazed me was how much effort it takes to change dietary habits. Just deciding to make a change is difficult enough. As author Dr. Dale E. Turner says, "Ours are busy lives, and no one can do everything; priorities are a must. But if we can't do everything at once, we can at least do *something* at once. The important thing is to begin." Yet often there's more to it than that. A woman on the program who lost 20 pounds told me, "I made good progress at the start, like having oatmeal instead of Danish pastry for breakfast or carrots instead of potato chips as a snack. But after a few weeks I had a candy bar for lunch! In the past, I'd have quit my healthy diet then and there. This time, I saw the candy bar for what it really was: a temporary setback to my normal, healthy eating pattern." That perspective will keep her on the road to achieving her goals.

Chapter Nine

Fruits, Vegetables, Beans, Nuts and Grains

THE SCIENCE BY ITSELF gives us good reasons to eat complex carbohydrates on a regular basis. After all, they've been shown time and again to promote cardiac health. But there's much more to these foods than the simple fact that they're good for us. If you make them central to your daily diet, you're in for a constant treat in terms of taste and satisfaction.

Fruits

Juicy, sweet and delicious . . . who can resist a piece of fresh fruit? The answer, it would seem, is most Americans! In the traditional Mediterranean diet, fresh fruit is the perfect finish to a delicious meal, but we'd rather eat store-bought cakes, pies and ice cream. This has to change if cardiac health is our goal.

Fruits are nutritional powerhouses, rich in fiber, antioxidants (particularly vitamin C), phytochemicals, flavonoids and minerals. In addition, most fruits are relatively low in calories and fat yet high in water content and bulk, so they make you feel more satisfied. For the equivalent of one chocolate-chip cookie, about 125 calories, you can enjoy:

1 whole cantaloupe	8 ounces of orange juice
1 whole grapefruit	3 peaches
1.5 cups of raspberries	2.5 cups of strawberries
6 apricots	1.5 cups of pineapple
4 figs	4 tangerines
1 cup of prunes	1 cup of pitted sweet cherries

Fruits also contain natural sugars that can satisfy a craving for sweetness without loading up on calories. Summer fruits are particularly well suited as substitutes for high-fat snacks. Eat a peach instead of potato chips, a wedge of cantaloupe instead of a brownie, and you'll cut fat, sugar, sodium and calories.

Choose from a variety of fruits— fresh, frozen, canned or dried—every day to meet the two-cup requirement. Try to emphasize those that contain fiber, soluble fiber, antioxidants and folic acid for cardiac benefit. Be sure to include blackberries, raspberries, strawberries and especially blueberries in your fruit choices. These fruits are little antioxidant and fiber jewels that can help lower the risk of cardiovascular disease.

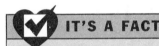 **IT'S A FACT**

According to Joanne Ikeda, codirector of the Center for Weight and Health at the University of California at Berkeley, you can eat seven servings (each one-half cup) of fruits and vegetables for only a dollar or so. That's a pretty big bargain compared with packaged food, snacks and meals.

SINGLE SERVINGS OF SOME COMMON FRUITS

Apple, 1 medium

Apricots, 3 medium

Banana, ½ medium

Blackberries, 1 cup

Blueberries, 1 cup

Cherries, 15

Fresh figs, 2

Grapes, 15

Grapefruit, 1 whole

Kiwis, 2

Mango, ½

Melon: cantaloupe, ½ medium;
honeydew, ¼ medium

Nectarines, 2 small

Orange, 1 large

Peaches, 2 small

Pear, 1 medium

Pineapple, ½ cup

Plums, 3 small

Raisins, currants, dried figs,
dates, dried apricots,
¼ cup

Raspberries, 1½ cups

Strawberries, 1½ cups

Tangerines, 2 small

Watermelon, 1¼ cup

Here are some additional ways to make fruit part of your diet:

■ Add berries or bananas to yogurt.

■ Keep dried dates, apricots, raisins and cranberries in your desk to snack on throughout the day.

■ Add raisins or other dried fruit to cereals. Stir applesauce into hot oatmeal.

■ Make a trail mix from dried fruit and a favorite dried cereal.

■ Bake apples and pears for dessert.

■ Make your grandmother's carrot-raisin salad.

■ Include fruit sauce on pork or cranberries with turkey.

■ Dice mangoes with red onions and cilantro to make a colorful and tasty fruit salsa.

■ Use apple butter instead of jam or jelly.

■ Add crisp slices of apples or pears to a green salad. Dried cherries or currants are also good salad additions.

■ Spice up rice or couscous by adding currants, diced apricots or raisins.

■ Add fruit to your favorite smoothie or yogurt shake.

■ Include strawberries or orange slices in your spinach salad.

Fresh fruits provide better nutrition than canned fruits because vital nutrients are lost in the canning process. If you do buy canned fruits, look for those labeled "unsweetened," "packed in its own juices" or "packed in fruit juice"; these products will not have added sweeteners. Frozen fruit generally does not have added sugar. If you're watching your weight, eat dried fruits sparingly—they're a concentrated source of calories.

The American Dietetic Association recommends substituting juice for no more than one of your daily servings of fruits and vegetables. That's because the whole orange also contains fiber, minerals and phytochemicals that are not found in the juice.

And finally, if you have discretionary calories to spend, consider a fruit dessert such as our Very Berry Cobbler or Poached Pears in Raspberry Sauce.

Vegetables

For any diet designer, vegetables would be the centerpiece both from a scientific standpoint and for their aesthetic value. Like fruits, vegetables are an important source of fiber, antioxidants, phytochemicals, vitamins and minerals. Among the vegetables considered "functional foods" for health are broccoli, cabbage, garlic, spinach, butternut squash, soybeans, kale, onions and tomatoes. The most colorful vegetables often confer the greatest cardioprotection.

Vegetables can also help with weight control. One-half cup of watery vegetables such as asparagus, green beans, tomatoes, summer squash and broccoli contains less than 25 calories. Lettuce, radishes, celery and raw greens are so low in fat that they can be eaten freely. But vegetables are more than their science. When you try our savory Minestrone, Christmas Salad or Roasted Asparagus with Parmesan, you won't be thinking about nutrition. You'll simply appreciate their vibrant color, their texture and, of course, their taste.

SINGLE SERVINGS OF SOME COMMON VEGETABLES

Asparagus, cooked, ½ cup

Artichokes, cooked, ½ cup

Bamboo shoots, 1 cup

Bean sprouts, 1 cup

Beets, cooked, ⅔ cup

Bell or other pepper, raw,
1 cup; cooked, ½ cup

Broccoli, cooked, ½ cup

Brussels sprouts, cooked,
½ cup

Carrots, 2 medium (or 12 baby),
cooked, ⅔ cup

Cauliflower, cooked, ½ cup

Celery, 1 cup

Cucumber, 1 cup

Cabbage (red, green, Chinese),
raw, 1 cup; cooked, ½ cup

Chives, onion, leeks, garlic,
raw, 1 cup; cooked, ½ cup

Dilled beans, asparagus or
pickles, ½ cup

Eggplant, cooked, ½ cup

Green beans, cooked, ½ cup

Greens, cooked: bok choy,
escarole, Swiss chard, kale,
collard greens, spinach,
mustard or beet greens, ½ cup

Lettuce/mixed greens: romaine,
red and green leaf, endive,
spinach, arugula, radicchio,
watercress, chicory, 1 cup

Mushrooms, cooked, ½ cup; raw,
1 cup

Okra, cooked, ½ cup

Parsnips, cooked, ½ cup

Radishes, 1 cup

Snap peas, cooked, ½ cup

Snow peas, cooked, ½ cup

Squash: acorn, butternut, yellow,
zucchini, crookneck, spaghetti,
cooked, ½ cup

Sweet potatoes or yams, cooked,
½ small

Tomato juice, vegetable juice,
1 cup

Turnips, cooked, ½ cup

Water chestnuts, 5 whole

Look for new ways to eat vegetables or combine them with what you already eat on a regular basis. Here are some ideas:

■ Snack on raw veggies and hummus, tahini or salsa.

■ Pack your sandwiches with tomatoes, lettuce and spinach. Accompany with baby carrots, sliced cucumbers and pieces of red and yellow peppers.

■ Make vegetables the entrée: stuffed peppers, cabbage rolls, eggplant parmigiana, vegetarian chili.

■ Top a homemade pizza with fresh tomatoes, mushrooms, artichokes and peppers.

■ Add tomatoes, onions and asparagus to an omelet.

■ Make a stir-fry with garlic, broccoli, mushrooms, onions, snow peas and peppers.

■ Don't forget soups such as minestrone, vegetable, tomato and gazpacho.

■ Make a pasta sauce from roasted red pepper, sun-dried tomatoes and marinara.

■ Drink vegetable juice—tomato, carrot or whatever catches your fancy. (Be aware of high sodium content.)

■ Serve red and green salsa on fajitas and eggs, as a dip for vegetables or on salads instead of dressings.

■ Roast firm vegetables such as zucchini, Brussels sprouts, butternut squash, carrots and asparagus.

■ Add corn kernels to green salads, salsa and soups.

■ Top a baked potato with fresh diced tomatoes, salsa, fat-free sour cream, broccoli or another vegetable.

■ Top spaghetti squash with marinara sauce.

■ Add broccoli, peas or snap peas to couscous, rice and stir-fries.

■ For an instant salad, drizzle sliced cucumbers with seasoned rice vinegar.

■ When eating out, ask for fresh (not fried) vegetable spring rolls as an appetizer.

■ Turn baby corn, cherry tomatoes, yellow and red peppers, sliced cucumbers or asparagus spears into a garnish.

■ Prepare cabbage slaw, pea salad or a marinated vegetable antipasto as a side dish.

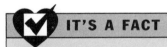

IT'S A FACT

In general, the deeper the color, the more nutritious the vegetable. Dark green spinach packs more nutritional punch than light green iceberg lettuce.

■ Grill portobello mushrooms instead of hamburgers. Make room on the grill for zucchini, red and yellow peppers, corn, eggplant and sweet onions.

■ And don't forget to use pasta as a vehicle for the vegetables you like best. Make macaroni and peas; pasta salad with baby corn, broccolini and roasted peppers; marinara sauce with garlic and onions.

The best way to eat vegetables is raw. I eat a cup of raw vegetables just as a predinner snack. If you decide to cook them, do it quickly; in general, the shorter the cooking time, the greater the health benefits. Whenever possible, cook vegetables with the skin on for better nutrition. For best results, steam them in a vegetable steamer in a pot with a lid; make sure the water level is well below the vegetables, since many of the vitamins leach into the water. If you stir-fry, cook the vegetables lightly in a nonstick pan or with a small amount of oil or cooking spray. Microwave in a dish or bowl with a glass lid. (There is some evidence that microwaving plastic releases chemicals into the food from the plastic wrap.)

 IT'S A FACT

The way vegetables are stored can affect their nutritional value. Keeping them whole until you're ready to use them is a good way to preserve vitamins.

Fresh regional vegetables contain the most nutrients. Frozen vegetables are the next best thing to fresh. Canned vegetables are usually not as tasty or nutritious. They also tend to have a high sodium content and need a thorough rinsing.

POTATOES

By far the most popular vegetable in America (we average over 135 pounds a year), potatoes can provide high nutritional value at a low caloric cost, particularly when eaten with the skin. A medium-size potato with only 90 to 100 calories is bursting with vitamins, minerals, trace nutrients and about 3.2 grams of high-quality protein. But how that potato is cooked makes a huge difference. French fries can get 85% to 90% of their calories from fat. And one ounce of commercial potato chips has more grams of fat than an ounce of Brie. To offset the calories in that one ounce, you'd have to walk for 25 minutes at a pace of 4 mph or cycle for 19 minutes at 10 mph.

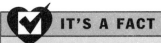 **IT'S A FACT**

Brimming with beta-carotene, fiber, folate and vitamins E and C, the sweet potato has been rated by *Nutrition Action Newsletter* as the number one healthiest vegetable.

Food (5 oz.)	Total Calories	Calories per Ounce
Baked potato	135	27
w/ 2 tbsp. butter/margarine	335	67
w/ 3 tbsp. sour cream and 2 tbsp. butter	425	85
w/ bacon and cheese	330	66
Potato salad	220	44
Hash browns	265	53
French fries	435	87
Potato chips	750	150

A good alternative is to select four large potatoes, slice them thin, toss with one tablespoon of olive oil and fry in a nonstick pan. Sliced or French-fry cut potatoes can also be cooked in the oven on a nonstick baking sheet as a low-fat alternative to French fries. (Try Bernie's recipe for Jumbo Oven Fries.)

Here are a few additional suggestions:

■ Top baked potatoes with fat-free yogurt, fat-free or low-fat sour cream, cottage cheese, salsa, black pepper, chopped dill, chopped Italian parsley and chives.

■ Use a baked potato as a base for stir-fried vegetables—bell peppers, carrots, broccoli and celery. Or try a filling of corn, black beans, fat-free sour cream and salsa.

■ Make lower-fat mashed potatoes by using margarine and fat-free milk in place of butter and cream.

■ For boiled, microwaved or steamed red potatoes, use a vinaigrette of equal parts fresh lemon juice and olive oil, and a dash of coarse salt and pepper. Toss with potatoes while still hot.

■ Peel and cube a sweet potato, toss with olive oil, salt and pepper, spread on a baking sheet and roast in a 450°F oven, stirring every 10 minutes until browned. Delicious!

Beans and Other Legumes

The ultimate health food, chock-full of protein, complex carbohydrates, fiber, B vitamins, iron, phytochemicals, potassium, zinc and magnesium, legumes such as beans, peas and lentils are cholesterol-free and low in fat, calories and sodium. Many also contain soluble fiber, which is effective in lowering blood cholesterol.

Legumes have been used as rich sources of protein since they were first cultivated in ancient times. Today, they continue to serve as a main source of protein for millions of people throughout the world. Good examples include black beans and rice (Cuba), pasta e fagioli (Italy), chili and refried beans (Mexico), falafel and hummus (Middle East), dal (India) and edamame (Japan). Still, despite the twin virtues of rich nutrition and taste, beans in particular have yet to take their proper place in the American diet. People think they're fattening, when in fact one-half cup of most cooked beans has only about 100 calories. Also, it used to take 2 to 12 hours of soaking to get dried beans ready to cook; now you can buy canned and frozen beans at the supermarket.

 IT'S A FACT

People who eat beans and other legumes at least four times a week have a 21% lower risk of heart disease than those who eat legumes less than once a week, says a 19-year study of nearly 10,000 people.

The new guidelines counsel eating at least one serving of legumes every day.

GO LEAN WITH LENTILS

Be sure to include lentils in your diet. They offer a bonanza of heart-protective nutrients, including folate and fiber, and their protein and iron content makes them a reasonable alternative to meat. To top it off, they're a cinch to prepare since they require no presoaking and cook up in 15 to 20 minutes. Try our French Lentil Salad and French Lentil Soup.

SINGLE SERVINGS OF BEANS AND OTHER LEGUMES

Beans: garbanzo, pinto, fat-free refried, kidney, black, mung, lima, cannellini, navy, cooked, ½ cup

Bean soup, 1 cup

Edamame (green soybeans), cooked, ⅓ cup out of pods

Green peas, cooked, ¾ cup

Hummus, ¼ cup

Lentil soup, 1 cup

Red or green lentils, cooked, ½ cup

Soy nuts, ¼ cup

Split peas (yellow and green), cooked, ½ cup

Split-pea soup, 1 cup

Tofu, ½ cup

A good way to include beans, peas and lentils in your diet is to mix them with other foods. Dietitian Bev Utt recommends a Tex-Mex salad using greens as a base. Just add black beans, canned corn, green onions and sautéed chicken, drizzle with a light ranch dressing and serve with a warm whole wheat tortilla.

Some other good suggestions:

■ Add black or pinto beans to ground beef in tacos and burritos.

■ Order whole pinto or black beans instead of refried beans in a Mexican restaurant

■ Make homemade chili and pea, lentil and multibean soups.

■ Buy fat-free commercial refried beans.

■ For a quick meal, spread no-fat refried beans with chicken, avocado, lettuce and salsa.

■ Serve vegetarian baked beans as a side dish.

■ Add red beans, black beans, cannellini beans and garbanzo beans to salads and soups.

■ Use red pepper hummus as a dip for raw vegetables and as a spread on pita bread.

■ Add tofu to your stir-fries.

Nuts and Seeds

In the hierarchy of healthy foods, nuts and seeds are coming into their own. A number of international studies show that people who eat nuts regularly cut their risk of high cholesterol, heart disease and diabetes, compared with those who rarely or never eat them. In the Nurses' Health Study, women who ate more than 5 ounces of nuts a week had a 35% reduction in their heart attack risk compared with women who ate only an ounce of nuts a week or none at all. The evidence has been so positive that the American Heart Association now allows packages of nuts to carry the health claim that they "may reduce the risk of heart disease."

Many types of nuts, including walnuts, almonds, Brazil nuts, cashews, filberts/hazelnuts and pecans, are rich in monounsaturated and polyunsaturated fats, vitamin E, omega-3 fatty acids, fiber, B vitamins and phytochemicals. In 2002 the Food and Nutrition Board of the National Academies' Institute of Medicine issued dietary guidelines for omega-3 fatty acids, calling for 1.6 grams and 1.1 grams daily for men and women, respectively. This quota can be satisfied with just 1.5 ounces of walnuts.

The recommendation is to eat one serving of nuts and seeds on most days, but watch out for the calories in nuts. One ounce of nuts can contain 160 to 200 calories, so don't go overboard. Think handfuls, not bowlfuls. A good rule is to consider a "shot glass" or one closed handful as one serving.

 IT'S A FACT

Studies have shown that consuming 2 ounces of walnuts a day can lower LDL cholesterol by 5.9%.

SINGLE SERVINGS OF NUTS AND SEEDS

Almonds, cashews, hazelnuts (filberts), pistachios, 10–12

Ground flaxseed, 4 tbsp.

Sunflower, pumpkin, sesame seeds, 2 tbsp.

Walnut, pecan halves, 7–8

Here are some simple ways to add walnuts to your diet:

■ Top fruit-sweetened fat-free yogurt with crushed walnuts.

■ Add chopped walnuts to sautéed vegetables.

■ Instead of chips or pretzels, reach for walnuts, almonds and other nuts and seeds.

■ Sprinkle walnut halves onto salads.

■ Add chopped walnuts to poultry stuffing.

■ Stir crushed walnuts into hot or cold cereals.

■ Toast walnut halves and toss with rice.

■ Add chopped walnuts to bran muffin and bread recipes.

■ Be adventurous. Season walnuts in the oven with spices to make your own trail mix.

■ Just enjoy walnuts as a snack.

Flaxseed, traditionally known as linseed, is a wonderful plant source of omega-3 fatty acids; in addition, it contains soluble fiber, which can help to lower cholesterol and protein. Many experts suggest adding about two tablespoons of ground flaxseed to your daily diet. You can sprinkle it on yogurt, cereals and salads or add it to applesauce, muffin batters, pancake mixes and casseroles. Or drizzle flaxseed oil over steamed vegetables or use it in salad dressings. (Flaxseed oil oxidizes, so it should never be heated.)

Grains

The new guidelines emphasize the importance of grains in a balanced diet. Of the six recommended servings of grains per day, three should come from whole grains. A Harvard University study of 42,850 men showed that those who ate more than 25 grams (about three servings) of whole grains daily cut their risk of heart disease by about 15%. And it gets better . . . Those who ate more than 11 grams of bran (the highest-fiber part of whole grains) every day cut their risk by 30%.

SINGLE SERVINGS OF GRAINS

Amaranth, teff, quinoa, cooked, ½ cup

Basmati and brown rice, cooked, ½ cup

Barley (whole), cooked, ½ cup

Bread: whole-grain or 100% whole rye, 1 slice

Buckwheat, groats, cooked, ½ cup

Bulgar (cracked wheat), cooked, ⅔ cup

Cold cereal: All-Bran, ½ cup; Grape-Nuts, 4 tablespoons; Fiber One, ½ cup; Optimum or Kashi GOLEAN, ¾ cup

Millet, cooked, ⅓ cup

Oatmeal, cooked, ¾ cup

Oats (whole), raw, ⅓ cup

Whole-grain crackers: Ry-Krisp, Ak-Mak, Ryvita, Wasa, 3

Whole wheat pasta, ½ cup

Whole wheat spelt or kamut berries, ½ cup

Whole wheat pita, ½

Whole wheat tortilla, 1

Wild rice, cooked, ½ cup

Scientists are still trying to determine specifically how whole grains boost cardiac health. It may be that fiber, plant sterols or other nutrients lower cholesterol. It may be that antioxidants protect arterial health. Or it may be simply that eating them makes you feel full and thus may help to prevent obesity, a cardiac risk factor. Whatever the reason, whole grains should be central to your heart-healthy diet.

It's easy to get sufficient grains in your diet, since serving sizes are small (one slice of bread, one cup of dry cereal, one-half cup of cooked oatmeal). Check to see that grains such as wheat, rice, oats and corn are described as "whole" in the list of ingredients.

BREAD

Whole-grain breads, a mainstay of Mediterranean eating, are nutritionally rich, high in fiber and low in calories. The best choices are 100% stone-ground whole wheat bread, pumpernickel multigrain bread, rye bread (dark), whole wheat pitas, whole wheat or corn tortillas, whole wheat pizza crust, oat bread with whole wheat, cracked-wheat bread, whole wheat bagels and whole wheat English muffins.

Choose carefully. Some breads are far lower in fiber and higher in calories, as shown in the table below:

Type of Bread (1 slice)	Grams of Fiber	Calories
Whole wheat	70	3.2
Pumpernickel	70	3.0
Rye	70	2.4
Cracked wheat	70	2.2
Bagel (3-inch diameter)	195	1.5
White, enriched	80	1.1
French, enriched	75	.1

Unless you read the label, you won't know what the bread contains. Always look for the word "whole." The words "wheat flour" instead of "whole wheat flour" tell you that the wheat bran and germ have been removed. Also, don't be fooled by color. Some manufacturers use caramel coloring or raisin juice to transform white bread into brown bread without adding any nutrients or fiber.

Most bread contains about one gram of fat per slice, which means the big problem in a sandwich is what you spread on the bread or put between the slices. (The exception is a croissant sandwich, which can have 15 grams of fat—the equivalent of four pats of butter.) Ethnic breads, such as French or Italian, contain minimal fat and are a good choice, but their crunchy crusts supply little more fiber than white bread does. Don't think bread is only for sandwiches. Try our Tuscan Bread with Olives and Tomatoes or Caprese Salad on Rustic Bread.

BREAKFAST CEREALS

The primary cereal grains found in the American diet are made from wheat, corn, oats, barley, rye and rice. They contain about 70% to 80% complex carbohydrates, some 23% to 15% protein and very little fat. Cereal grains can be great sources of fiber as well as vitamins and minerals.

In general, whole-grain cereals are the best nutritional buy, providing up to 12 grams of fiber—nearly half a day's worth of the recommended amount. Choose a cereal with at least 8 grams of fiber in a cup, such as Kashi's Good Friends or Kellogg's All-Bran. Other good choices include Kellogg's All-Bran with Extra Fiber and Bran-Buds, Post Grape-Nuts, General Mills' Fiber One, Kashi's GOLEAN and Nabisco's 100% Bran and Shredded Wheat. Serve them with fat-free milk and berries or other fresh fruit.

IT'S A FACT

Researchers have found that cinnamon can help to lower blood sugar, total and LDL cholesterol, and triglycerides. Sprinkle it on oatmeal or other hot cereals.

Some whole-grain cereals are made from refined grain (i.e., the nutritious bran and/or germ has been removed in the milling process) and many have refined sugar added, so it's important to read the Nutrition Facts. A good rule of thumb is to make sure each serving contains at least 3 grams of fiber (5 grams is better) per 100-calorie serving with no added fat and 5 grams or less of added sucrose or other sugars. Remember, 4 grams of "sucrose and other sugars" equals one teaspoon of sugar. Be aware that granola is usually high in fat and sugar.

A last piece of advice: *Don't buy "junk" cereals.* Be cautious about manufacturers' advertising claims that their cereal is "whole grain" if the amount of fiber per serving is only a gram or two. And reconsider your choice if the second ingredient is sugar and the third is high-fructose corn syrup. Stick with cereals whose Nutrition Facts indicate high fiber.

RICE

Rice can be either an excellent choice or a food to watch out for. Unfortunately, polished white rice—the type of rice favored by the western palate—diminishes in nutritional value during processing and contains virtually no fiber in a half-cup serving. Instant and "minute" rice are the poorest nutritional varieties of white rice. A better choice is whole-grain brown rice; not subject to processing, it has about 2 grams of fiber per half-cup. Wild rice has 3 grams of fiber per half-cup. If your family just can't do without white rice, mix it with brown rice to improve its nutritional value.

The benefits of rice are often adulterated by fatty toppings. For example, one cup of cooked brown rice has 230 calories, but those calories will soar if you drench the rice in butter, butter sauce or gravy. You're better off topping a bowl of rice with beans or a low-fat vegetable stir-fry, or serving rice on the side with a few drops of sodium-reduced soy sauce. Watch out for packaged rice dishes that contain added fat. All rice can be prepared without the butter, margarine or oil suggested in the directions on the box. Don't be tricked into thinking that a rice dish is fat-free just because the Nutrition Facts list the fat content as zero. Some manufacturers give nutritional information for their products "as packaged" so they don't have to include the fat called for in cooking directions.

PASTA

A while ago, I heard on the news that Italy is the only country that doesn't publish low-carbohydrate/high-protein diet books, because anyone who doesn't eat pasta is *pazzo,* or crazy. I agree. Sure, you can gain weight on pasta (or any other food) if you eat too much of it, but in the proper amount it's a great source of nutrients. Two ounces of enriched dry pasta provides starch, riboflavin, iron, niacin, thiamin and 10% of the USRDA for protein—all for less than one gram of fat and just over 200 calories. Whole wheat pasta has considerably more fiber than regular pasta and can be higher in protein and iron as well.

IT'S A FACT

Spinach pasta contains little spinach—the equivalent of less than a tablespoon per cup of cooked pasta. Don't count it in your vegetable quota.

Available in over 600 shapes and sizes and almost every color in the rainbow, pasta lends itself to an assortment of dishes. Spaghetti, linguine, rigatoni, penne, fettuccine and vermicelli make delicious, low-fat main dishes. Rotelle, fusilli, rotini and shells make tasty salads with fresh vegetables. Tortellini, pastina and orzo are good for hearty soups. Many types of pasta today come flavored and colored with vegetables, including spinach, carrots and tomatoes.

The type of pasta you choose is less important than how you serve it. Drenched in Alfredo sauce or served with a half-dozen meatballs, even the most healthful pasta will become a dish with 40 to 80 grams of fat. A better choice is a simple marinara sauce or a red seafood sauce, each with less than 10 grams of fat. Don't overlook Oriental noodles such as soba (buckwheat) and saifun (cellophane); they're particularly good in chicken broth with vegetables and make a tasty main course. Avoid canned, dehydrated and frozen foods and meals with noodles. Many come in fatty sauces or smothered with cheese.

How much you eat is also important. One cup of pasta with a quarter-cup of marinara sauce and a tablespoon of grated Parmesan cheese contains about 260 calories, or about the same as a cup of yogurt sweetened with fruit preserves, but most restaurant plates contain six or more cups of pasta! Learn what a one-cup serving looks like on your plate. It's easy to overeat this favorite food if you don't manage your serving size.

Chapter Ten

Seafood, Poultry and Meat

O NE OF THE GOALS OF THIS BOOK is to demonstrate that smart choices allow us to eat certain favorite foods that generally would be restricted in a diet intended to promote healthy living. While there certainly is too much animal food in the current American diet, many of us would find it discouraging to limit fish or chicken or even red meat to a weekly or monthly treat. For this reason, such foods are included in our Mediterranean-style diet with a frequency that takes into account all their pluses and minuses. Complex carbohydrates remain at the core of our healthy eating program, but moderate amounts of seafood, poultry and meat can still be enjoyed.

Seafood

F ish ranks high on the list of heart-healthy foods. For starters, it's rich in nutrients such as protein, niacin, vitamin B_{12} and zinc, and oily fish contains vitamins A and D. But most importantly, the oil in fish and other seafood is low in saturated fat and high in polyunsaturated omega-3 fatty acids.

A number of studies have noted the benefits of fish as part of a regular diet. A study conducted in Greenland found that men who ate fish two or three times a week were much less likely to suffer heart attacks than men who did not eat fish. More recently, in the Physicians' Health Study, men who ate fish at least once a week were 52% less likely to die of a heart attack than men who ate fish no more often than once a month.

While there may be a number of factors at work in fish to produce cardiac protection, the evidence so far points to the omega-3 fatty acids. Omega-3s have been shown to lower cholesterol and reduce triglycerides. They also help to prevent blood clots, which can trigger heart attack and stroke. And they contribute to the body's production of prostaglandins, chemicals that have an anti-inflammatory effect that reduces cardiac risk.

This positive connection to cardiac health seems to hold true for all types of fish—from oily salmon to leaner cod, from ocean fish to freshwater varieties—and applies to shellfish as well. According to Dr. William Castelli, former director of the Framingham Heart Study, shellfish are no longer condemned for their high-cholesterol content. "The omega-3s contained in shellfish tend to offset their higher cholesterol content," he says. As a result, shrimp, lobster, crab, scallops, mussels, clams, oysters and squid can now be included in a healthy diet.

IT'S A FACT

A report in the *New England Journal of Medicine* suggests that eating only two fish dishes a week may cut the risk of dying from heart attack in half.

Because of fish oil's positive effect on the prevention of heart attacks, the new dietary guidelines call for eating about 8 ounces of seafood (about two meals' worth) a week. On the Mediterranean-style diet, we eat fish about four times a week. "Fish is very hard to beat as a food item," says Dr. Castelli. "There's something about fish and fish oil that is extremely beneficial and protects against degenerative cardiovascular diseases. In fact, I think people who have had a heart attack or know they have a cholesterol problem would be crazy not to eat fish at least twice per week."

Some seafood is richer in omega-3s than others. The figures for a 3.5-ounce serving are as follows:

Type of Seafood	Grams of Omega-3 Fatty Acids
Atlantic mackerel	2.5
Lake trout	1.7
Salmon	1.2
Tuna	0.5
Pacific halibut	0.4
Channel catfish	0.3
Shrimp	0.3
Dungeness crab	0.3
Swordfish	0.2
Red snapper	0.2
Sole	0.1

USE HEALTHY COOKING METHODS

Cooking methods make a considerable difference in fat content. Grilling, baking, broiling, poaching and microwaving are among the healthiest ways to cook seafood. Frying or deep-frying fish can add more than a gram of fat per ounce, which can quickly turn a healthy food into an unhealthy meal. If you do fry, be sure to use a nonstick pan with a small amount of olive oil. Avoid using butter, stick margarine or lard.

MANAGE PORTION SIZE

If weight control is an issue, you should be aware of the fat content of your selections. Most types of seafood contain no more than 5 grams of fat in a typical 3.5-ounce serving before cooking, but the range is wide. Dover sole has just one gram of fat, while oily fish such as Chinook salmon can have 10.5 grams.

FAT CONTENT OF SEAFOOD

**Low-Fat Seafood
(less than 5% fat)**

Black sea bass	Perch	
Catfish	Pollack	
Clams	Red snapper	
Cod	Rockfish	
Crab (Alaskan and	Scallops	
blue)	Sea trout	
Crayfish	Shark	
Flounder	Shrimp	
Grouper	Skate	
Haddock	Smelt	
Halibut	Sole	
Mahimahi	Squid	
Monkfish	Striped bass	
Mussels	Swordfish	
Orange roughy	Tilefish	
Oysters	Whiting (hake)	

**Moderately
Fat Seafood
(5% to 10% fat)**

Bluefish
Butterfish
Carp
Lobster
Trout
Tuna
Whitefish

**Fatty Seafood
(over 10% fat)**

Herring
Mackerel
Pompano
Salmon
Sardine

A WORD ABOUT CANNED TUNA

Fancy or chunk, flaked or grated, canned tuna is particularly suitable for sandwiches, salads and casseroles. The downside is that it provides so many opportunities for heavy calories. A 6.5-ounce can of tuna in oil has 300 calories more than the same amount of tuna packed in water.

And what about all that mayonnaise in tuna salad? Make the salad with 3 tablespoons of mayonnaise and you add 300 calories. I *never* order a tuna sandwich in a restaurant, since it's often the highest-fat sandwich on the menu. Instead, I make mine at home, using light mayonnaise or a mixture of light and regular. Bernie's recipe for The Big Tuna sandwich has only 251 calories.

HEALTH CONCERNS

Like any other food, seafood is subject to health concerns. A "red tide" can contaminate shellfish. Raw seafood such as sushi can harbor parasites. And some large, long-lived fish, such as tuna, shark, king mackerel and swordfish, may be contaminated by mercury. During pregnancy, women should either avoid these fish completely or eat them no more than once a month.

In addition, some species of fish show high levels of PCBs and other industrial pollutants. A recent study found that farm-raised salmon contain up to 10 times more PCBs than wild salmon do. But that's still 40 to 50 times below FDA levels that cause concern. As a heart patient, I am going to eat fish regularly, so how do I protect myself against high PCB levels? First, I ask at the store if the fish I intend to buy is wild or farm-raised. Next, I peel off the skin before cooking. According to Dr. Michael Gallo of the Cancer Institute of New Jersey, removing the skin takes away up to 75% of the PCBs in each serving.

Poultry

According to the USDA, over 70% of our households serve chicken at least once every two weeks; about 35% serve turkey. In general, this is a positive step because most poultry is higher in protein and lower in fat than red meats and contains vitamin A, many B vitamins, calcium, iron, potassium and zinc. However, it often falls short of its potential because of all the added fat in fast-food chicken nuggets, fried chicken and turkey hot dogs. Smarter choices need to be made when it comes to cuts, cooking methods and portion size.

One simple rule will lead you to the leanest cuts of chicken and turkey: *Choose a skinless white breast.* The fat is concentrated just beneath the skin, so by removing the skin before cooking, you'll save about 5 grams of fat per piece of chicken. If you do leave the skin on during cooking, be sure to remove it before serving. A little bit of skin contains a tremendous amount of fat. Three ounces of roast chicken skin, about the amount that covers a small breast, is equal in calories to 11.5 ounces (almost three-quarters of a pound) of roast breast meat.

The same relationship exists between light (white) and dark meat. Light meat contains about a third less fat than dark meat, so a skinless breast is a much better choice than a drumstick or thigh. The table below shows that while a serving of skinless, light poultry will not break anyone's fat budget, dark meat with the skin on can put a real dent in it.

Poultry Meat (3.5 oz.)	Total Calories	Grams of Fat	Grams of Saturated Fat
Chicken			
Light meat, skinless, roasted	165	3.5	0.9
Light meat w/ skin, roasted	194	7.7	2.1
Dark meat, skinless, roasted	207	10.8	2.6
Dark meat w/ skin, roasted	245	15.4	3.5
Turkey			
Light meat, skinless, roasted	155	3.1	1.1
Light meat w/ skin, roasted	220	10.1	2.3
Dark meat, skinless, roasted	185	7.1	2.4
Dark meat w/ skin, roasted	219	11.4	3.5

 IT'S A FACT

Half a rotisserie chicken (the kind usually found in the deli department of a grocery store) has 41 grams of fat and 665 calories.

Poultry fat is about 30% saturated. Consequently, of the 3.5 grams of fat in a 3.5-ounce serving of roast chicken breast, about one gram is saturated.

The leanest cut of turkey is the boneless tenderloin from the center of the breast half. A 3.5-ounce serving is about 130 calories and about one gram of fat. Of course, whole turkeys continue to be a favorite at holidays, and here a word of caution is needed. Do not choose a self-basting whole bird, since the basting solution contains added fat (usually in

A WORD ABOUT GROUND TURKEY

If only skinless white breast went into ground turkey, this would be a very low-fat product. But commercial ground turkey often includes fatty, dark meat and skin, so 4 ounces of some brands contain as much as 13 to 16 grams of fat. A much better choice is ground turkey breast. Made from skinless white meat, it has just 3 to 4 grams of fat per serving.

the form of coconut oil, soybean oil, corn oil or butter) as well as added sugar and sodium.

Read the food labels when you buy processed poultry products such as chicken hot dogs, turkey bacon, turkey sausage and turkey ham. Some brands contain dark meat and skin and are as fatty as their beef and pork counterparts. Others are low enough in fat to be acceptable in small amounts. The bottom line: Don't buy a product just because it's made from poultry. Check the Nutrition Facts first.

USE HEALTHY COOKING METHODS

Frying a skinless chicken breast in a cup of oil or smothering it in fatty gravy will offset any low-fat benefit. Use cooking methods that allow fat to drip off, such as roasting, broiling, grilling, baking, steaming, stewing and sautéing. Or cut the breast into strips and stir-fry with vegetables. Don't add fat when cooking. Frying flour-coated or batter-dipped chicken in oil, lard, vegetable shortening or grease can add approximately 3 grams of fat per ounce of meat. In general, turkey lends itself to the same preparation methods used with chicken, particularly roasting, broiling and grilling.

MANAGE PORTION SIZE

Just because poultry is lower in fat and saturated fat than red meat, don't make the mistake of thinking it's a free ride. "People have been heavily blitzed with the message to eat less fat," says Dr. Walter

Willett, chief of nutrition at the Harvard University School of Public Health. "But instead of replacing fatty animal foods with grains, beans, vegetables and fruit, as they should, they're eating more low-fat animal foods. A huge chunk of chicken breast has replaced the 12-ounce steak in our culinary repertoire. This might appear to be a sensible exchange, but it's only sensible if the steak is replaced by a moderate amount of chicken—say, 3 or 4 ounces—surrounded by rice, pasta, vegetables and other foods rich in complex carbohydrates and fiber."

Beef and Other Meats

Obviously, no one would ever recommend a steady diet of marbled meat, but I was happy to learn that I didn't have to become a vegetarian for my heart's sake. Beef is not necessarily high in fat and calories. A slice of apple pie has more than double the amount of fat and calories contained in one serving of lean meat. In addition, beef is a good supplier of high-quality protein, iron, zinc and B vitamins, and is particularly effective in building and repairing muscle tissue, aiding metabolism and satisfying hunger.

So red meat *can* be included in a healthy eating plan if several factors are taken into account. First and foremost, some cuts are so fat that they have to be ruled out. T-bone steak and prime rib can have as many as 30 grams of fat per 3.5-ounce serving. (And few of us limit ourselves to such small servings!) Keep in mind also that about 40% of beef fat is saturated fat. A 3.5-ounce portion of top sirloin has just 7.1 grams of fat . . . but 2.8 grams are saturated. (You can multiply the fat-grams in beef by 0.40 to estimate saturated fat content.)

As a rule, beef cuts labeled "loin" or "round" are the leanest choices; for veal, look for cuts labeled "leg" or "cutlet." Choose "Select" grade over "Choice" and "Prime" grades. Some of the best choices, according to the Beef Council, are shown in the table on the facing page.

THE SKINNIEST SIX

Cut of Beef (3.5 oz.)	Total Calories	Grams of Fat	Grams of Saturated Fat
Top round, broiled	179	4.9	1.6
Eye of round, roasted	166	4.9	1.8
Round tip, roasted	183	6.9	2.3
Top sirloin, broiled	192	7.1	2.8
Top loin, broiled	205	9.3	3.5
Tenderloin, broiled	208	9.9	3.7

A number of supermarkets are offering meat from animals raised on grass. Not only is this "pasture-raised" meat leaner, but it contains large amounts of omega-3 fatty acids and a cancer-fighting fat called CLA. By contrast, meat from grain-fed animals increases cholesterol and may contain hormones, herbicides and pesticides; it's also full of omega-6, which may contribute to coronary inflammation.

PORK AND LAMB

Although pork isn't really a white meat, many lean cuts are close to skinless poultry in fat and calorie content. Some low-fat choices include the tenderloin, center-cut leg, loin chops, Canadian bacon and fresh ham. A 3.5-ounce serving of lean pork roast has about 215 calories, with substantial amounts of high-quality protein, B vitamins and iron. Keep in mind that pork fat is about 35% saturated, so high-fat pork products such as sausages and bacon should be eaten only in moderation. *A good suggestion:* Cook one piece of bacon and crumble it on your salad; it's very satisfying without contributing excessive fat.

Lamb is another high-quality, nutritious meat, rich in essential vitamins

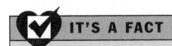 **IT'S A FACT**

If you have access to wild game, meats such as buffalo, deer, elk and moose are low in fat. Meats to avoid include duck, pheasant with skin, quail with skin, goose and domesticated rabbit.

and minerals. Often, much of the fat is found on the outside of the meat and can be trimmed before cooking. Two of the leanest selections of lamb are loin chop and leg. A 3.5-ounce portion of roast lamb has about 230 calories.

GROUND BEEF

While it's easy to choose leaner cuts of fresh meat and trim visible fat, ground beef continues to be an issue because the grinding process mixes meat with fat. It's important, then, to read labels to find the leanest ground beef available. Past descriptions like "lean" and "extra lean" weren't always accurate, so labeling laws have banned them. Instead, ground beef is now described in lean/fat ratios by weight. For a package to carry a ground beef label, the meat must be at least 70% lean and no more than 30% fat. "Regular" ground beef, for instance, must be 73% lean/27% fat. Try to select ground beef with no more than 10% of calories from fat. (But remember, a better option is to replace ground beef with ground turkey breast or chicken breast.) The table below refers to medium-broiled 4-ounce servings of ground beef:

COMPARING GROUND BEEF

% Lean / % Fat by Weight	Calories	Grams of Fat
73% lean / 27% fat	291	21
80% lean / 20% fat	268	18
85% lean / 15% fat	240	14
90% lean / 10% fat	199	11
95% lean / 5% fat	155	6

PROCESSED MEATS

Hot dogs at the ballpark, bologna sandwiches for lunch, pepperoni pizza on a Saturday night . . . there's no arguing about the good taste of processed meats. Sadly, however, most are too high in fat to be a regular part of a heart-healthy diet.

FAT CONTENT OF PROCESSED MEATS

Over 60% Fat	Over 70% Fat	Over 80% Fat
Beer salami, pork	Bratwurst	Beef and pork hot dog
Chicken hot dog	Chopped ham	Beef bologna
Corned beef	Italian sausage	Beef sausage stick
Turkey bologna	Kielbasa	Beer salami, beef
	Pastrami	Bockwurst
	Pork bologna	Knockwurst
	Salami	Liverwurst
	Smoked link sausage	Pepperoni
	Summer sausage	Polish sausage
	Turkey hot dog	

If you just can't give up processed meats altogether, make them a very occasional treat. Fortunately, many national and local brands offer lower-fat versions. Read the labels. Low-fat pastrami, for instance, has one gram of fat per ounce, while regular pastrami has 8 grams.

The fattest cold cuts are the drier ones such as pepperoni and hard salami, which run about 12 grams of fat per ounce. Sausages have 15 to 30 grams of fat per link. In general, poultry versions of cold cuts are lower in fat than their beef and pork counterparts. But be aware that they're not necessarily "low-fat"; they're just lower in fat than the beef and pork versions. Better choices for sandwich fillings include roast turkey breast, roast chicken breast, lean roast beef, lean boiled or baked ham and water-packed tuna.

USE HEALTHY COOKING METHODS

Be sure the meat you choose is trimmed of all visible fat before cooking. The difference can be significant, even in low-fat cuts. By trimming the fat from 3.5 ounces of beef, you can save 7 grams of fat and about 60 calories. (You can't do much about marbling, the fat that runs through the muscle, except perhaps not to select a well-marbled cut in the first place.)

IT'S A FACT

When asked in a government survey to list their favorite and most frequently eaten meals, women did not include meat in their top five choices. Men, however, listed meat in three of their top five choices: steaks, hamburgers and pizza with meat topping. This is something to consider when planning family meals.

Frying sears fat in, so it's the least desirable method. Cooking methods that allow fat to drip off include roasting, broiling, baking, grilling, stewing and barbecuing. In general, the longer meat cooks, the more fat is lost, so "medium" and "well done" are preferable to rare. When preparing ground beef, sauté it in a nonstick pan and drain it on paper towels to defat it as much as possible. Be sure to pour off juices before adding other ingredients to browned meat.

MANAGE PORTION SIZE

It's clear that there's no room in a heart-healthy diet for a 16-ounce T-bone steak or a huge slab of prime rib, each with some 800 to 1,000 calories and half or more of these calories coming from fat. Even too large a portion of a leaner choice can produce excessive fat intake. But a three- or four-ounce serving of lean meat will not upset a healthy diet. Since this amount of cooked lean meat often contains fewer than 200 calories, it's easy to offset the fat in these calories by including other foods in the meal that are lower in fat, particularly fruits and vegetables. A good rule of thumb is to reduce meat portion size to one-quarter of your plate.

A Word About Protein

Much of the emphasis on animal foods is the result of an over-emphasis on protein, a nutritional building block essential to every cell in the human body for growth or repair. Unfortunately, in our society, the term "protein-rich" is usually used in reference to red meat, poultry and seafood rather than soy foods and beans. As a result, our protein-rich diet contains a high level of artery-clogging saturated fat.

The fact is, only 12% to 15% of daily calories should come from protein. The table below shows the USRDA for protein compared with average protein consumption:

Sex and Age	USRDA for Protein (grams)	Average Protein Consumption (grams)
Males		
11–14	45	92
15–18	59	122
19–24	58	105
25–29	63	105
30–59	63	93
60–69	63	79
70+	63	69
Females		
11–14	46	66
15–18	44	63
19–24	46	65
25–49	50	65
50–69	50	55
70+	50	49

For adults, the USRDA for protein is no more than 0.36 grams per pound, or 0.8 grams per kilogram (2.2 pounds) of body weight. (Endurance athletes need 0.54 to 0.64 grams of protein per pound, or 1.2 to 1.4 grams per kilogram of body weight.) To put normal needs into perspective, a 154-pound person with a daily allowance of 56 grams of protein could consume more than 50% of that amount in a lunch consisting of a turkey sandwich (4 ounces of turkey breast, two slices of whole wheat bread) and an 8-ounce glass of fat-free milk.

The point is, there's more to protein than just the usual animal foods. Pour a cup of soy milk on your breakfast cereal and you'll get

7 grams of protein. A quick, easy snack of celery stalks spread with 2 tablespoons of peanut butter will provide you with 9 additional grams. Add a half-cup of tofu to a vegetable stir-fry for dinner and you'll gain another 10 grams.

The bottom line: Far too much of our protein comes from high-fat animal foods. It's time to start thinking in terms of other, healthier sources.

Chapter Eleven

Dairy Foods

D AIRY FOODS OFFER A DELICIOUS WAY to get high-quality protein, vitamins and minerals. They're also a primary source of calcium, which not only helps to prevent osteoporosis, but also protects against high blood pressure and may spur weight loss. The new guidelines recommend three servings of fat-free or low-fat milk or other dairy foods daily. The biggest difference among these foods is fat content. By making smart choices, you can receive the full nutritional benefit without overloading on fat and saturated fat.

SINGLE SERVINGS OF DAIRY FOODS

Fat-free or low-fat milk, 1 cup

Low-fat soy milk, 1 cup

Fat-free or low-fat yogurt, 1 cup

Fat-free or light cream cheese, 4 tablespoons

Fat-free or low-fat cottage cheese, ¾ cup

Fat-free or low-fat cheese (such as mozzarella), 1½ ounces

Milk

The dairy industry has done a great job of promoting milk, from the ads of the 1950s linking milk to strong bones and healthy teeth to the more recent "milk mustache" celebrity campaign. A catchphrase such as "Got milk?" might make you think of this product as a single entity, but in reality there are many kinds of milk—some good for cardiac health and some not so good.

The best choice is fat-free milk (also called "nonfat" and "skim"). (I recommend fat-free organic milk because it contains no antibiotics, growth hormones, pesticides or herbicides.) One cup of fat-free contains just 0.4 grams of fat and 0.3 grams of saturated fat but has all the calcium and protein benefits of whole milk. Three cups a day, which almost supplies the USRDA for calcium, contributes only 1.2 grams of fat to your diet. The same amount of whole milk, however,

---

A WORD ABOUT CALCIUM

Mention calcium, and most people think of dairy foods. But many of these foods are also great sources of fat, so it's important to know how much calcium you really need each day. The National Institutes of Health recommends the following:

Age	Milligrams of Calcium
1 to 5	800
6 to 10	800 to 1,200
11 to 24	1,200 to 1,500
Women 25 to 50	1,000
Women 50 to 65 taking estrogen	1,000
Women 50 to 65 not taking estrogen	1,500
Pregnant or lactating women	1,200 to 1,500
Men 25 to 65	1,000
Men or women over 65	1,500

The daily requirement of calcium for most people can be met by two glasses of fat-free milk. Indeed, a cup of fat-free milk has more milligrams of calcium (302) than the same amount of whole milk (288). Other good sources include nondairy foods such as calcium-fortified orange juice and cereals, soybeans, dried beans and peas, tofu, nuts and dark green leafy vegetables (but not spinach).

contains 25.5 grams of fat for virtually the same amount of calcium. A difference of about 65 calories per cup may not seem like a lot, but if you're a three-cups-a-day milk drinker like me, it's enough calories saved in one year to equal 20 pounds!

FAT CONTENT OF MILK

Type of Milk (8 fl. oz.)	Calories	Grams of Fat	Grams of Saturated Fat
Whole chocolate milk	210	8.5	5.3
Whole milk	150	8.1	5.1
2% chocolate milk	180	5.0	3.1
2% milk	125	4.7	2.9
1% milk	100	2.6	1.6
Fat-free milk	85	0.4	0.3

While it's easy for me to recommend fat-free milk based on its nutritional breakdown, you might be put off at first by its taste. The secret to success is to take small steps. Gradually move from whole milk to 2%, then to 1%, and finally to fat-free over a period of four to six weeks. Your taste buds will adapt over time, and you'll come to enjoy it. When we started to make dietary changes, my initial instinct was to switch from whole milk to "reduced fat" 2% milk. But in checking the Nutrition Facts, I was amazed to learn that "2%" refers to what fat weighs in the carton; in other words, only 2% of the milk's total weight comes from fat. Big deal! Your heart doesn't care how much fat weighs in the carton. It wants to know how many calories in the milk come from fat. And at almost 5 grams of fat per 8 ounces of milk, 2% milk is practically full fat!

Not everyone should be a milk drinker. Many Asians, Hispanics and African Americans lack the enzyme lactase, which is needed to digest milk; this means they can experience indigestion, nausea or bloating. Some lactose-intolerant people can tolerate small amounts of other dairy products, such as cheese or yogurt. For those people, calcium-enriched soy or rice milk may be a good choice.

Cheese

Americans love cheese. And why not? It tastes great as a snack, melted on a hamburger or sprinkled on a salad. It's also a particular favorite among women. Remember the government survey of favorite foods in the section on red meat? While men listed meat in their top five favorites, women ranked cheese (along with chocolate and ice cream) much higher than meat.

About 8 pounds of milk is concentrated in a pound of cheese. The upside of this ratio is that cheese is a good source of calcium, protein and other nutrients. The downside is that it's rich in fat, saturated fat, sodium and calories. Most regular cheese is between 60% and 80% fat, two-thirds of which is saturated. One ounce of cheddar cheese, for example, has about 115 calories and 9 grams of fat. The fact is, cheese can be as fat as or even fatter than meat. If you eat just three of those little cubes of cheese at a cocktail party, you'll take in more fat than if you'd eaten a 3.5-ounce serving of flank steak!

Use the Nutrition Facts as a guide to learn how much fat and calories come in different cheeses. The fat content of most types of cheese is as follows:

Type (1 oz.)	Total Grams of Fat	Grams of Saturated Fat
Regular, or full-fat	9–11	6–7
Reduced-fat, or part-skim	5–7	3–5
Light	2–4	1–3
Fat-free	Less than 0.5	Trace

Once again, the key is to make smart choices. Cheese is an excellent food and can be part of a healthy diet. But if you choose high-fat varieties, and you eat too much too often, cheese can be highly problematic, particularly for those watching their weight or cholesterol levels.

■ Research shows that an average-size serving of Brie in France is far smaller than a serving in the United States. Move away from those large hunks of cheese and opt for smaller servings. Grate and sprinkle cheese to flavor vegetables, salads, soups and pasta. A small amount of sharp cheese

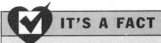

IT'S A FACT

In general, hard cheese is fatter than soft cheese because it has less moisture and a higher concentration of fat solids.

(Parmesan, Romano, feta) added at the last moment will season your meals with a minimum of added fat. This way, you'll be getting it by the teaspoon, not by the cup.

■ Choose from the great range of tasty lower-fat cheeses on the market, but be sure to read the food labels. Be aware that some products are "lower in fat" than the original version, but not necessarily "low in fat." An ounce of reduced-fat cheddar, for instance, contains about 6 grams of fat. That's less than regular cheddar at 9 grams per ounce, but it's not truly low in fat for one ounce of food.

■ If you don't like the taste of a particular cheese, don't buy it just because it will save on fat and calories. Go for the best taste, even if it means eating a higher-fat cheese. Just make portion size reasonable. In many of our recipes, we mix light and reduced-fat cheese to increase taste without overloading on fat.

Yogurt

Eaten as a snack or dessert and used as a condiment or in cooking, yogurt is a staple in many countries that eat the traditional Mediterranean diet. It's also a favorite food on the American diet. Not long ago, it was considered a product for health-food faddists. Now there are several generations of Americans who couldn't conceive of a supermarket dairy case that didn't have row upon row of yogurt in all its myriad forms and flavors.

Yogurt comes in fat-free, low-fat and full-fat varieties. Low-fat yogurt typically contains 2 to 5 grams of fat per 8-ounce serving; the

IT'S A FACT

Yogurt has been touted as a cure for insomnia and yeast infections, as a cancer preventive and as a life extender. Whether or not such claims have any validity, this dairy food is an excellent source of calcium (one cup provides 20% to 25% of the USRDA), protein, riboflavin, phosphorus and vitamin B_{12}.

same amount of whole-milk (full-fat) yogurt may contain 6 to 8 grams.

Plain yogurt, the original and most versatile variety, contains 110 to 140 calories per cup. Most varieties, however, are flavored. These yogurts fall into two categories: sundae-style, with the fruit at the bottom of the container, and blended, custard-like Swiss- or French-style, with the fruit distributed throughout. One other variety of yogurt is flavored with vanilla, coffee or fruit juice (but no fruit solids). Fruited and flavored yogurts range from about 100 calories per cup (for artificially sweetened nonfat vanilla) to 310 calories (for some whole-milk sundae-style yogurts). If you're looking for the most nutritious yogurt, skip the fruit-flavored varieties; most of these products contain fruit jam, which is not a significant source of nutrients and which adds the equivalent of 8 or 9 teaspoons of sugar per cup. You can get the same taste by stirring fresh fruit into plain yogurt.

Hard and soft-serve frozen yogurts can be a healthy treat, but be aware that servings are not standardized. One brand might list the serving size as 3 ounces, which makes it look lower in fat than other brands of frozen yogurt and light ice cream that use 4 ounces as a standard serving. Fat-free frozen yogurt is the best choice. Although it has plenty of added sugar, it still has half the calories of some premium ice creams and, of course, no fat. Low-fat versions are next best. Other types of frozen yogurt may be enriched with whole milk or cream, raising their calorie and fat content significantly but still leaving it far below that of most ice cream. Sauces, toppings or mix-ins like nuts, cookies and candies can also increase the calorie and fat content.

Butter

Long the king of American table fats, butter has gone through two shifts in our eating habits. For many years, it was a staple used to improve the flavor, moistness and "mouthfeel" of many foods. Then in the 1980s, with the emphasis on cholesterol and heart disease, the spotlight fell on butter's major drawback: saturated fat. The experts told us to stay away from butter, but the alternative—margarine—was no panacea. Many types were hydrogenated and contained trans fatty acids, making them more harmful to heart health than butter. So now there has been a rethinking of recommendations. Butter has been taken off the "banned foods" list and put on the "use very sparingly, from time to time" list.

Still, there's no denying that butter is 100% fat and 63% saturated fat. A single pat has 4 grams of fat; a tablespoon has 11 grams. Ounce for ounce, butter has more fat than prime rib. For a better understanding of what that means, consider the following:

1 teaspoon of butter = 1 teaspoon of regular mayonnaise

= 2 teaspoons of French or Italian salad dressing

= 3 teaspoons of mayonnaise-type salad dressing

= 3 teaspoons of cream cheese

= 3 teaspoons of reduced-calorie mayonnaise

= 4 teaspoons of table cream

= 5 teaspoons of sour cream or whipped cream

If you must use butter, do so sparingly. A little goes a long way. You'll find a few instances where butter is used in our Mediterranean-style way of eating, but mostly we rely on olive oil and other healthy oils, balsamic vinegar and seasoned rice vinegar, lemon juice and spices.

A good suggestion: Dip your bread in olive oil instead of butter or spread it on toast to save saturated fat and calories.

WHAT ABOUT EGGS?

This is a good place to consider eggs, even though they're not a dairy item. Eggs are a nutritional powerhouse rich in protein and vitamins A, B$_{12}$ and D, as well as zinc, selenium, choline (important for memory and brain development), iron, essential amino acids and the antioxidant lutein. They're also low in saturated fat and calories (about 70 per egg).

But eggs are also rich in cholesterol. The American Heart Association recommends no more than 300 milligrams of dietary cholesterol a day; if you're a heart patient or have high blood cholesterol, the recommendation is for no more than 200 milligrams a day. The traditional view was that since most eggs contain from 200 to 250 milligrams of cholesterol, you could easily overdo it. Today, however, we know that for most people dietary cholesterol has far less impact on cholesterol than saturated and trans fats. This means that the fat you cook your eggs in and the foods you eat with those eggs (toast with butter, fried hash brown potatoes, sausage or bacon) may be more significant than the eggs themselves. It makes more sense to have a poached egg with veggies than to cook an egg-white omelet in butter or to scramble Egg Beaters with fatty cheese.

Those who wish to reduce dietary cholesterol should avoid egg yolks in favor of egg whites or commercial egg substitute. Egg yolks contain 90% of the cholesterol and 80% of the fat; egg whites contain most of the protein. If you limit daily cholesterol intake to 300 milligrams, the American Heart Association allows one egg a day.

Cream

Unlike most other dairy foods, cream doesn't come in reduced-fat, lower-calorie versions and must be relegated to the "too rich to be regularly eaten" list. If you drink three cups of coffee a day, using half-and-half or table cream can add from 5 to 9 grams of fat (and 3 to 9 grams of saturated fat) to your daily intake. Better choices are fat-free or 1% milk, evaporated skim milk or soy creamer.

Type (1 tbsp.)	Grams of Fat	Grams of Saturated Fat
Half-and-half	1.0	1.1
Heavy whipping	5.0	3.5
Light table	5.5	3.4
Medium	7.1	4.4

Watch out for nondairy creamers and liquid flavored coffee creamers. Many of these products contain the same amount of fat as table cream and are rich in fructose corn syrup. Some are made with coconut oil, palm oil or hydrogenated fat, all heavily saturated.

Instead, choose creamers made with unsaturated vegetable oils. But keep in mind that, while the oil used may be more heart-healthy, these products have the same fat and calories as half-and-half.

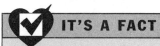 **IT'S A FACT**

Two tablespoons of full-fat sour cream can carry 5 grams of fat (3 saturated). Look for "light" and fat-free versions to use as a topping or as an ingredient in recipes. Some brands taste better than others, so keep trying until you find one that you really like.

Ice Cream

Finally, let's take a look at ice cream, that very American favorite food. Ice cream actually has substantial amounts of calcium and protein, but it comes with a high price—an enormous amount of artery-clogging saturated fat.

Again, there's a wide range of choices. Government standards decree that ice cream must be made with a minimum of 10% cream, milk or butterfat. Premium ice cream contains the most butterfat, generally about 30 grams of fat per cup. One cup of Häagen-Dazs Vanilla Swiss Almond, for instance, has 580 calories and a whopping 38 grams of fat, 18 of which are saturated. Regular ice cream contains less fat (about 12 to 20 grams per cup) but is definitely not *low* in fat. The best option for heart health is light ice cream, which has 6 to 8 grams of fat per cup.

The point is that with ice cream there are many ways to balance taste preference with dietary concerns. Light or fat-free ice cream can save you 25 grams of fat (much of it saturated) or more over a cup of the premium stuff.

A word of caution: Don't use low-fat or fat-free choices as a license to load up on high-fat, high-calorie toppings such as sprinkles.

IT'S A FACT

Generally speaking, the least expensive ice creams contain the minimum 10% fat while premium brands have double the fat. (Where do you think the fat from fat-free milk ends up?)

Chapter Twelve

Table Fats and Oils

T ABLE FATS AND OILS ARE OFTEN GIVEN short shrift because we eat them in dribs and drabs. But those dribs and drabs add up to about 55 pounds of fat a year for the average person. And too many can not only contribute to weight gain but also increase cholesterol and cardiac risk.

Vegetable Oils

V egetable oils have been around almost as long as civilization itself. Before refrigeration, they were essential to preserving foods. Today, particularly in Mediterranean cooking, they're valued for their flavor, aroma and texture. All vegetable oils contain about 120 calories and 14 grams of fat per tablespoon. These oils provide a concentrated form of energy and play a role in the body's absorption of fat-soluble vitamins A, D, E and K. They're also cholesterol-free, although some may have a profoundly negative impact on blood cholesterol levels.

The guidelines recommend 6 tablespoons of vegetable oil a day. However, as covered in some detail in Chapter Five, vegetable oils differ significantly in their fatty acid makeup. While we tend to classify oils as one of the three types of fatty acids, in fact no oil is made up of just one type.

THE MAKEUP OF COMMON OILS

Type of Oil	Monounsaturated%	Polyunsaturated%	Saturated %
Olive	76	10	14
Hazelnut	75	14	11
Avocado	69	11	20
Almond	65	26	9
Canola	62	32	6
Peanut	48	35	17
Sesame	41	41	18
Walnut	28	56	16
Corn	25	62	13
Soybean	25	61	14
Sunflower	22	66	12
Cottonseed	21	53	26
Grape seed	17	70	13
Safflower	15	76	9
Palm kernel	12	5	83
Coconut	8	3	89

Oils rich in monounsaturated fat, particularly olive oil and canola oil, are the best choice for your heart. "These oils contain omega-3 fatty acids that lower harmful LDL without reducing protective HDL," says Dr. Scott Grundy at the University of Texas Southwestern. Polyunsaturated oils, such as safflower, soybean, sunflower, corn, cottonseed and sesame oil, are another good choice. Rich in omega-6 fatty acids, these oils also lower total and LDL cholesterol when they're substituted for saturated and trans fats. However, this benefit is somewhat blunted by the fact that polyunsaturated oils can lower beneficial HDL cholesterol. And there is an emerging concern that processed foods may be supplying too many omega-6s, which some experts believe can contribute to coronary inflammation. Says Judith Shaw, former director of The Family Institute of

Berkeley, "A healthy dietary ratio of omega-6 fatty acids to omega-3 fatty acids is four to one. But the American diet has 15 times more omega-6s. This can lead to structurally damaged blood vessels and inflammation."

Recent studies suggest that two new polyunsaturated oils confer cardiac benefit. Many experts are recommending the addition of about 2 tablespoons of ground flaxseed to your daily diet, since the oil in flaxseed has high levels of cardioprotective omega-3 fatty acids. It can be sprinkled on yogurt, cereal and salads, mixed with juice and added to baked goods and soups. Flax oil can be added to salad dressings 50-50 with olive oil (but remember, don't cook with flax oil). The oil in walnuts also benefits cardiac health by protecting coronary artery walls. Add a handful of walnuts to salads or eat them as a replacement for chips, crackers and less healthy snacks. Or substitute walnut oil in recipes utilizing cooking oils.

Oils rich in saturated fat are the nutritional "bad guys," since they raise LDL cholesterol. But certain tropical oils are also sources of saturated fat and should be avoided. Palm oil, palm kernel oil and coconut oil are found mainly in processed foods such as nondairy creamers, frozen meals, salad dressings, cake mixes, pie crusts, soups, cheese-flavored snacks, chips and crackers. Read the food label and avoid foods made with these oils.

Whenever possible, buy single-source oils such as pure olive oil or pure canola oil. These are the oils you'll find in our recipes, and they should be a pantry staple, ready for daily use. In processed foods, however, blended oils are often used. Generally, a blended oil has an overwhelming proportion of the cheapest and probably least healthful oil mentioned on the label, with only a small amount of better-quality oil. Be sure to read the ingredients list on the food label. If you see the words "made with one or more of the following oils," you won't know from the description which oil was actually used. If palm, palm kernel, palm fruit or coconut is listed, leave the food on the shelf.

ANOTHER BENEFIT OF OLIVE OIL

Long recommended as the healthiest oil because of its impact on cholesterol, clotting and inflammation, olive oil has also been shown to benefit blood pressure. In one study, people with high blood pressure who ate a diet rich in complex carbohydrates that included 3 to 4 teaspoons of extra-virgin olive oil each day were able to reduce their blood pressure medications by 48%; others in the study who ate the same diet but used sunflower oil instead were able to reduce their medication by just 4%.

Margarine

Doubts about margarine as an alternative to butter were first raised in the early 1990s, when research conducted at Harvard University suggested that some types might be even riskier than butter in terms of cardiac health. The main difference lies in their fat makeup. All margarines use a liquid vegetable oil, usually unsaturated corn, safflower, canola, sunflower or olive oil, as the basic ingredient. As long as the oil in the product remains "soft," as it does in tub types and liquid squeeze types, the margarine is considered more healthful than butter. In a study conducted by the USDA, participants who ate these types of margarine significantly improved their cholesterol levels, while participants who consumed butter did not. A second type of margarine that can benefit cardiac health is made from plant sterol esters, such as Benecol and Taking Control. Clinical trials show that these margarines can lower total cholesterol by 10% and LDL cholesterol by 14% when eaten regularly.

One of the downsides of all margarines, including those that lower cholesterol, is the extra calories supplied to your diet. But there's an even greater problem. When liquid oil is hydrogenated in order to produce stick margarine, trans fatty acids are created. And it's worth repeating here that trans fats raise LDL cholesterol and lower HDL cholesterol. From a cardiac standpoint, stick margarine is as bad as butter. Either way, your cholesterol can go up. So, if you use spreads, a better choice is soft or tub margarine made with liquid oil and free of hydrogenated fats.

To sum up, all margarines are about the same in fat content (100%), calories (100) and fat-grams (about 11) per tablespoon. In this respect, margarine is the same as butter and should be used very judiciously. If you're trying to cut calories, it doesn't make much sense to switch from butter to margarine as a spread on both pieces of bread in a sandwich. A smarter choice is to spread margarine lightly on one piece of bread and mustard on the other, cutting the fat and calories in half. The smartest choice, of course, would be to use mustard on both pieces of bread and eliminate any added fat-calories.

Hydrogenated shortenings are also problematic. Used extensively in food preparation to improve the shelf life and stability of baked goods and processed foods, they are an additional source of trans fats. Foods most likely to contain these fats include fried fast foods as well as cookies, crackers, potato chips, doughnuts, breakfast waffles, pastries and other processed foods. According to Dr. Helen Brown of the Cleveland Clinic, trans fats make up 24% to 35% of the fat in fast-food French fries. And just one doughnut has as much of this cholesterol-raising fat as a double cheeseburger.

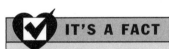

IT'S A FACT

The labels on canned shortenings often boast that the content is "100% all-vegetable oil" but fail to tell you that palm oil is used. If the food label isn't specific, assume the worst.

Mayonnaise

Oddly enough, mayonnaise has a plus side even apart from its taste and texture. It's a good source of vitamin E, an antioxidant that's often hard to get on a low-fat diet. The chief downside is that few foods are richer in fat and calories. One tablespoon of mayonnaise has about 12 grams of fat, 2 grams of saturated fat and 110 calories. Ounce for ounce, it's fatter than spareribs.

Mayonnaise is made from vegetable oil and egg, so the quality of the oil is a key consideration. Choose a mayonnaise made from heart-healthy oils such as canola or safflower oil. ("Cholesterol-free" mayonnaise does not include egg yolk.) The next consideration is caloric contribution. This can be managed by simply eating less. When making a sandwich, put mayonnaise on one slice of bread and mustard on the other. Also, you can cut calories by using "light" or "calorie-reduced" mayonnaise in place of regular.

Salad Dressings

Most regular commercial salad dressings are about 90% fat, which means they contain about 9 grams of fat per tablespoon. This makes them richer in fat than an equal amount of hot fudge. To put this in perspective, 2 tablespoons of salad dressing can have:

- As many calories as a chocolate bar.
- As much fat as two pieces of pizza.
- As much sodium as a handful of taco chips.

I used to use "light" or "low-fat" versions of commercial dressings, but now I avoid them because they're so rich in fructose corn syrup. Instead, I choose dressings primarily for the quality of the fat used (most often olive oil) and watch how much I use. A good tip is to serve dressing on the side and dip your fork first in the dressing, then in the salad. It takes only a small amount of a high-quality dressing to satisfy your taste buds.

Making your own salad dressing at home provides a lot more taste. We make a delicious dressing by blending a good-quality olive oil with balsamic or red wine vinegar.

Chapter Thirteen

Sugar and Other Sweeteners

IT WOULD BE HARD TO FIND ANYONE who never enjoyed the taste of sweet foods. In fact, at least in early childhood, there seems to be a biological basis for craving sweets. But the foods that satisfy this desire today are no longer healthy first choices. Until the Industrial Revolution, people relied on the natural sugar found in foods such as fruits and berries. Then, after the advent of sugar refining in the early 1800s, fruits and berries slowly gave way to pastry, cakes and candies, and the American "sweet tooth" was born. By 1875, the average American consumed 40 pounds of sugar (mostly white table sugar) per year; by 1910, consumption had reached 70 pounds.

But, of course, it didn't stop there. The development of the processed food and beverage industries in the second half of the 20th century caused the consumption of refined sugar and other sweeteners to skyrocket. And now, after the turn of the century, sweeteners have replaced sodium as the most popular food additive. Every day, the average American consumes over one-third of a pound of added sugar—more in a week than our forefathers consumed in an entire year.

This level of consumption is a source of great concern to health professionals. Not only does it contribute to the twin epidemics of overweight and heart disease, but it also leads to lower amounts of needed nutrients. Research shows that women over age 50 who take in 10% of their calories as sugar average only about 650 milligrams of calcium a day, or some 550 milligrams less than the recommended amount. Raise their sugar level to 25% of calories, and the average calcium consumption drops another 100 milligrams. And across all age groups, for both sexes, intakes of vitamins A and E, iron, magnesium and zinc are minimized.

The Main Problem

Let's get something straight. When used judiciously, as in the Mediterranean-style diet, table sugar does not pose a problem. The trouble lies in the amount of added sugars we eat, and that amount has soared primarily because of the inclusion of high-fructose corn syrup in products such as soft drinks, jams and jellies, commercially baked goods, milk products, cured meats, cereals, canned fruit, salad dressings, ketchup and candy. Manufacturers favor liquid high-fructose corn syrup because it's cheaper, sweeter and easier than table sugar to transport and mix into foods and because its sweetness and thickness can be regulated. It can also be used in place of more nutritious ingredients.

MAJOR SOURCES OF ADDED SUGARS AND SWEETENERS

Food	% of Sugar Calories
Regular soft drinks	33.0%
Table sugars and candy	16.1
Cookies, cakes and pies	12.9
Fruit drinks, fruit ades and fruit punch	9.7
Dairy desserts and milk products	8.6

Some 70% of added sugars and sweeteners currently come in the form of high-fructose corn syrup. I would rank it right up there with trans fat, saturated fat and sodium as a significant nutritional ill. And I would certainly add it to the list of reasons for avoiding a steady diet of processed foods.

Weight Control

The impact of added sweeteners on overweight is a major concern of health professionals. Again, we need to look at sources. At just 16 calories per teaspoon, table sugar is no more fattening than protein or carbohydrate and less than half as fattening as fats or oils. Moreover, the fructose in a moderate amount of fruit eaten each day doesn't penalize weight. But concentrated high-fructose corn syrup is an altogether different matter. Because it's a liquid, it allows small quantities of food to contain a large amount of sugar calories.

In addition, foods rich in high-fructose corn syrup generally provide very little mass, which means there's no signal that you've had enough to eat. You can consume virtually an unlimited amount of candy bars (and a large number of calories) without feeling full. This is particularly true with liquid calories. In a study at Purdue University, participants ate 450 calories' worth of jelly beans every day for four weeks and 450 calories' worth of soft drinks every day for another four weeks. On the days they ate jelly beans, the participants ate about 450 fewer calories of other foods. But on the days they drank soft drinks, they ended up eating 450 calories more than normal. "Liquid calories don't trip our satisfaction mechanism," says Dr. Richard Mattes, author of the study.

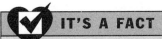 **IT'S A FACT**

Artichokes contain an organic acid that stimulates sweetness receptors in the taste buds. After eating an artichoke, you may find that everything else tastes sweet for a while.

Researchers have found that too much concentrated fructose can change the levels of two hormones that help to regulate appetite. Fructose not only tends to lower levels of leptin, which lets us know when we're full, but also triggers a rise in levels of appetite-stimulating ghrelin. The net result: You may still feel hungry after consuming high-fructose foods and end up overeating.

According to the World Health Organization and the Food and Agricultural Organization, two United Nations agencies, the excessive consumption of added sugars and other sweeteners, when it displaces other nutrients in the diet, is a major contributor to the worldwide obesity epidemic. The WHO recommends restricting calories from added sweeteners to no more than 10% of total calories. If you eat 2,000 calories a day, that works out to 200 calories, or 50 grams of sugar. (That may sound like a lot until you realize that one-half cup of commercial applesauce has 22 grams!) The current dietary guidelines give no recommendation for how many calories should come from sugar in a healthy diet. Some government agencies say that up to 25% of our total daily calories can come from sugar, but Dr. John Yudkin of London University strongly disagrees with that figure: "Added sugar in soft drinks and processed foods are causative of obesity. If only a fraction of what is already known about the effects of sugar were revealed in relation to any other material used as a food additive, that material would promptly be banned."

IT'S A FACT

Foods that contain refined sweeteners often result in the simultaneous extremes of being overfed and still feeling hungry. But foods containing natural sugar—fruits, berries, vegetables and grains—do just the opposite. These low-calorie foods are fiber-rich. At 55 calories per cup, you'd have to eat a mountain of strawberries before you took in too many calories.

Heart Health

Too many sweeteners can also penalize heart health. Studies in the United States and in Japan and South Africa show that a diet high in sugary refined carbohydrates can elevate artery-clogging triglycerides. An estimated 20 million Americans have a genetic predisposition to high triglycerides, so this is an important consideration. In addition, the combination of high triglycerides and low HDLs produces metabolic syndrome, which affects an estimated 60% of American adults. Also, foods rich in refined sweeteners tend to produce "empty" calories. If you satisfy your sweet tooth with a candy bar, you take in virtually zero nutrients. But if you choose a piece of fruit instead, you consume beneficial vitamins, minerals, fiber and phytochemicals in addition to natural sugars.

Positive Steps

Left unchecked, refined sweeteners can contribute a substantial amount of calories to the American diet. There are, however, a number of simple actions that can be taken to manage sugar consumption.

READ FOOD LABELS

Refined sweeteners, the number one additive in processed foods, are found not only in sweet-tasting foods such as candy, cakes and cookies, but also as a surprise ingredient in frozen dinners, nondairy creamers and ketchup. They can even be found in pipe tobacco! Since processed foods are the chief contributor to the 30-teaspoons-a-day habit of most Americans, it's important to read the Nutrition Facts on food labels to determine sweetener content. Remember that food labels lump all sweeteners into the sugar category, but most of that sugar comes in the form of high-fructose corn syrup.

Also, the Nutrition Facts give you grams of sugar per serving, but what does that number mean in practical terms? What you want to remember is that *4 grams of sugar equals 1 teaspoon.* So, if the label tells you that a breakfast cereal has 12 grams of sugar per serving, you know that it contains 3 teaspoons of added sweeteners. This is a more graphic and practical way to view sugar content.

And don't be misled by the other names for sugar. If you see any fo the following ingredients listed on a food label, it's considered an added sugar, regardless of its form.

Barley syrup	Evaporated cane juice	Maltose
Beet sugar	Fructose	Malt syrup
Brown sugar	Fruit juice concentrates	Maple syrup
Cane sugar/syrup	Glucose	Molasses
Confectioners' sugar	High-fructose corn syrup	Raw sugar
Corn sweetener	Honey	Rice syrup
Corn syrup	Invert sugar	Sucrose
Crystallized cane juice	Lactose	Sugar
Dextrose	Maltodextrin	Turbinado

Look for the number of times sugar appears on the ingredients list. If you find two or more, especially near the beginning of the list, the product probably contains a significant amount of added sugar. Also be particularly aware of how much high-fructose corn syrup is in the food. You might expect a high level in soft drinks and other sweet-tasting foods. But what's amazing—and even scary—is the amount of high-fructose corn syrup found in other foods:

- Two tablespoons of ketchup have 1 teaspoon of added sugar;
- A half-cup of baked beans has 3 teaspoons;
- Six ounces of fat-free yogurt has 4 teaspoons.

A MISLEADING LABEL

In a study conducted by Washington State University and the Department of Agriculture, a cereal being test-marketed was shown to contain sucrose, brown sugar and corn syrup. It also contained four cereal grains: white flour, corn flour, cornmeal and rice flour. The food manufacturer circumvented the listing of sugar as the main ingredient by grouping the four flours into a single "cereal grain" category and by listing the three sugars separately, giving the impression that the cereal was primarily made up of grain. This only served to confuse consumers about the real sugar content of the product.

CUT BACK ON SOFT DRINKS

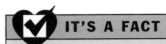

IT'S A FACT

Many popular foods, such as jams and fruit drinks, are sweetened with concentrated grape or apple juice—sucrose-free, yes, but high in fructose.

Soft drinks, the single greatest source of high-fructose corn syrup, have replaced water as America's most consumed beverage. The amount of added sweeteners (and consequently calories) that come in a can or bottle ranges from 8 to 14 teaspoons in a standard 12-ounce serving (often promoted as a "kid's size") to 40 teaspoons and beyond for some supersize varieties such as 7-Eleven's 64-ounce Double Gulp.

Soft Drink (12 oz.)	Calories	Teaspoons of Added Sweeteners	% of Calories from Sugar
Coca-Cola	144	9.3	100
Mountain Dew	178	11.0	100
Pepsi-Cola	158	11.0	100
Shasta Orange	172	11.8	100
Sprite	142	19.0	100

In addition, sit-down restaurants often offer free refills, making it easy to take in excessive sugar calories in the course of a meal. And while soda pop earns most of the negative comments, don't overlook lemonades and other "ades," juice drinks and cocktails. Most are extremely high in added sweeteners.

This is particularly salient in light of results from the Harvard Nurses' Health Study, which found that participants who drank at least one sugary soft drink a day were at about twice the risk for type 2 diabetes as those who drank soda pop and other sweetened beverages less often than once a month. Part of the reason for this result may come from the contribution of soda pop to overweight. Sugar-sweetened soft drinks contribute more than 7% of Americans' calories, making them the largest single source of calories in our diet. In addition, research

IT'S A FACT

British researchers compared children from two schools, one of which set up a program to discourage kids from drinking soda pop. The percentage of overweight and obese children dropped by 0.2% in the school with the program. Obesity increased by 7.5% in the school that did not participate.

indicates that people perceive liquid calories differently from those in solid foods. Drinking a 150-calorie can of soda won't make you less apt to consume 150 fewer calories at some other point in the day, the way a solid 150 calories would, because it doesn't appear to trigger any satiety mechanism.

Whatever the link, sugary soft drinks contribute to excess calories and overweight, which can lead indirectly to diabetes. However, some experts believe there may be a direct link as well. Dr. JoAnn Manson, who worked on the Nurses' Study, says it's "biologically plausible that high-fructose corn syrup increases the risk for diabetes beyond its effect on weight gain." In a nation where a lot of people get at least 20% of their calories from sugar but treat fruits, vegetables and whole grains as condiments, treating soda pop as a dietary staple is nutritionally unsound.

The smart thing would be to cut out sugary soft drinks altogether and make water your first choice. Not only is it a better thirst-quencher, but it also helps to keep you feeling full and satisfied and to avoid overeating. Keep a pitcher of ice water and sliced lemons or limes in the refrigerator. Drink bottled mineral water on your "coffee breaks." Fruit juice diluted with club soda or mineral water is also refreshing and cuts calories in half.

LIMIT SUGARY SNACKS AND DESSERTS

Americans eat almost 21 pounds of candy each year. And when we're not snacking on Snickers, we're indulging in other sugar-rich desserts. But keep these figures in mind: A 4-ounce serving of iced chocolate cake contains about 10 teaspoons of sugar. One ounce of fudge has 4.5 teaspoons of sugar. There is no way to reconcile this amount of sugar

WHAT ABOUT ARTIFICIAL SWEETENERS?

The popularity of artificial sweeteners, also called sugar substitutes or noncaloric sweeteners, has soared as we've tried to cut down on refined carbohydrates, especially sugar. Today, a wide array of such sweeteners exists, among them saccharin (Sweet'N Low), aspartame (NutraSweet and Equal) and sucralose (Splenda). But are they safe?

According to the FDA, the answer is yes. At one time, saccharin carried a warning label because it was linked to an increase in bladder cancer in animals; however, investigations exonerated it as a risk for humans. Aspartame, which has been in wide use for 30 years, is safe for everyone except people born with a rare genetic condition called phenylketonuria (PKU). (A number of rumors have surfaced on the Internet that aspartame causes headaches, dizziness and even brain tumors, but there are no data to back up these claims.) Sucralose, a synthetic compound made from sugar, is 600 times sweeter than sugar and can be used anywhere regular sugar is used; unlike aspartame, it can be used in cooking.

A second question concerns weight loss. The fact that most sugar substitutes are calorie-free hasn't seemed to help in the battle against overweight. According to the Eating Disorder Clinic of Brigham Young University, sweet-tasting drinks (including those made with artificial sweeteners) often cause a craving for more sugar and may be responsible for the increased consumption of snack foods. In addition, some people have trouble understanding that the calories they save by drinking a diet soda instead of a regular soda are offset by the pepperoni pizza that goes along with it.

(not to mention calories) with a healthy diet pattern. The best approach is to treat such foods as "discretionary calories," which means you can have them in small amounts from time to time. When the craving strikes, opt for a packet of fun-size M&M's (100 calories), a fun-size Snickers bar (85 calories) or four squares (a third of a bar) of Hershey's Special Dark Chocolate (73 calories). In other words, you don't have to give up chocolate altogether. Instead, eat your nutritionally rich foods, be physically active and enjoy chocolate as a special treat.

Speaking of chocolate, the dark variety (not milk chocolate) is now being considered a functional food because some studies show that it promotes cardiac health. However, before you buy stock in a candy company, understand that not all experts recommend adding chocolate to your diet. "It's simply too rich in sugar, fat and calories," says Dr. Jeffrey Blumberg of Tufts University. "It's a delightful treat and should be enjoyed as such, not as a health food."

EAT FRESH FRUIT

Always keep a good supply of seasonal fruits on hand. Fresh fruit is central to the Mediterranean-style approach to balanced eating. It provides a much better way to satisfy your sweet tooth with the natural sugar found in a ripe peach, a crisp apple or an ice-cold watermelon wedge.

HIDE THE SUGAR BOWL

Most people use table sugar far too liberally. Get rid of the sugar bowl, and within a few weeks your taste buds will become acclimated to the natural taste of foods. You'll begin to relish new flavors and textures. A bowl of blueberries will be appreciated for its natural sweetness; the nutty flavor of breakfast cereal can be discovered. The true flavor of foods more than compensates for the loss of added sugar.

Chapter Fourteen

Salt and Sodium

N OT TOO LONG AGO, WE BEGAN TO QUESTION the amount of salt we consumed on the American diet. We had learned about dangerous levels of sodium intake, and we had to deal with the fact that about 40% of salt is sodium. Study after study recommended a reduction in our consumption of salt, but scientific advice has landed on deaf ears. Says Dr. Jeremiah Stamler of Northwestern University Medical School, "Over 95% of American men and 75% of American women eat more than a teaspoon of salt daily. In fact, the average person consumes 2 to 4 teaspoons of salt a day, which translates to 4,000 to 8,000 milligrams of sodium, or a yearly consumption of about 15 pounds per person."

The most recent dietary guidelines advise limiting daily sodium intake to no more than 2,300 milligrams, or about a teaspoon of salt. But even this amount is well above the body's actual sodium requirement. About 500 milligrams of sodium daily is all you need for your body to function properly. Indeed, a new report by the U.S. Institute of Medicine recommends consuming even less sodium:

Age	Daily Maximum Intake of Sodium (milligrams)
19–50	1,500
51–70	1,300
70 +	1,200

People with kidney ailments, high blood pressure and certain heart conditions, or those who are sodium-sensitive and retain fluids, may want to keep their intake below the levels shown in the preceding table; at the very least, they should consult their physician for guidelines.

What's the Problem?

A high-salt diet is also high in sodium, and the amount of sodium consumed is a health issue. Sodium, which is essential to life, has both positive and negative characteristics. On the positive side, sodium is the chief regulator of the fluid balance of the body. Our tissues must constantly be bathed in a saline solution, and the correct sodium-to-fluid ratio in this solution is critical to proper metabolic functioning. Sodium regulates this balance by triggering a thirst sensation when body fluid is too low or sodium content too high. For example, when you lose fluid by sweating, the ratio of sodium is increased, causing you to become thirsty. By drinking liquids to satisfy your thirst, you also replace the fluid necessary to restore the proper balance. This relationship of excess sodium to thirst has long been understood by savvy bartenders who offer free salted peanuts or popcorn to their patrons.

When the concentration of sodium in the body is constantly high, as it often is as a result of a high-salt diet, the fluid-balance mechanism can be perverted to produce negative health results. A characteristic of sodium is that it holds liquid, which places more strain on the kidneys and can cause kidney damage or failure.

Excessive amounts of sodium and fluid also tax the heart. In order to move additional fluid in the bloodstream, the heart has to pump harder to create more pressure. At the same time, sodium causes the small blood vessels to constrict, thereby increasing resistance to blood flow. The heart is forced to respond by further increasing blood pressure. Although a cause-and-effect relationship between high salt intake and high blood pressure is difficult to prove conclusively, numerous studies have established a link. Research shows that in low-salt societies, such as those in New Guinea, the Kalahari desert and parts of Brazil, hypertension is virtually nonexistent. However, in high-salt societies, such as those in Japan and the United States, hypertension is rampant. In Japan, where salt consumption can be 20 times that in the west, areas can be found where over 40% of the adult population suffers from serious hypertension; in fact, it's that country's leading cause of death.

Not everyone with an excessive sodium intake is susceptible to hypertension; in many people, the excess is promptly excreted no matter how much is consumed. But in about 10% to 30% of the American population, there exists a genetic predisposition to hypertension. For these people, a diet rich in salt and therefore in sodium can increase the risk of high blood pressure and heart disease. Unfortunately, there are no tests that will let you know whether or not you're sodium-sensitive; consequently, people with sodium-rich diets are playing Russian roulette with their health.

Positive Steps

There is no natural affinity for salt. Says Dr. Lot Page, a Harvard Medical School hypertension specialist, "Salt appetite is determined by early dietary habits and has no relationship to salt need." In other words, we learn to like the taste of salt in childhood when we're fed salty food. But this means that a taste for salt can be *un*learned. After a period of consuming foods with less salt, our taste buds can be freed to savor the natural flavors of food.

EAT FEWER PROCESSED FOODS

About 12% of our sodium intake comes from natural sources such as meat, fish, dairy products, vegetables and drinking water. Another 11% is table salt used as a condiment and as a cooking spice. But fully 77% is derived from processed foods containing MSG, garlic salt, onion salt and sodium-containing preservatives. With such foods making up so much of the modern American diet, it's easy to exceed the recommended daily allowance of 2,300 milligrams a day of sodium or one teaspoon of salt.

SOURCES OF SODIUM

Food	Milligrams of Sodium
Salted cashews, 1 oz.	230
White bread, 2 slices	240
Bacon, 1 strip	300
Tomato juice, 6 oz.	600
Deli frankfurter, 1	675
Vinaigrette salad dressing, 1.5 fl. oz.	730
Spaghetti sauce, 4-oz. serving	740
Chicken noodle soup, 1 cup	940
Salted popcorn, 2 oz.	1,100
Ham, 3-oz. slice	1,177
Meat lasagna, 2 cups	1,380
Sauerkraut, 1 cup	1,755
Dill pickle, 1 large	1,940
Soy sauce, 1 oz.	2,075

Many of the foods in the list above *taste* salty, so their sodium content should come as no surprise. What might come as a shock is the amount of sodium in foods that we don't identify as salty. According to *Consumer Reports*:

■ One ounce of cornflakes has nearly twice the sodium as an ounce of salted peanuts.

■ Two slices of white bread contain more sodium than 14 potato chips.

■ One-half cup of prepared chocolate pudding has more sodium than three slices of bacon.

Sodium is also found in such diverse sources as cereals, pancakes, ketchup, barbecue sauce, mustard, breakfast drinks, cooking wines and antacids.

There are three reasons for adding sodium to processed foods. First, it's a cheap filler that adds weight and mass to food. Second, it adds a semblance of recognizable flavor to bland-tasting food. And third, the fact that most consumers like the taste of salt is not lost on food companies. A basic way to reduce sodium consumption, then, is to replace as many processed foods as you can with fresh, whole foods. Since this is done quite naturally on the Mediterranean-style diet, whole foods are central to most of the recipes in this book.

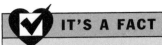

IT'S A FACT

Draining off the liquid from canned salted beans or vegetables and rinsing them thoroughly is a good way to reduce sodium intake.

READ FOOD LABELS

One of the keys to restricting salt and sodium is to read the Nutrition Facts on food labels. This will tell you how many milligrams of sodium come in one serving of the food and allow you to determine whether or not it fits your diet. Familiarize yourself with the most commonly used advertising descriptions:

- *Low sodium* means 140 milligrams or less per serving.
- *Very low sodium* means 35 milligrams or less per serving.
- *Sodium free* means less than 5 milligrams per serving.
- *Reduced sodium* means at least a 25% reduction of the sodium in the regular food.
- *Unsalted* means no salt (but not necessarily no sodium) has been added to the food.

Also, be sure to read the ingredients lists on food labels for sources of sodium other than salt. These include baking soda, baking powder and any ingredient with the word "sodium" in its name, such as monosodium glutamate (MSG). Remember, ingredients present in the greatest amount are listed first and those in the smallest amount come last. So, if you find salt or sodium as one of the first three ingredients, it would be prudent to avoid the food.

HIDE THE SALT SHAKER

Do you salt your food even before you taste it? In order to change this habit, keep the salt out of sight. Or, if this seems too drastic at first, consider using a one-hole salt shaker or pouring the salt into a pepper shaker, which has fewer holes. Give yourself enough time to allow your taste buds to get used to less salt. If you need to zip up flavor, use non- or low-sodium spices such as black pepper, garlic, garlic powder, tarragon, chili powder, chili flakes, lemon juice or commercial dried herbs and seasonings.

IT'S A FACT

You're better off using coarse (or kosher) salt. Because its crystals are larger than normal salt crystals, each teaspoonful contains less sodium.

EAT MORE POTASSIUM

For years, doctors have recommended cutting back on sodium to avoid or manage high blood pressure, but the guidelines now say that isn't enough. We have to add potassium to our diet to maintain correct fluid balance. Experts recommend consuming at least 4,700 milligrams of potassium every day. Many of the foods found on the Mediterranean-style diet are good sources of potassium: tomatoes and tomato products, beans, fish, lentils, nuts, seeds, oranges, melons, dark leafy greens, soybeans and dairy foods.

COMMON SOURCES OF POTASSIUM

Food	Milligrams of Potassium
Fruits	
Apricots, 3 medium	272
Avocado, 1 medium	976
Banana, 1 medium	422
Cantaloupe, cubed, 1 cup	427
Honeydew melon balls, 1 cup	404
Kiwi, 1 medium	252

Nectarine, 1 medium	273
Orange, 1 medium	355
Orange juice, ¾ cup	355
Prunes, 10	615
Raisins, ⅔ cup	717

Vegetables

Artichoke, boiled, 1 medium	425
Broccoli, chopped, 1 cup	278
Carrot juice, ¾ cup	517
Potato, baked with skin, medium	926
Spinach, boiled, ½ cup	419
Sweet potato, baked, 1 medium	542
Tomato, 1 medium	426
Tomato juice, 6 oz.	417
Tomato paste, ½ cup	1,328
Tomato sauce, ½ cup	405
Winter squash, cooked, ½ cup	448

Dairy

Fat-free milk, 8 oz.	382
Chocolate milk, low-fat, 8 oz.	425
Yogurt, 8 oz.	531

Protein Sources

Clams, canned, 3 oz.	534
Halibut, cooked, 3 oz.	490
Kidney beans, cooked, ½ cup	358
Lentils, boiled, 1 cup	731
Lima beans, boiled, 1 cup	969
Navy beans, boiled, 1 cup	708
Pinto beans, boiled, 1 cup	746
Pork chop, center loin, cooked, 3 oz.	382
Tuna, canned, 3 oz.	201

REDUCE SALT IN COOKING

Begin by questioning whether salt is really needed in a recipe. If you can't do without it, reduce the amount called for by at least a quarter. If a recipe specifies one teaspoon of salt, use just three-quarters of a teaspoon. You'll find there is very little change in taste. After a few months, make a second reduction by another quarter. Again, you won't notice the difference. Then make a final cut of another quarter. The result will be a dramatic reduction in sodium intake with virtually no change in the taste of the food.

It's especially worthwhile to reduce the amount of salt when you cook with processed foods such as canned tomatoes, tomato sauce, tomato paste, and chicken and beef broth, since these foods are already rich in sodium. To bring out natural flavors, rely on lemon juice, flavored vinegars, and herbs and spices that are low in sodium and avoid salty condiments such as sea salt, garlic salt and soy sauce. (Reduced-sodium soy sauce, with about 160 milligrams per teaspoon, can be used in moderation.)

The recipes in this book have been analyzed for sodium content. Most are well within the guidelines. Where the sodium content of a recipe is high due to a necessary ingredient, we advise eating less sodium at other meals that day. It's all a question of balance.

IT'S A FACT

Salt substitutes, technically potassium chloride, are not necessarily a good alternative. They can trick your taste buds into thinking you're still eating salt, so the craving doesn't go away.

Chapter Fifteen

Water

H EALTHY EATING IN THE MEDITERRANEAN STYLE is mostly about, well, eating! But the evolution of beverage choices has had a definite impact on our diet. We've already discussed some beverages with cardioprotective functional qualities: black tea, wine, fat-free milk and soy milk. And we've warned against sugary beverages, mainly soda pop, that can penalize health. This chapter will examine the most important beverage: water.

Most people today are aware of the need for an adequate intake of water. Ask the man on the street what it takes to stay hydrated, and chances are his answer will be "eight glasses of water a day." While science has not established a definitive daily level, this rule of thumb is probably in the ballpark. And judging by the number of people walking around with bottles of "designer" water, you're likely to think just about everyone is drinking that amount. In reality, however, the average individual intake of water falls woefully short of the recommended eight glasses a day. (A serving of water is one eight-ounce glass.)

This shortfall is important because an adequate intake of water is necessary for good overall health. Water regulates body temperature, transports nutrients and oxygen, dissolves vitamins and minerals, and promotes effective exercise. Of particular significance is the kidneys' need for water in order to function properly. When that supply is short, the liver is forced to pick up some of the kidneys' function, impairing its ability to metabolize body fat into usable energy. As a result, the body burns less fat as fuel and more fat is stored for future use.

Sufficient water in the diet also relieves fluid retention, the cause of unattractive "puffiness." The body sees insufficient water as a threat to survival, so it tries to hold on to every drop, storing emergency rations that show up chiefly in swollen feet, ankles, legs, wrists and hands. Diuretics, which force the body to eliminate some of the stored water, can provide relief but are not a healthy long-term solution. Nutrients are expelled along with the water, and worse, the body "sees" the loss of water as a threat of insufficiency and redoubles its effort to retain it.

Another problem is that insufficient intake of water has a negative impact on eating habits. Have you ever found yourself at ten o'clock in the evening in front of an open refrigerator door, thinking, *What am I doing here?* When you're dehydrated, your brain receives a message that your body needs more water, but this message is often misinterpreted as a hunger cue and you reach for a snack instead of a drink of water.

Water is also filling, so it helps with weight control. In analyzing people's lack of success in restricting calories to lose weight, experts found that dieters weren't getting enough food to feel satisfied. They felt deprived and soon reverted to their old way of eating. Water (along with complex carbohydrates and fiber) helps to maintain satisfaction without adding calories.

IT'S A FACT

Drinking eight glasses of water a day will not only keep your stomach feeling full but will actually decrease hunger pangs.

And finally, water contains no calories. You can drink it all day long without adding extra calories to your diet. This is not true of other beverages. Drink a cola (144 calories), a beer (regular, 150 calories; light, 90 calories) or a glass of apple juice (120 calories), and those liquid calories will add up. Every one glass of whole milk,

BURNING OFF CALORIES

Researchers in Germany measured the resting metabolism of 14 men and women both before and after they drank just over 16 ounces of water. Within 10 minutes of drinking the water, their metabolism began to rise. After 40 minutes, the average calorie-burning rate was 30% higher, and it stayed elevated for more than an hour.

From these results, the researchers calculated that drinking eight 8-ounce glasses of cold water a day can burn off almost 35,000 calories a year, or about 10 pounds.

generally not considered "diet-busting," is 150 calories; a brownie, which everyone knows is high in calories, contains just 97! For some people, beverages, rather than solid food, may be their greatest calorie problem.

Here are a few suggestions for increasing water intake:

■ Figure out your own hydration plan and then stick to it. If drinking water is not part of your regular routine, chances are slim that you'll take in as much as you need. My own plan is to drink two glasses each with breakfast, lunch and dinner, and follow each workout with two more.

■ Spread out your water consumption over the entire day. It's a good idea to take a drink before you get the urge; don't wait until you're thirsty. By the time you get the signal, you might already be slightly dehydrated.

■ Fill your office coffee mug with hot water and sip from it during business meetings or while you're at your desk.

■ Carry a bottle of water around with you and sip from it steadily throughout the day. Experiment with bottles of different sizes. (A 32-ounce bottle might seem more intimidating to you than two 16-ounce bottles.)

■ Keep a pitcher of water laced with fresh lemons in the refrigerator. Cold lemon-flavored water is a satisfying alternative to soda pop and fruit drinks.

■ Try different water temperatures. Some people like their water to be room temperature; others like it icy cold. Cold water burns more calories.

And What About Coffee?

The average American consumes about 450 cups of coffee a year, causing concern among medical experts who believe that a high level of caffeine can elevate blood pressure and cause an increase of fatty acids in the bloodstream. In fact, a Johns Hopkins study of over a thousand men found that those who drank five or more cups of caffeinated coffee every day had nearly three times the risk of heart disease as those who drank decaffeinated coffee or no coffee at all.

Strong caffeinated coffee is part of the traditional Mediterranean diet, but the amount consumed in a day is generally less than Americans drink. And that may be the key point. Research to date has not linked a *moderate* consumption of caffeinated coffee to heart disease. Still, a good rule of thumb is to keep caffeine intake to no more than 300 milligrams a day. For me, a morning espresso gives the best of both worlds: a great cup of coffee without adding a lot of caffeine to my day.

Type of Coffee (1 cup)	Milligrams of Caffeine
Drip	150
Brewed	135
Espresso (1.5 to 2 oz.)	100
Instant	95
Decaffeinated	5

There may be another upside to moderate consumption of coffee. One study suggests that coffee is the number one source of disease-fighting antioxidants in the American diet. "Nothing else comes close," says Dr. Joe Vinson at the University of Scranton. "But the *best* sources are still antioxidant-rich fruits and vegetables, and they offer more in terms of total nutrition due to their higher content of vitamins, minerals and fiber."

So don't increase your daily java dose just yet. A lot more study is needed.

Chapter Sixteen

Discretionary Calories

YOU CAN DESIGN the perfect heart-healthy diet on paper, bursting with fruits, vegetables, whole grains and other functional foods, but that doesn't mean you'll follow it to the letter. There are times when a piece of chocolate cake just *feels* right. And according to the new dietary guidelines, such discretionary calories are acceptable from time to time as long as you manage 99% of your diet well and stay physically active. This chapter will take a hard look at snacks and restaurant foods, with an eye to making smarter choices.

Snacks

Despite the increase in nutritional awareness, virtually everyone snacks. According to the *National Eating Trends Report,* the average American consumes snack foods over 200 times a year. The figures for candy consumption alone recently jumped from 19 to 25 pounds per person.

Today's most popular snacks—chips, candy, cookies and ice cream—are usually rich in fat, sodium and sugar. They're also high in "empty" calories. Potato chips, the all-American favorite, are indicative of the problem. Eating 8 ounces of chips is tantamount to adding 12 to 20 teaspoons of vegetable oil to a baked potato.

The table below shows how a one-cup serving of a favorite snack, a mere handful or two during a TV program, can penalize your healthy eating efforts.

Item	Calories	Grams of Fat
Cheese combos	510	21
Cheese puffs/twists	235	15
Corn chips	230	14
Corn nuts	375	12
Potato chips	150	10
Potato sticks	190	12
Tortilla chips	180	9

So, should we do away with all chips and sweets? No. Salty and sugary snacks can be a nice occasional treat. If you'd like to include such snacks in your diet, you need to do two things. First, be sure to eat an adequate amount of nutritious foods and keep physically active. Next, choose healthier snacks most of the time. If you're eating fruits, vegetables and nuts as your regular snacks, an occasional dish of ice cream will not undermine your healthy eating efforts.

Below are a few tips for making better choices:

■ *Change your grocery list.* Potato chips are hard to resist if they're around when a craving hits. But if all you have on hand is fresh and dried fruits, peanut butter, cut-up vegetables, nuts or juice bars, these snacks will do the trick most of the time. As Dr. David Katz of Yale University says, "Eating well becomes the easy choice because it's the *only* choice."

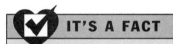

IT'S A FACT

"Crunchiness" is one of the main reasons that potato chips and similar snack foods are so popular. But that same satisfying crunch is a characteristic of apples, broccoli, carrots, celery, green, red and yellow peppers, pears and radishes.

■ *Choose fruits and vegetables.* These foods satisfy without adding extra calories. Watery vegetables like cucumbers and radishes are less than 10 calories per ounce. Fresh fruits in season are one of the best deals around. An apple, a banana, half a cantaloupe, 29 grapes, 2 peaches, 2 cups of strawberries . . . each snack is less than 100 calories. But be prepared. Baby carrots with salsa make a great snack, but if you have to wash and peel the carrots and run to the store for salsa, it might be easier just to tear open a bag of chips. Have the carrots or a plate of cut-up fruit and vegetables washed, trimmed and ready to go when you come home hungry.

IT'S A FACT

Peanuts and peanut butter reduce hunger for a longer time than other types of snacks. In one study, participants who ate peanuts and peanut butter lowered their calorie intake spontaneously for the rest of the day.

■ *Eat nuts.* People who eat nuts regularly cut their risk of high cholesterol, heart disease and diabetes, compared with those who rarely or never eat nuts. In the Nurses' Health Study, women who ate more than 5 ounces of nuts a week had a 35% reduction in their heart attack risk compared with women who ate one ounce of nuts a week or none at all. So, instead of chips or pretzels, help yourself to some walnuts, almonds, Brazil nuts, cashews, filberts/hazelnuts and pecans.

■ *Satisfy with cereal.* Try cereal in place of a snack when an after-dinner craving hits. In a study of 58 overweight nighttime snackers at Wayne State University, half had a 150-calorie bowl of cereal and low-fat milk at least 90 minutes after dinner; the other half ate their customary evening snacks. After four weeks, the cereal eaters had lost two pounds and ate 140 fewer calories than usual after dinner.

■ *Don't wait until you're hungry.* Plan healthy snacks ahead of time so you won't make unhealthy choices.

To help you make the right choices, we've included a comprehensive list of snacks starting on the facing page.

SNACK SUGGESTIONS

Vegetables
baby carrots
celery sticks
cucumber sticks
edamame
mushrooms
radishes
red, green, yellow and
    orange peppers

Dips
black-bean dip
guacamole
humus
peanut butter
three-bean dip
tomato salsa

Fruits
apples
apricots
bananas
blackberries
blueberries
cantaloupe
cherries
dates
dried apricots,
    peaches or plums
figs
frozen berries, grapes
    or watermelon
grapes
honeydew
nectarines
papaya
peaches
pears
pineapple
plums
raisins
raspberries
satsumas
strawberries
tangerines
watermelon

Accompaniments
Gouda cheese
Laughing Cow light creamy
    Swiss cheese
Laughing Cow Mini Babybel
    cheese
mozzarella cheese sticks
organic nonfat or low-fat yogurt
part-skim mozzarella cheese
reduced-fat cheddar cheese
peanut butter

Kashi Original 7 Grain
    Crackers
Kashi TLC Crackers
Rye Crisps
Wasa crackers

(continued on pages 200–201)

Soups (Be sure to watch for sodium.)

black bean	minestrone
chicken broth	noodle (chicken, beef or vegetarian)
five-bean or pasta-and-bean	split-pea
lentil	vegetable

Beverages

black tea	lemon spritzer
coffee	mineral water
fresh orange juice and other	nonfat smoothies
whole water fruit juices	(yogurt or milk with berries)
fresh organic juices	sparkling water
green tea	water

Munchies

2–3 cups air-popped popcorn, plain or with a little sea salt. (Watch for unhealthy saturated fats in stove-popped popcorn; use nonhydrogenated canola, olive, soybean, safflower oil.)

Kashi GOLEAN cereal, Kashi GOLEAN Crunch!, Cheerios or Kashi Heart to Heart

¼ cup fat-free pretzels

¼ cup (separate or mixed):

	almonds	other unsalted, roasted
	hazelnuts	raw nuts or seeds
	pecans	dried apricots
	pistachios	dried peaches
	soynuts	dried plums
	sunflower seeds	raisins
	walnuts	

Now and Then

2 small chocolate-covered strawberries

5 gingersnaps

4 squares heart-healthy graham crackers and 2 chocolate kisses

1 frozen fruit juice bar

½ cup unsweetened fruit sorbet

2 Oreos

2 fig bars

1 sugar-free fudgesickle

½ cup vanilla frozen yogurt topped with 1 cup fresh or frozen raspberries or strawberries

½ cup orange sherbet topped with ¾ cup freshly squeezed orange juice

½ cup lemon sorbet topped with ¾ cup homemade lemonade

To Tide You Over . . .

½ toasted whole wheat English muffin with tomato slice and
    1 tablespoon shredded reduced-fat cheddar or part-skim mozzarella cheese
¼-inch whole wheat tortilla with 1 tablespoon fat-free refried beans
    and 1 ounce reduced-fat cheddar cheese (microwave for 30 seconds)
½ whole wheat bagel with 1 teaspoon of fat-free cream cheese
    and 1 ounce of smoked salmon (lox)
½ warm whole wheat pita and 2 tablespoons hummus
1 slice whole wheat toast with 1 teaspoon apple butter
1 ounce reduced-fat cheese with 2 Ak-Mak, rye crisp, soy crisp
    or Wasa crackers and apple slices
6 ounces V-8 juice and 1 ounce string cheese
1 whole wheat pita with 2 tablespoons hummus
½ cup cottage cheese with ½ cup pineapple
1 slice (1 ounce) angel food cake with ½ cup berries
½ cup whole-grain cereal with ½ cup nonfat milk
1 slice whole-grain toast with 1 tablespoon peanut butter
1 whole-grain frozen waffle with small amount of all-fruit jam

Again, be realistic. Occasionally, it's reasonable to have a higher-fat dessert or snack. There will be times when your "fat tooth" kicks in and nothing but chocolate will do. Then have the food and enjoy it without guilt, but go small and have less of it. And understand that it's discretionary eating.

Restaurant Food

Gourmet, ethnic, family-style, fast-food, deli . . . restaurant meals are part of the fabric of modern American life. Indeed, more of us are eating out than ever before. According to the American Restaurant Association, over half of all meals in the United States are eaten in restaurants. Fast-food restaurants alone serve more than 60 million Americans daily.

There are many reasons for the shift toward increased restaurant meals. Eating out is often a social event with friends and family. It's more convenient than shopping for food, preparing and serving it, then cleaning up afterwards. Restaurant food is usually delicious. And many restaurants are moderately priced or, in the case of fast-food restaurants, even inexpensive. But the overriding reason for the popularity of restaurant meals is "lack of time." The fast-paced modern lifestyle just doesn't leave enough hours in the day for shopping and cooking.

But dining out can pose a serious problem for cardiac health and weight because of what many restaurant foods contain: liberal amounts of fat, salt, sugar and calories. Even if they see baked chicken on the menu, most people will still order their chicken fried. In addition, many restaurant foods and meals are served in oversize portions. The amount of rice served with your kung pao chicken can be as much as three servings. The Enormous Omelet Sandwich at Burger King, with two slices of cheese, two eggs, three strips of bacon and a sausage patty, has 730 calories and 47 grams of fat. In keeping with this trend, Ben & Jerry's recently introduced a wider cone to hold two scoops of ice cream instead of one.

Restaurant meals can also be a problem because of what they *don't* contain: foods rich in complex carbohydrates and fiber. Fruits, vegetables and whole grains are normally in short supply in restaurant offerings, particularly fast food.

THE RIGHT MIND-SET

Too often we practice "souvenir eating," treating each restaurant meal as if it were a special occasion that allows extra indulgences. This might have been a valid concept 25 years ago, when people went to restaurants less frequently, but it doesn't apply to the way we live and eat today. Now most people eat in restaurants so often that once-in-a-while treats have become regular fare.

■ *Choose your restaurant carefully.* It's more difficult to make good choices stick at a rib restaurant that specializes in oversize portions or at a fried chicken or fish-and-chips fast-food restaurant. So it makes sense to have a game plan. One way to keep from being caught off-guard is to go online to check out the menu at the restaurant of your choice. Then you can decide what to order even before you get there. For example, I learned online that T.G.I. Friday's has a Barbecue Jack Chicken with black beans and corn salsa, herbed rice, grilled vegetables and steamed broccoli . . . with just 500 calories and 10 grams of fat. P.F. Chang's is an example of a restaurant chain that provides complete nutrition information for every dish on its Web site. The Chili's chain, for instance, offers a Guiltless Grill menu of low-calorie choices.

■ *Don't set yourself up to overeat.* If you skip meals all day long to "save calories" for a restaurant dinner, chances are that you'll overeat. You'll arrive at the restaurant famished, so your resistance to tempting foods high in fat and calories will be low. It's also easier to rationalize eating *anything* when you're ravenous. A high-protein snack in the afternoon, such as almonds, peanut butter or an apple with a little cheese, will keep the edge off of your hunger at dinner. You might want to have a glass of mineral water or orange juice, a piece of fruit or some raw vegetables an hour or so before dinner. Alcohol can increase your hunger, so be aware of your predinner cocktail choices. A Virgin Mary (nonalcoholic Bloody Mary) is a good alternative.

■ *Ask the right questions.* Is the dish made with butter, margarine, cream, oil or animal fat? Is it fried or deep-fat fried? Is the dressing made with cream? Can I get the sauce on the side? Questions like these can keep a restaurant meal from turning into a disaster with respect to your dietary plan. These days, restaurant personnel, particularly at sit-down restaurants, are very knowledgeable about meal content and cooking methods, so don't hesitate to ask. I remember an eye-opening visit to a restaurant soon after I began to change my diet. Being more conscious of the fat content of marbled meats, I avoided the prime rib, New York steak and spareribs in favor of a broiled salmon fillet. But when the fish arrived, it was swimming in butter sauce! And the same fatty sauce covered the rice and vegetables! I hadn't reduced fat consumption by one whit. This discouraging episode took place because I didn't ask how the dish was prepared. Had I known about the butter sauce, I would have asked them to "hold" it.

Be prepared for suggestions from the server and your dining companions. Others may try to tempt you away from your sound choices. Simply say, "I prefer it that way" or "I enjoy healthy eating" and stick to what you know is best for you.

■ *Look for key words on the menu.* Avoid foods described by the following terms: buttery, butter sauce, sauté, fried, pan-fried, crispy, creamed, cream sauce, aioli, pesto, in its own gravy, au gratin, in cheese sauce, escalloped, au lait, à la mode, au fromage, marinated, basted, prime, béarnaise, beurre blanc, hollandaise. Better choices are: steamed, in broth, in its own juice, poached, garden-fresh, roasted, broiled, stir-fried and lean.

■ *Be innovative.* Ask for olive oil instead of butter for your bread. Order a side dish of fresh fruit, sliced tomato, a side salad, wild rice or grilled vegetables instead of French fries or onion rings. If you're out for a weekend breakfast and want eggs, order them poached or soft boiled, not fried.

TAKE YOUR TIME

Mediterranean people take more time to eat their food than we do. They appreciate the simple act of sitting down to talk and eat with friends and family, which allows them to get more enjoyment out of less food.

In a study that compared eating habits in France with those in the United States, it was found that the average French person takes 22 minutes to eat a McDonald's burger and fries, compared with 14 minutes for the average American. Overall, the French spend 100 minutes a day eating, while we spend just 60. The study suggests that this may partly explain why just 7% of the French are obese compared with 30% of Americans.

Many enjoyable restaurant foods conform to healthy principles. Instead of taking a "gloom and doom" approach when you go out to eat, open your mind to all the possibilities. If you're mentally and emotionally committed to healthy eating, neither the menu choices offered nor the food selections of others will keep you from ordering a nutritious meal.

MANAGE YOUR PORTIONS

Go lean if you can. But, above all, go easy. Restaurants typically serve portions that are much larger than what would normally be served on a Mediterranean-style diet. A transatlantic comparison of serving sizes found that portions of similar foods were twice as large in Philadelphia as they were in Paris; in fact, a single portion in Philadelphia provided enough calories *for at least two meals*. Since most restaurant portions are large enough for at least two people, sharing the grilled fish, chicken or lean-meat entrée (or taking one-half home) will save on calories.

What else can you do to avoid overeating?

■ Skip buffets and "all you can eat" restaurants.

■ Make a meal out of appetizers and sides.

■ Order smaller portions when they're offered (look for "half sizes" or "light menu").

■ Leave one-half to one-third of your meal to be brought home in a doggie bag.

■ Develop a mental picture of what size a serving should be. Three ounces of fish or meat is about the same size as the palm of a woman's hand. Three ounces of chicken is equal to about one-half a chicken breast.

■ If you order dessert, share it. One piece of chocolate cake shared among four people will give everyone a taste without destroying anyone's healthy diet.

Another way to manage portion size is to skip the entrée and instead focus on a number of courses. For example, in my favorite

Asian restaurant, I might start with hot-and-sour soup, then order a salad and, as my entrée, an appetizer portion of fresh (not fried) spring rolls. Or I might have soup followed by an appetizer portion of chicken satay and a cup of rice topped with steamed vegetables. Planning ahead keeps food choices healthy and portion sizes realistic.

BEST CHOICES

Too often, we focus on the entrée and pay little attention to appetizers, salads and side dishes. Low-calorie grilled fish in the same meal with a cup of New England clam chowder or a salad with Thousand Island dressing doesn't make much sense (not to mention the bread sticks at 14 calories apiece!). If nothing will do but clam chowder, make it Manhattan. Have a green salad with dressing on the side or order sliced tomatoes with balsamic vinegar. Make smarter side choices: wild rice and sliced fruit, for example, or sautéed or stir-fried vegetables without added fat. A good question for your waiter is "What are your best vegetables today?"

■ *Appetizers.* Stay away from all those appetizers that are fried or deep-fried, drenched in oil, butter or cheese, or served with creamy dips. Nachos with guacamole and cheese, meat and cheese antipasto, deep-fried mozzarella sticks, fried egg rolls, tempura vegetables, fried calamari, mussels in butter sauce, and buffalo wings are good examples. Think Mediterranean for more acceptable choices: oysters (raw, baked or steamed); steamed mussels with lemons; clam, crab, oyster and lobster cocktails; fresh spring rolls; chicken satays; seviche; steamed pot stickers; sushi and sashimi; steamed, grilled or raw vegetables; and edamame.

■ *Soups.* Skip the cream-based soups such as clam chowder and lobster bisque, meat soups, and soups with melted cheese (French onion soup is a good example). Instead, order gazpacho, minestrone, vegetable soup, beef or chicken consommé with pasta or pastina, riboletto, miso, cioppino and bouillabaisse (fish soup) and black bean soup (hold the sour cream).

■ *Salads.* Stay away from salads with strips of meat and cheese. A chef's salad, for instance, can have 800 calories and 65 grams of fat. A simple green salad is virtually fat-free and runs about 10 calories per ounce, but pour on a few tablespoons of dressing and fat/calories

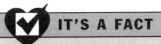

IT'S A FACT

Salad dressing ladles at salad bars generally hold 2 to 6 tablespoons of salad dressing!

skyrocket. Avoid regular dressings, especially creamy dressings such as sour cream, Thousand Island and blue cheese. Ask for "light" and "fat-free" versions of salad dressings.

■ *Entrées.* Maximize whole grains, fruits and vegetables. Use Mediterranean-style principles as your guide with animal foods. Broiled, poached, blackened, in marinara sauce, in light wine sauce, grilled, marinated, barbecued, stir-fried and steamed seafood are excellent choices, as are seafood stews such as cioppino. Watch out for fish and chips, and any seafood that is fried, deep-fried, breaded or batter-dipped and fried, served with a cream or cheese sauce, cooked en casserole, Newburg or thermidor, or baked, stuffed, or stuffed and rolled.

If it's a red meat night, the best choices for beef include round steak, roast (round eye, top round, bottom round, round tip), top loin or top sirloin; for pork, choose loin, tenderloin, center loin and ham. Avoid all fatty meats. Ask for meat to be lean, well trimmed and cooked in a low-fat manner with no butter or fatty sauce used in its preparation.

Avoid any chicken that is fried, batter-dipped and fried, or served smothered with gravy. Always order chicken that is baked, broiled, roasted or barbecued without skin. Make sure any sauces are served on the side. If chicken comes with the skin, remove it yourself before you eat it. In ethnic restaurants, baked or broiled skinless chicken topped with tomato-based or vegetable sauces and minimal cheese are acceptable. Examples include chicken cacciatore (Italian) and arroz con pollo (Mexican). In Asian restaurants, ask for chicken stir-fried in canola oil. And, of course, don't forget that roast turkey dinners with gravy and stuffing can break your fat budget.

Pasta dishes with low-fat sauces, such as marinara, are excellent entrée choices; just watch the serving size. Linguine in a marinara sauce is about 550 calories and 8 grams of fat.

The real challenge is to make smarter, more nutritious choices in restaurant settings. Remember, the road to a healthy heart doesn't just run through your own kitchen; it runs through restaurant kitchens as well.

Chapter Seventeen

Exercise

W ITH PHYSICAL ACTIVITY RANKING SO HIGH on the list of smart things you can do for your heart, you'd think the American landscape would be full of people jogging and biking in earnest. But all we do is put up a good front. As one physician put it, "Americans don't exercise. We just buy exercise stuff."

To be fair, there are people out there who actually *do* exercise, but fewer than 15% of them do it often or vigorously enough to produce cardiovascular benefits. The sad truth is that physical activity has been engineered out of our modern society and 50% of American adults are completely sedentary. It isn't that we don't know better. The media are full of reports showing that physically active people have health benefits such as increased cardiovascular stamina, lower resting heart rate, lower blood pressure, reduced body fat, increased metabolism, better ability to cope with stress and greater longevity. Those benefits are at the root of the guidelines that counsel us to:

■ Exercise at a moderate intensity on most days for at least 30 minutes for overall health.

■ Aim for 30 to 60 minutes on most days to prevent weight gain.

■ Exercise 60 to 90 minutes daily to lose weight.

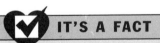

IT'S A FACT

People who are out of shape in their twenties run a high risk of developing high blood pressure, diabetes and other heart disease risk factors by the time they reach their thirties.

Exercise for Your Heart

The connection between physical inactivity and coronary heart disease is paramount. "Since couch potatoes run nearly twice the risk of coronary heart disease as people who are physically active," says Dr. William Haskell of Stanford University, "a sedentary lifestyle just doesn't pay. Sedentary people are at the same risk for heart attacks as the obese and heavy smokers."

Conversely, people who gain cardiovascular fitness through exercise reduce their risk of a heart attack by up to 50%. A study of more than 16,000 Harvard University alumni revealed that active men had one-third fewer heart attacks than their sedentary counterparts; in addition, the study demonstrated that fit persons who suffer heart attacks are more likely to survive. The study also found that benefits accrued in a bell-shaped curve, beginning to appear with 500 calories expended a week (less than two hours of brisk walking) and peaking between 2,000 and 3,500 calories a week (about a daily 20-minute run). But benefits tapered off after 3,500 calories, thereby making moderate, regular exercise the best prescription.

The following table shows how many calories are expended in different activities by weight category:

CALORIES BURNED PER MINUTE

Activity	Weight in Pounds				
	Up to 130	131–152	153–170	171–187	188+
Badminton/volleyball	4.4	5.4	6.1	6.8	7.4
Baseball	3.6	4.5	5.0	5.6	6.1
Basketball	5.5	6.7	7.5	8.4	9.2
Bowling (nonstop)	5.2	6.3	7.1	7.9	8.7
Calisthenics	3.9	4.8	5.4	5.9	6.5
Cycling					
5.5 mph	3.9	4.8	5.4	5.9	6.5
13 mph	8.3	10.2	11.5	12.7	14.0

EXERCISE STRENGTHENS YOUR HEART

Like all muscle tissue, cardiac muscle responds to exercise by increasing in size and strength. As Dr. Steven Blair of the Aerobics Institute in Dallas has observed, "If you exercise, what you get is a bigger, better, stronger pump." This increased efficiency can greatly reduce strain on the heart, as measured in changes in resting pulse. The "average" resting pulse is 72 beats per minute or 103,680 beats a day. When less effort is needed, however, the resting pulse might be reduced to 58 beats per minute, or just 83,520 beats a day, saving a considerable amount of wear and tear on the heart.

EXERCISE CONDITIONS YOUR HEART

Everyone has a maximum heart rate, the most heartbeats per minute that can safely take place. Maximum heart rate is regulated by a mechanism within the heart itself that keeps it from overbeating. A conditioned heart generally responds well to this mechanism, but in a deconditioned heart the regulator may not work the way it's supposed to. Then, when called upon to beat faster because of a strenuous activity like shoveling snow, the heart may speed up to 180 beats a minute or more in an effort to supply blood to the muscles. This can strain the heart to the breaking point and cause plaque to rupture, which may lead to a heart attack.

It's the same for emotional stress. We've all experienced near-misses on a highway and that "heart in your throat" feeling. A deconditioned heart may refuse to slow down and instead speed up dangerously. But in a conditioned heart the slowdown mechanism will help to keep racing heartbeats in check.

EXERCISE IMPROVES CHOLESTEROL

Regular aerobic exercise, such as brisk walking, cycling, swimming or step classes, can boost protective HDL cholesterol. Studies show that by walking two miles a day, three times a week, you can raise your HDL level by up to 10%. Greater increases may occur

Dancing					
Moderate	3.3	4.0	4.4	5.0	5.5
Vigorous	4.4	5.4	6.1	6.7	7.4
Golf					
Twosome	4.2	5.2	5.8	6.4	7.1
Foursome	3.2	3.9	4.4	4.8	5.3
Handball/squash/ racquetball	7.6	9.3	10.4	11.6	12.7
Housework	3.2	3.9	4.4	4.8	5.3
Rope skipping					
70 counts/minute	6.0	7.4	8.3	9.2	10.0
100 counts/minute	9.9	12.0	13.6	15.0	16.5
Rowing					
Leisurely	3.9	4.8	5.4	5.9	6.5
Vigorous	10.6	13.0	14.6	16.2	17.8
Running					
5.5 mph	8.3	10.2	11.5	12.7	14.0
7 mph	10.8	13.3	14.9	16.6	18.0
9 mph	12.9	14.8	16.6	19.9	20.
Skating	4.4	5.4	6.1	6.6	7
Soccer	6.9	8.5	9.6	10.6	1
Swimming					
Crawl (moderate)	3.8	4.6	5.1	5.7	
Crawl (vigorous)	8.3	10.1	11.4	12.6	
Sidestroke	6.5	7.9	8.9	9.9	
Tennis					
Moderate	5.4	6.6	7.4	8.2	
Vigorous	7.6	9.3	10.4	11.6	
Walking					
2 mph	2.7	3.3	3.8	4.2	
4.5 mph	5.0	6.3	7.1	7.9	
Up/down stairs	9.3	11.4	12.8	14.1	
Weight lifting	6.0	7.2	8.2	8	

with more extensive training. Does that mean you have to run marathons to acquire HDL protection? The answer is no. Several studies suggest that joggers who average 11 miles a week exhibit significantly higher HDL cholesterol levels than do their inactive counterparts. The message here is that moderate exercise can provide optimal benefit.

EXERCISE REDUCES BLOOD PRESSURE

A number of studies show that regular exercise lowers blood pressure by about 11 and 9 points for systolic and diastolic pressures respectively, particularly in people with borderline hypertension. Moderate-intensity exercise such as walking seems to be as effective as more intense activities. The mechanism for reducing hypertension risk is not clear. It may simply be that exercise promotes weight loss, a factor in blood pressure. But exercise may work in other ways as well. Studies at Boston University have shown that regular exercise can cause blood vessels to dilate over time, thereby helping to reduce blood pressure.

EXERCISE REDUCES INFLAMMATION

Exercise is one of the best ways to reduce arterial inflammation, possibly because of its positive impact on stress and/or its ability to reduce blood pressure. Research suggests that blood concentrations of C-reactive protein (CRP), a measuring stick of inflammation, drop as levels of physical activity rise. In one study, 21% of sedentary adults had high CRP levels, while just 13% of moderately active and only 8% of very active exercisers had elevated CRP.

 IT'S A FACT

In one study, 377 men and women who ate healthy meals were divided into two groups: those who exercised and those who did not. After a year, the LDL levels of those who exercised had dropped 15% (for men) to 20% (for women) lower than those of the nonexercising group.

OTHER BENEFITS

Strengthened muscles require less oxygen and therefore reduce the demands on the heart. In addition, exercise can produce the growth of small blood vessels in the heart, forming collateral circulation pathways that reduce heart attack risk.

Exercise for Weight Control

Weight loss—and more importantly, keeping weight off—has more to do with physical activity than with diet. Experts say that in about 70% of instances, being overweight is related to inactivity; in only about 30% is it linked primarily to increased food intake. Says Dr. Haskell, "Lack of exercise is the major culprit in the weight gain of most Americans. There has been an overemphasis on caloric intake, with too little emphasis placed on the role of energy expenditures."

Indeed, recent studies have shown that many overweight people do not consume more calories than people of normal weight. A study of runners in the San Francisco area showed that male participants who consumed about 3,000 calories a day weighed 20% less than inactive men of the same age who ate only 2,300 calories a day. Women runners averaged 570 calories more per day than their inactive counterparts but weighed 30% less.

EXERCISE BURNS CALORIES

Although much of our concern is focused on being "overweight," the real problem is being "overfat," i.e., carrying an excess of body fat. When you take in more calories than you use, the excess is stored as body fat. It takes 3,500 extra calories to create a pound of fat and an energy expenditure of 3,500 calories to burn up that pound of fat. Daily exercise draws on fat for fuel, which over time will lead to weight loss. Most health professionals recommend balancing a low-fat diet (to decrease caloric intake) with a regular program of moderate exercise (to burn stored body fat) as the most effective method of permanent weight loss. Walking 30 to 45 minutes a day, for example, burns 200 to 300 calories in a person who weighs 150 pounds.

EXERCISE RAISES METABOLISM

Losing even one pound of body fat requires hours of physical activity. A 150-pound person would have to walk more than 9 hours at an aerobic pace of 4 miles per hour to burn 3,500 calories. A fit runner burns fewer than 1,000 calories on a 10-mile run, which barely covers a hot fudge sundae with whipped cream and nuts. Indeed, the winner of the Boston Marathon loses only about three-quarters of a pound of fat. It doesn't take a trained mathematician to conclude that losing weight exclusively through calories burned is painfully slow.

Fortunately, regular exercise also raises metabolism, the rate at which the body burns calories, even after the activity stops. Many experts consider this to be more important than calories burned directly. People who exercise vigorously experience a 7.5% to 28% increase in metabolic rate for up to four to eight hours after the activity is concluded. By causing the metabolic furnace to burn at a higher level, regular exercise makes it harder for the body to conserve energy (calories) and easier for it to lose weight. Says Dr. Jack Wilmore, an exercise expert at the University of Texas, "If exercising regularly changes your metabolism even slightly, so that you burn an extra 100 calories a day, that small change can add up to 10 pounds of weight loss a year."

EXERCISE BUILDS AND MAINTAINS MUSCLE

Regular exercise creates and maintains muscle tissue, a critical factor because muscle is what burns fat. Think of your body as a car. Muscle is the engine, and fat is the fuel burned. The more muscle you have, the bigger your engine and the easier it is to burn fat. Studies show that every added pound of lean muscle burns an additional 30 to 50 calories a day. Perhaps more important is the impact of muscle on metabolism. Quite simply, the more muscle, the higher the resting metabolic rate. So, the more muscle you have, the easier it is to burn fat even while you're sitting down. Health professionals recommend moderate exercise, such as walking, in combination with resistance training (such as light weight lifting, rowing, push-ups and aerobic dance) and core exercises (such as yoga and Pilates) to build and preserve muscle tissue.

EXERCISE RELIEVES STRESS

As an old saying goes, "When you're under stress, all roads lead to the refrigerator." When we feel pressured, anxious about the future or depressed about the past or present, we tend to make poor lifestyle decisions. And that's when we overeat, binge, or live for days on a diet of fast food and snacks.

Fortunately, exercise dissipates stress. Described as nature's own tranquilizer, exercise may be the most effective method of managing pressure, reducing tension and increasing endorphins. Research at Duke and Stanford has revealed that people who exercise demonstrate less anxiety and a more positive sense of well-being than those who exercise little or not at all. And this affects eating habits. Case Western Reserve University conducted a study of the dietary habits of sedentary and physically active people that clearly showed the active participants choosing to eat more healthful foods and fewer foods high in fat. Says Dr. Kenneth R. Pelletier, "When people take time out to exercise regularly, they're demonstrating a psychological stance that in itself is going to give them better control over their food choices."

Exercise also creates an environment for success. Dietary change can be frustrating when it involves giving up favorite, comfortable foods. Exercise, however, helps to shed a positive light by emphasizing what we can do rather than what we can't have. In addition, unlike dietary change, an exercise program is easy to start and progress can be made quickly. This often produces a feeling of success that carries over to other aspects of life, including making more healthful food choices. Indeed, regular exercise is the first step to a permanent change in dietary habits.

A Balanced Program

All types of physical activity have a beneficial effect on cardiovascular health, weight and appearance. In creating a program for yourself, however, it's important to practice balance. Most experts counsel four components to maintaining exercise equilibrium: 1) daily physical activities as part of everyday life; 2) aerobic exercise for cardiovascular endurance and fat burning; 3) resistance (weight) training for building strength; and 4) flexibility exercises to prevent injury and to allow daily movement and other exercise to be more enjoyable.

DAILY PHYSICAL ACTIVITIES

This isn't even about exercise; it's about daily movement. Anything you can do to increase physical activity is beneficial, even everyday activities such as walking up stairs instead of taking the elevator, doing errands on foot, washing your car, walking the dog, parking at the far end of the lot, raking leaves, gardening and doing household chores such as vacuuming. These daily tasks add up in a way that can help you to improve your fitness level. You don't have to put on special exercise clothes, go to a fitness center or buy exercise equipment. You simply aim to be more active in your daily life.

Both the surgeon general and the USDA guidelines recommend a minimum of 30 minutes of these activities every day at a moderate intensity for

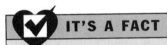

IT'S A FACT

The Nurses' Health Study, the first large study to look at women and exercise, found that regular, moderate exercise (such as three hours of brisk walking a week, or 1.5 hours per week of aerobic dance or jogging) reduced the risk of heart disease by 35% to 40%.

general health. One big difference from past recommendations is that these activities do not have to be continuous. They can be 5 minutes here, 10 minutes there, as long as they add up to at least 30 minutes and are of moderate intensity. Studies show that this level of daily physical activity is effective in reducing body fat, improving blood pressure and boosting aerobic fitness in sedentary people.

These activities burn more calories than you might think. A 160-pound person expends 175 calories in 30 minutes of gardening, 210 calories mowing the lawn, 150 raking the lawn and 135 cleaning the house.

AEROBIC EXERCISE

While mild-to-moderate-intensity daily activities are beneficial, it takes moderate-to-high-intensity aerobic exercise to create cardiovascular strength and stamina and boost metabolism and fat-burning. Aerobic exercise is simply continuous, rhythmic physical activity that makes the large muscles work hard—but not so hard that the heart and lungs can't keep up with the oxygen demand. According to the American Heart Association, to be sure that an activity qualifies as aerobic, you should be able to answer "yes" to the following questions:

■ Does it use the large muscle groups of your body, such as those in your buttocks, thighs and back?

■ Does it increase your heart rate? And can you continue the activity for more than a few minutes?

■ Does it cause you to feel warm, perspire and breathe heavily without being really out of breath and without feeling any burning sensation in your muscles?

Some of the most effective aerobic exercises include:

Brisk (power) walking	Running in place
Cycling (stationary and spinning)	Stair climbing
Aerobic dancing (high-impact, step)	Jogging
Cross-country skiing (indoor)	Skipping rope

Stair stepping	Swimming
Rowing (indoor)	Elliptical exercise

The following exercises and activities can be aerobic if performed at a continual vigorous pace for a period of time:

Aerobic dancing (medium-impact)	Jumping rope
Basketball	Rowing (outdoor)
Cross-country skiing (outdoor)	Skating
Cycling (outdoor)	(ice, roller, in-line)
Handball/squash/racquetball	Soccer
Hiking	Tennis (singles)

It's a good idea to perform more than one type of aerobic exercise in any given week. This is called cross-training. Not only does it produce a higher level of fitness because a greater number of muscles are used, but it also reduces the risk of injury due to overuse of the same muscles.

In order to be classified as aerobic, an exercise must conform to the so-called F.I.T. criteria: frequency, intensity and time. Many health professionals counsel an aerobic exercise program of *at least* three or four days a week. This takes into account the recommendations of the American College of Sports Medicine, which suggests the following:

- Fitness is *improved* if you exercise more than three days a week.
- Fitness is *maintained* if you exercise three days a week.
- Fitness is *lost* if you exercise less than three days a week.

Exercising every other day is very effective for cardiovascular conditioning. (People who need to lose weight may require daily exercise.) However, anyone who exercises more than four days a week should be certain to alternate jarring and nonjarring activities, such as brisk walking and swimming, to minimize strain and other injuries.

Intensity is the second determinant of effectiveness. Golf, casual walking and similar forms of light exercise may improve general health but simply do not stress the heart muscle sufficiently to improve cardiovascular fitness or problems. You have to raise your heart rate to get results, and the most effective way to do this is to exercise at a moderate-to-vigorous pace. (I think of it as "training," which creates a mental picture for me of greater effort than just "exercise.") If you're walking, be sure to keep up a "brisk" pace with your arms pumping. Brisk walking means covering 3.5 to 4 miles within an hour, certainly not a leisurely pace, as if you're running late for a doctor's appointment. On the other hand, it's important to exercise at a safe intensity level. Unless you're a competitive athlete, sprinting and other intense exercise may result in injury or fatigue rather than fitness.

Checking your pulse is the most common way to tell if you're in the zone. There are many places where a pulse can be taken: chest, neck, temple, wrist, groin, inside of the elbow. Pressing in gently, you can feel the "throb" of rushing blood. Each throb is one beat. The "normal" resting pulse rate is between 60 and 90 beats per minute, with an "average" of 72 beats per minute. Practice taking your pulse when you're not exercising. Count it for 10 seconds (be sure to count the first beat as zero), then multiply by six to estimate your pulse for a minute.

Next, determine your maximum heart rate. Ideally, this should be done by a doctor supervising an exercise stress test. However, you can use the following formula:

$$220 - \text{your age in years} = \text{maximum heart rate}$$

How hard you should exercise is determined by your target heart-rate zone, defined by the American Heart Association as between 70% and 85% of your maximum heart rate—the parameters within which you can safely train your cardiovascular system. The chart on the facing page offers a quick way to determine your target zone. Individual ranges may differ from 10 to 20 beats per minute. Beginners should work at the lower end of this zone; only competitive athletes should work at the high end.

HEARTBEATS PER MINUTE

Age	Estimated Maximum Heart Rate	Estimated Target Heart-Rate Zone
20–24	200	140–170
25–29	195	137–166
30–34	190	133–162
35–39	185	130–157
40–44	180	126–153
45–49	175	123–149
50–54	170	119–145
55–59	165	116–140
60–64	160	112–136
65–69	155	109–132
70–74	150	105–128
75–79	145	102–123
80 +	140	98–119

Cardiac patients, particularly those on medication, should check with their doctor regarding the target zone. Many medications can cause changes in heart rate that preclude the use of the standard target zone formula.

To determine whether or not you're in your zone, wait until you're about 5 or 10 minutes into the exercise, then stop and locate your pulse on the side of your neck or on the thumb side of your wrist. If your pulse rate is below your target zone, you probably need to increase effort; if it's above, you can ease off a bit.

An alternative method of monitoring your exercise intensity, and one that I prefer, is to use the Rating of Perceived Exertion scale, or the Borg RPE scale, shown on the following page. Based on the simple concept that the mind is an excellent judge of how much work the body is doing, the RPE scale grades exercise levels according to the individual's overall feeling of exertion and physical fatigue. These ratings correspond well with metabolic responses to exercise, such as heart rate and oxygen consumption.

BORG RPE SCALE

6	*No exertion at all*
7	*Extremely light*
8	
9	*Very light*
10	
11	*Light*
12	
13	*Somewhat hard*
14	
15	*Hard (heavy)*
16	
17	*Very hard*
18	
19	*Extremely hard*
20	

After you've been exercising for 10 minutes or so, ask yourself the question "How hard am I working?" If the level feels "extremely light" or "very light," the intensity is probably too low and you'll need to increase it in order to be in your target zone. But if the response is "very hard" or "extremely hard," your exercise is probably too vigorous and needs to be adjusted. Exercise rated as "light" to "hard" is generally appropriate for cardiovascular conditioning, corresponding to 70% to 85% of maximum heart rate. For more general health benefits, it may be enough to exercise at a perceived level of only "very light."

Pay attention to signs of overexertion, such as pounding in your chest, dizziness, faintness or profuse sweating. If you're very tired during the exercise or if it takes you more than an hour to recover, you may be working too hard regardless of your heart rate. On the other hand, if the exercise doesn't take any effort and there's no hard breathing or sweating, your pace probably needs to be increased. If you feel that you're performing the exercise at an appropriate level of intensity, stay there—even if you're not in your target zone. Listening to your body is of prime importance.

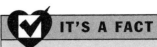

IT'S A FACT

According to researchers at the University of Wisconsin at La Crosse, the "talk" test can be as accurate as a heart rate monitor in gauging exercise intensity. If you can respond to conversation, your intensity level is just about right. If you can't talk, slow down.

Clinical studies have shown the necessity of keeping your heart rate in the target zone for at least 20 continuous minutes in order to promote cardiovascular fitness. *Remember, this is a minimum.* An ideal duration would be 30 minutes to an hour, depending on the activity. Warm-up and cool-down activities such as stretching are not part of the 20-minute minimum. Be sure to give yourself time to build up a tolerance for exercise. Don't expect to walk briskly for an hour your first day out. Take it slow and easy, build up your stamina and endurance, and you'll be able to go as long as you like without harm.

STEPPING OUT

Walking is one of the simplest yet most effective aerobic activities. Researchers are finding evidence that 10,000 steps in a day represent a significant threshold for physical fitness. The 10,000-steps regimen first took hold in Japan in the 1960s after researchers there noticed that people who walked that much every day were noticeably healthier than those who walked less. Studies in the United States have come to the same conclusion. At the University of Tennessee, pedometers were used to measure the walking habits of 80 women aged 40 to 60. After a short time, a clear pattern emerged: the women who walked more than 10,000 steps a day lost more weight, had a lower percentage of body fat and experienced lower blood pressure than did the women who walked fewer than 6,000 steps a day.

Six thousand steps add up to about three miles, which is the walking distance covered by the average adult during a typical day of working, doing chores or taking care of children. Adding 4,000 more steps requires conscious exercise such as taking regular brisk walks, walking the dog or making an effort to walk instead of drive. It's no coincidence that this added activity takes about 30 minutes a day, the recommended minimum to achieve fitness. "While there may not be a magic step recommendation for everyone, right now 10,000 steps looks like a very good target," says Dr. Dixie Thompson, director of the University of Tennessee's Center for Physical Activity and Health. According to Dr. James Hill, an obesity researcher at the University of Colorado in Denver, getting to that level takes some time for most people. Data show that the average office worker takes about 5,000 steps a day, and Dr. Hill contends that adding an extra 2,000 steps while eating 100 fewer calories a day is a good first effort. Then work your way up to the 10,000-steps-a-day goal, a level necessary for losing weight and keeping it off.

Counting steps is a great way to gauge the level of your normal activity. Inactive people take between 2,000 and 4,000 steps per day; moderately active people, between 5,000 and 7,000 steps per day; and active people, at least 10,000 steps per day. Following is a list of some rough targets.

 IT'S A FACT

It takes about 52,400 steps to cover a marathon distance of 26.2 miles. If you take just 5,240 steps a day, you'll complete your own marathon in 10 days. But boost your walking to 7,500 steps per day and you'll cover the distance in less than one week.

■ For long-term health and reduced chronic disease, take 10,000 steps a day.

■ For successful, sustained weight loss, take 12,000 to 15,000 steps a day.

■ To build aerobic fitness, make 3,000 or more of your daily steps fast ones.

Set your goal for 10,000 steps. This is a rough equivalent of the surgeon general's recommendation to accumulate 30 minutes of activity on most days of the week. One mile is about 2,000 to 2,500 steps. Walking nine holes of golf is about 8,000 steps. One city block is about 200 steps.

Not everyone should start right out trying to get 10,000 steps a day. If you have been inactive, are overweight or have a health condition, take a comfortable, gradual approach called the "20% Boost Program." First, invest in a pedometer and calibrate it to your average stride. Use the first week just to learn your baseline average daily step total. Then, for the next two weeks, try to boost that average by 20%. The goal is to measure your steps in a typical week. Each morning, reset the pedometer to "zero." Set it to show your steps. Keep it closed and attached to the front of your waist to the left or right of center. Wear it all day long. When you remove it at night, record the number of steps you've taken in a log like the one shown below, and make a note of any formal exercise you did, such as a 20-minute walk.

LOG

Date:	Mon.	Tue.	Wed.	Thur.	Fri.	Sat.	Sun.
Steps today:							
Exercise minutes:							
More or less than usual:							
Add steps for all 7 days	_____						
Divide by 7	_____						
Multiply by 1.2	_____ (This is your goal for Week 2.)						

Your goal is to boost your average daily steps by 20%. Use the above formula to set your goal for the second week. If you averaged 3,000 steps a day in Week 1, try for 3,600 a day in Week 2. How you reach your goal is up to you. Most physical activity counts, including formal workouts (a brisk walk) and informal activities (taking the stairs). Fill out another log for this week, then set your goal accordingly for Week 3. If you haven't reached 10,000 steps, or if your goal is substantial weight loss (for which many experts recommend 12,000 to 15,000 steps a day), then boost your steps again by 20%. If aerobic fitness is a goal, try boosting the speed of at least 2,000 to 4,000 of the steps you're already doing. Some people find that with just three weeks of effort they've gotten their daily step average close to or beyond 10,000. But many find that it takes several more weeks of boosting by 20% each week until they can create a 10,000 steps-per-day habit.

WEIGHT TRAINING

For years, the American Heart Association discouraged heart patients from weight training for fear it would increase heart attack risk. Now, the AHA acknowledges that weight training provides many cardiovascular benefits. It tones and maintains existing muscles, builds new muscles, increases the ability to burn body fat, increases metabolism, strengthens bones and prevents the loss of bone mass. In a study by the Harvard School of Public Health, men who engaged in weight training for 30 minutes or more weekly had a 23% lower risk of heart disease than men who did not pump iron.

How much exercise is necessary to achieve and maintain an adequate level of strength? This depends on the number of times a week you train, the amount of weight you lift and the

 IT'S A FACT

Without weight training, adults after age 40 typically lose a quarter to a third of a pound of muscle a year and gain an equal amount of body fat.

number of times you lift it. Many organizations recommend a minimum of 8 to 10 exercises involving the major muscle groups a minimum of two times per week. (Studies suggest that training one time per week can maintain muscle strength and endurance. Training two times a week can improve strength and maintain endurance. But training three

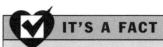

times a week can improve both strength and endurance.) Research shows that a three-month weight training program in previously sedentary adults can increase strength by 25% to 100% or more. The American College of Sports Medicine recommends biceps curls, triceps extensions, chest presses, shoulder presses, pull-downs, abdominal crunches, lower-back extensions, quadriceps extensions, leg curls and calf raises.

Good instruction is extremely important, since form and proper breathing are critical to success. *The correct form is more important than the number of pounds lifted.* Work with the instructor to tailor a program to your specific needs, establishing your individual goals, determining how much weight you should lift, teaching you the correct techniques, using free weights, machines or resistance tubing and bands, and covering all the muscle groups. Look for an instructor who has been certified by the American College of Sports Medicine (ACSM), the American Council on Exercise (ACE), the National Strength and Conditioning Association (NCSA) or the National Academy of Sports Medicine (NASM).

The key is to build muscle gradually. Start with relatively light weights that you use 20 minutes twice a week. Don't worry about getting through your entire routine. Add weight gradually over time and adjust the load until you can perform the entire routine. Traditionally, a weight training prescription called for 8 to 12 repetitions of each exercise, done three times to near fatigue, but new studies show that one set of 12 to 15 repetitions done slowly, with good form and using lighter weights, provides nearly the same improvement in muscular strength and endurance. This is great news for people who want increased muscular strength and endurance but don't want to spend hours in the weight room.

And finally, don't think strength training is just about lifting dumbbells and barbells or using weight machines. Elastic exercise bands can also be effective in building strength.

FLEXIBILITY EXERCISES

Stretching or flexibility exercises are essential for maintaining (or improving) range of motion and function. Unfortunately, they're one of the most neglected parts of a balanced fitness program. Having good flexibility reduces the likelihood of injury to muscles, ligaments and tendons. Without a specific program to maintain flexibility, many middle-aged and older adults become hampered by stiffness in the hamstrings, shoulders and back.

Stretching is simple to do and doesn't have to take a lot of time. Start by slowly and gently stretching the muscles of each major muscle group for about 10 to 30 seconds to the point of mild discomfort. At least four repetitions per muscle group should be performed a minimum of two to three days per week. Don't hold your breath while you stretch. Instead, maintain an even breathing rate, inhaling before the stretch and exhaling during the active phase of the stretch. Avoid bouncing, which can cause a muscle tear.

Activities that incorporate stretching are a great way to get your muscles ready for more strenuous activity. Many good books, audiotapes and videotapes are available on stretching, Pilates, yoga and tai chi. Private instruction is available, and classes are offered at many health clubs, YMCAs and community centers.

A good suggestion: Sign up for six weeks of a yoga class. If you don't like it after that time, nothing much is lost. But the probability is that you'll be hooked for life.

Before You Start

Get an okay from your doctor. The American Heart Association recommends a stress test before undertaking anything more strenuous than walking, particularly if you're over 40 years old, have high blood pressure or coronary disease, a family history of coronary disease or more than one coronary risk factor (e.g., obesity, smoking, elevated blood pressure, a sedentary lifestyle) or haven't had a checkup recently. Additional preliminary steps are outlined below:

■ *Select activities that match your fitness level and interest.* If you hate jogging, don't do it. Try brisk walking instead. Keep looking until you find an activity that suits you.

■ *Start slow and steady.* It takes a minimum of six to eight weeks, depending on age and condition, to begin to notice a difference. If you push yourself too hard at the beginning, you run the risk of injuring yourself.

■ *Listen to your body.* If it hurts, stop the activity. Never "go for the burn." Remember, the target heart-rate zone is just a guide. Take time to warm up and cool down. Always start your exercise routine slowly, gradually move into your target zone and end with a gentle slowing down. Build your fitness gradually. Don't try to undo years of sedentary habits in the first week of exercise.

■ *Keep an exercise journal.* Simply keep a record of your daily exercise on a calendar, then total it all up at the end of the week or month. Watching your miles and minutes build can bring enormous satisfaction.

■ *Drink enough water before you exercise.* It can help you keep at it longer so you'll have a better workout.

And finally, exercise should be a good time, not a grind. Look forward to enjoying yourself. Before bypass surgery, I always thought jogging was a drudge. Now, every morning run is a joy, a celebration of the fact that I'm still here and still fit.

Recipes

From My Heart to Your Heart

"Where healthy meals meet good taste" . . . that's an important theme in this book. As most cooks know, balancing health and taste is not always easy.

The best recipes are those that are tried and true, passed down in families or shared by friends. That's why in our cookbooks I've utilized my own favorites, inherited from my mother, and Italian family recipes from Joe's mother. But *The Road to a Healthy Heart* includes contributions by many other people. From the bottom of my heart I want to thank Mary Lou O'Grady and her mother, Maryanne Iandoli, for generously sharing and describing their old family recipes. Many of these recipes had been passed down orally, and we sat together for hours as I converted them into written form.

A number of recipes were contributed by my daughter Anne and son-in-law Pat and my son Joe and daughter-in-law Jill. Jill even had her mother, Pat Roberts, send me their family favorites. Many of my friends also shared their best recipes as well as their support and love: my sister and dear friend, Joan Imhof; my niece Michelle Eichten; my nephew Todd Imhof and his wife Heidi; and my good friends Bette Kirk, Sally Barline, Peggy Paradise, Sharon Iverson, Aija Ozolin, Kaye Bickford, Nancy Weaver and Melanie Goetz. The dietitians who worked on this project with us—Bev Utt and Deborah Robinett—also got into the spirit and offered recipes as well as advice.

Thus was born *The Road to a Healthy Heart* recipe collection that I pass from my heart to yours. My recipes are dedicated to Joe with loving gratitude for all the ways he took care of himself so that he is still with us—for all the times he ordered the grilled chicken when what he really wanted was a burger and fries and for all the times he got out of bed an hour early to fit in exercise when what he really wanted was another hour of sleep.

Bernie Piscatella

About the Recipes

I hope you'll use the recipes in this section as you begin to develop healthy eating habits that will benefit your heart. Each recipe was designed to fall well within the USDA dietary guidelines and those of the American Heart Association for fat, cholesterol and sodium. Bear in mind that on occasion, in order to give a particular recipe the proper taste and texture, the fat guideline may be exceeded. The great majority of recipes keep well below this percentage, and all of them are significantly below the fat content of conventional recipes; however, while accommodating as healthy a diet as possible, this must be balanced with foods that give pleasure as well.

PANTRY BASICS

Keep a selection of the following foods in your refrigerator or pantry, and you'll have the basic ingredients for our heart-healthy recipes and menus.

Breads	whole wheat bread	whole wheat English muffins
	whole-grain bread	whole wheat pizza crusts
	multigrain bread	whole wheat tortillas
	whole wheat pita bread	
Broth	chicken broth, beef broth, vegetable broth	
Canned and dried foods	artichokes packed in water	garbanzos/chickpeas
(Read the labels	cannellini beans	dried French lentils
and select heart-healthy,	kidney beans	couscous
reduced-sodium brands.	black beans	quinoa
Don't overlook the new	red pinto beans	green split peas
organic varieties.)	Great Northern beans	arborio rice
	cranberry beans	brown rice
	barley	

tomatoes: canned Italian-style plum tomatoes, tomato puree, tomato sauce, tomato paste

soup: split-pea, tomato, roast tomato vegetable, pasta-and-bean, black bean, minestrone, lentil

Cereals   whole-grain, high-fiber, low-sugar (Look for cereals with at least 3 grains of fiber per 100-calorie serving and sugar content below 5 grams.)

oatmeal	Kashi GOLEAN, Kashi GOLEAN
Cheerios	Crunch or Kashi Heart to Heart
raisin bran	Special K
shredded wheat	Grape-Nuts
all-bran	Flax Plus
	Total

Condiments   Dijon mustard, light mayonnaise (made with canola oil, soybean oil or safflower oil), Tabasco sauce, reduced-sodium soy sauce, Worcestershire sauce, Thai chili sauce

Crackers

Ak-Mak	rye crisps
Wasa Multigrain	soy crisps
rice crackers	Lavasch
Kashi TLC	Stoned Wheat Thins
Kavli 5 grain	

Dairy   low-fat or nonfat yogurt (be careful of added sugar) with whole fruit added
nonfat or low-fat fruit-sweetened yogurt
nonfat cottage cheese
eggs
nonfat milk or fortified soy milk
cheese: Parmesan, reduced-fat cheddar, part-skim mozzarella, mozzarella cheese sticks, Gouda, Laughing Cow, mini Babybel

Fruit
(Pick the season's best.)

apples	satsumas	cantaloupe
berries	bananas	watermelon
oranges	pineapple	apricots
grapefruit	papaya	plums
mango	kiwi	raisins
peaches	nectarines	dates
pears	grapes	figs
honeydew		

Nuts and seeds	almonds	hazelnuts
	soy nuts	pistachios in the shell
	walnuts	peanuts in the shell
	pecans	sunflower seeds
		flaxseed

Oils   olive oil, canola oil, safflower oil, soybean oil, sesame oil, flaxseed oil

Olives   kalamata olives, black olives, green olives

Pasta   penne, rigatoni, spaghetti, fusilli, lasagna, bow-tie pasta, wide egg noodles, orecchiette, soba noodles, acini di pepe or pastina, alphabets, macaroni

Spices   coarse salt, cracked pepper, crushed red pepper, basil, oregano

Spreads
black bean dip
three-bean dip
hummus
light or nonfat cream cheese
squeezable liquid and tub-type margarines made with
  canola or safflower oils
cholesterol-lowering margarines

Vegetables	mixed greens	tomatoes
(Pick the season's best.)	baby spinach	baby carrots
	radishes	English cucumber
	celery	edamame
	garlic	onion
	red, green, orange and yellow peppers	

Vinegars   balsamic vinegar, red wine vinegar, cider vinegar, rice wine vinegar, champagne vinegar

NUTRITIONAL ANALYSES

A nutritional analysis is provided for each recipe, usually on a per-serving basis and listing number of calories, grams of total fat, grams of saturated fat, milligrams of cholesterol, grams of carbohydrates, grams of dietary fiber, grams of protein and milligrams of sodium.

In the interest of consistency and clarity, the analyses were based on the following factors:

■ When a range is given for an ingredient, the midpoint amount is analyzed.

■ When the ingredients listing gives one or more options, the first ingredient is the one analyzed.

■ Figures are rounded off to whole numbers, so there might be slight discrepancies between an analysis for a whole meal and the sum of its parts.

■ Fat-grams are rounded off to whole numbers. A total of less than 0.5 grams of fat is considered a trace amount.

■ In many cases, salads and dressings have been analyzed separately. The amount of dressing, which is an individual choice, can greatly alter the calories and fat content of a salad.

■ We have used ground beef that is 90% lean/10% fat, which according to the USDA has no more than 11 grams of fat per 3.5 ounces cooked.

■ Recipes that call for "light" soy sauce use a soy sauce yielding 600 milligrams of sodium per tablespoon (about half that of regular soy sauce).

■ Recipes calling for a pinch of salt are analyzed using ⅛ teaspoon salt.

■ Recipes calling for chicken broth are analyzed using home-made broth with 275 milligrams of sodium per cup.

■ Recipes using a "reduced-fat" cheese call for a cheese containing 5 grams or less of fat and 80 calories per ounce.

■ Recipes that call for a "nonfat" cheese use a cheese containing 0 grams of fat and 30 to 40 calories per ounce.

■ In recipes using oil-based marinades, only a quarter to a half of the marinade was used in the nutritional analysis if the marinade is drained off before cooking.

■ Portions are based realistically on average-size servings and have not been shaved to make the numbers appear more favorable.

■ For most recipes, the decision was made not to measure the amount cup by cup, since this is not the way most families eat. The analysis per serving is to be understood as an approximation.

Although every effort has been made to ensure the accuracy of nutritional data, we cannot guarantee suitability for specific, medically imposed diets. People with special dietary needs should consult their physician and/or a registered dietitian.

Recipes have been analyzed for nutritional content by consultant Beverly Utt, M.S., M.P.H., R.D., using Nutribase Clinical Nutrition Manager V.5.18. The primary sources of values used in the analyses include the USDA Nutrient Data Base Standard Reference Release S.R. 18 and information from manufacturers. In the few cases where data are incomplete or unavailable, substitutions of similar ingredients have been made. Each analysis is based on the entry of nutritional data for all ingredients in each recipe.

While nutritional information is certainly important, it must be kept in perspective. Some of our recipes may be higher in fat or in sodium than recommended. In those cases, balance out those nutritional elements by picking foods lower in fat or sodium at your other meals. Balance is the key to long-term success.

Soups

Three-Bean Soup Makes 3 quarts (1-cup servings)

Preparing a hearty bean soup doesn't have to be a time-consuming effort if you start with canned beans.

> *2 cups macaroni*
> *1 28-ounce can plum tomatoes, diced*
> *1 tablespoon chili powder*
> *1/8 teaspoon ground cumin*
> *1/8 teaspoon cayenne*
> *1/2 teaspoon paprika*
> *1/2 teaspoon coarse salt*
> *1/8 teaspoon pepper*
> *2 15-ounce cans cannellini beans,*
>   *drained and rinsed*
> *1 15-ounce can red pinto beans,*
>   *drained and rinsed*
> *2 15-ounce cans black beans,*
>   *drained and rinsed*

Cook macaroni 15 to 20 minutes, or until al dente. Meanwhile, combine tomatoes, chili powder, cumin, cayenne, paprika, salt and pepper. Heat just to boiling; reduce heat and simmer 20 minutes. Add beans and pasta, and heat through.

PER SERVING
Calories - 182
Protein - 10 g
Sodium - 192 mg
Carbohydrates - 35 g
Cholesterol - 0 mg
Total Fat - 1 g
Saturated Fat - 0 g
Dietary Fiber - 8 g

Homemade Chicken Broth

Makes 5 to 6 quarts (1-cup servings)

Homemade chicken broth is worth the effort. Not only does it taste delicious, but the whole house smells wonderful while the broth is simmering on the stove. It also freezes well, so you can keep it on hand. Plus, the amount of sodium you cut by not using canned broth is truly amazing.

1 4-pound chicken, cut up, plus 2 whole chicken breasts
1 large onion, peeled and quartered
2 carrots, peeled
2 garlic cloves, peeled
1 tablespoon chopped fresh basil or ½ teaspoon dried
2 to 2½ tablespoons coarse salt or to taste
½ teaspoon pepper
6 quarts cold water or enough to cover chicken

Place chicken in a 10-quart stockpot. Add onion, carrots, garlic, basil, salt, pepper and water. Heat gradually just to boiling, but do not allow to boil (boiling makes broth cloudy). Reduce heat and simmer 3 hours, or until chicken falls easily away from the bone. Strain stock; discard bones and vegetables. Refrigerate broth overnight. Use a slotted spoon to skim off fat that rises to the top.

PER SERVING
Calories - 33
Protein - 4 g
Sodium - 275 mg
Carbohydrates - 0 g
Cholesterol - 2 mg
Total Fat - 1 g
Saturated Fat - 0 g
Dietary Fiber - 0 g

Return broth to stockpot. Simmer, uncovered, 1 hour, or until broth is reduced by about a third. Test seasonings; sparingly add more salt if needed. Use broth at once or store in refrigerator or freezer for later use.

A WORD ABOUT CHICKEN BROTH

Chicken broth is an essential ingredient in a number of our recipes. The nutritional analyses in these recipes are based on the numbers for homemade chicken broth. If, because of time constraints or preference, you use canned broth, be sure to check the sodium level. National brands generally run from about 380 to 980 milligrams of sodium, although broth with about 60 milligrams of sodium is available in some areas.

Country-Style Chicken Noodle Soup

Makes 8 2½-cup servings

Curl up with a bowl of this comforting soup and enjoy the depth of flavor only a homemade broth can bring.

> *3 quarts Homemade Chicken Broth*
> *(page 240)*
> *1 skinned and boned chicken breast,*
> *diced (2 cups)*
> *8 carrots, diced*
> *½ pound wide egg noodles, cooked*
> *(6 cups)*

In a small stockpot, bring broth, chicken and carrots to a boil. Immediately reduce heat to medium and cook 10 minutes, or until chicken is done. Stir in noodles and heat through.

PER SERVING
Calories - 198
Protein - 11 g
Sodium - 454 mg
Carbohydrates - 26 g
Cholesterol - 42 mg
Total Fat - 3 g
Saturated Fat - 0 g
Dietary Fiber - 3 g

French Lentil Soup 6 servings

Lentils require no presoaking and are an easy first step toward including heart-healthy plant proteins in your meals. We've found that French lentils hold their shape better than the regular varieties; they're available in specialty food stores or by mail order.

1 cup French lentils
1 tablespoon olive oil
2 cups chopped yellow onion
3 cloves garlic, chopped
1 cup chopped white portion of leek
2 cups diced carrots
8 cups chicken broth, preferably homemade
    (page 240)
¼ teaspoon coarse salt
¾ teaspoon black pepper
1 tablespoon fresh lemon thyme leaves
    or ½ teaspoon dried
½ teaspoon cumin
1 8-ounce can tomato sauce
¼ cup tomato paste

Place lentils in a large bowl and cover with 2 cups boiling water. Let stand 15 minutes. Drain.

Heat olive oil in a nonstick skillet. Add onion, garlic and leek; sauté 10 minutes over medium heat. Add carrots; sauté 10 minutes longer.

In a stockpot, combine broth, salt, pepper, thyme and cumin. Bring to a boil. Add lentils, tomato sauce and tomato paste, and sautéed vegetables; bring to a second boil. Reduce heat and simmer, uncovered, 1 hour, or until lentils are tender.

PER SERVING
Calories - 304
Protein - 17 g
Sodium - 804 mg
Carbohydrates - 47 g
Cholesterol - 3 mg
Total Fat - 5 g
Saturated Fat - 0 g
Dietary Fiber - 18 g

Tuscan Bean Soup Makes 2½ quarts (5 main-dish servings)

Fiber-rich cannellini beans, known as white kidney beans, are also excellent in salads or served by themselves with a splash of olive oil.

3 15-ounce cans cannellini beans

1 28-ounce can plum tomatoes, including liquid, diced

2 cups chicken broth, preferably homemade (page 240)

1 fresh rosemary sprig

1 fresh thyme sprig

2 teaspoons olive oil

1 medium onion, chopped

1 clove garlic, minced

1 large carrot, diced

¼ pound extra-lean ham, diced

½ teaspoon coarse salt

¼ teaspoon freshly ground black pepper

8 drops Tabasco sauce

¼ cup freshly grated Parmesan cheese

Place cannellini beans in a colander; rinse with cold water and drain thoroughly.

In a 6½-quart stockpot, combine tomatoes, broth, rosemary and thyme; heat just to boiling. Reduce heat and let simmer.

In a nonstick skillet, heat olive oil; add onion and sauté 3 to 4 minutes. Add garlic and carrot, and sauté until carrot is tender and onion is soft. Add vegetables to tomato mixture. Stir in beans and ham. Heat through. Season with salt, pepper and Tabasco sauce. Serve into individual soup bowls. Sprinkle with cheese.

PER SERVING
Calories - 471
Protein - 34 g
Sodium - 898 mg
Carbohydrates - 48 g
Cholesterol - 16 mg
Total Fat - 6 g
Saturated Fat - 2 g
Dietary Fiber - 28 g

Sodium Alert: Choose low-sodium foods at other meals throughout the day to offset the higher sodium in this recipe.

Great Northern Bean Soup 10 servings

This soup freezes well. Make a double batch and save it for a quick-to-fix weekday dinner.

1 pound dried Great Northern beans
3 tablespoons olive oil
3 yellow onions, chopped
4 cloves garlic, chopped
2 quarts chicken broth, preferably homemade
(page 240)
2 bay leaves
2 fresh rosemary sprigs
1½ teaspoons coarse salt
½ teaspoon white pepper
½ teaspoon crushed red pepper

Place beans in a large bowl and cover with water. Soak 6 hours or overnight, or use quick-cook method (page 376). Drain and rinse.

Heat olive oil in a nonstick skillet over medium heat; add onion and sauté 8 to 10 minutes. Add garlic and sauté 2 to 3 minutes longer.

In a large stockpot, combine beans and broth; bring just to boiling. Reduce heat to simmer. Add bay leaves and rosemary. Cover and cook 40 to 45 minutes, or until beans are tender.

Pour soup in batches into a food processor and whirl until beans are coarsely pureed. Return to stockpot and heat to serving temperature. Season with salt, white pepper and red pepper.

PER SERVING
Calories - 224
Protein - 14 g
Sodium - 517 mg
Carbohydrates - 31 g
Cholesterol - 2 mg
Total Fat - 5 g
Saturated Fat - 1 g
Dietary Fiber - 8 g

Split-Pea Soup   Makes 4½ quarts (1-cup servings)

Who would have thought an old favorite comfort food could fit so well into today's heart-health goals? The dark green color of this soup tells you it's packed full of antioxidants and vitamin A.

1 tablespoon olive oil
2 cups chopped yellow onion
4 cloves garlic, finely chopped
4 quarts chicken broth, preferably homemade
    (page 240)
2 cups diced carrots
2 cups unpeeled, diced Yukon Gold potatoes
2 16-ounce packages green split peas
1 teaspoon coarse salt
⅓ pound thickly sliced ham, diced

Heat olive oil in a nonstick skillet. Add onions and garlic, and sauté over medium heat 10 minutes, or until onions are translucent.

In a large stockpot, combine broth, carrots, potatoes and 1 pound of the split peas; bring to a boil. Reduce heat; stir in onions and garlic. Simmer, uncovered, 45 minutes. Skim off and discard white foam that rises to the top. Add remaining 1 pound of split peas. Cook 45 to 50 minutes longer, or until peas are tender. Season with salt.

Preheat a small nonstick skillet over medium-high heat; add diced ham. Cook 2 to 3 minutes. Stir into soup.

PER SERVING
Calories - 239
Protein - 16 g
Sodium - 475 mg
Carbohydrates - 36 g
Cholesterol - 6 mg
Total Fat - 3 g
Saturated Fat - 0 g
Dietary Fiber - 14 g

Tortilla Soup Makes 3 quarts stock (6 2-cup servings)

The fun part of this soup is that everybody gets to share in adding the final touches.

> *2 28-ounce cans crushed tomatoes in heavy puree*
> *8 cups chicken broth, preferably homemade*
> *   (page 240)*
> *1 tablespoon ground cumin*
> *1 tablespoon olive oil*
> *1½ cups diced onion*
> *2 jalapeño peppers, minced*
> *1 boned and skinned chicken breast, diced*
> *4 corn tortillas, cut into ¼-inch strips*
> *1 cup grated reduced-fat sharp cheddar cheese*
> *2 cups chopped fresh cilantro*
> *2 avocados, peeled, seeded and diced*
> *6 tablespoons nonfat sour cream*

In a large stockpot, combine tomatoes and 6 cups of the broth. Bring to a boil; reduce heat and simmer uncovered 1½ hours. Stir in cumin.

Heat oil in a nonstick skillet over medium heat. Add onion and jalapeño; sauté 10 minutes, or until onions are tender. Add to soup.

PER SERVING
Calories - 405
Protein - 19 g
Sodium - 963 mg
Carbohydrates - 34 g
Cholesterol - 40 mg
Total Fat - 16 g
Saturated Fat - 6 g
Dietary Fiber - 8 g

In a small saucepan, bring remaining 2 cups of the broth to a boil. Add diced chicken and reduce heat to medium. Cook 5 to 7 minutes, or until chicken is done. Remove chicken from broth and set aside. Add broth to soup.

Arrange tortilla strips in a single layer on a nonstick cookie sheet. Bake at 400°F for 6 to 7 minutes, or until crisp.

Pour soup into bowls. Let each person add chicken, cheese, cilantro, avocado, a dollop of sour cream and tortilla strips. (Serve leftover soup as a first course with Pan-Seared Tuna, page 399.)

Nutrition Note: The fat content in this recipe may appear high; however, it's predominantly heart-healthy monounsaturated and polyunsaturated fat.

■

Get-Well Soup Makes 2½ quarts (6 servings)

This is a perfect soup to take to a friend who's under the weather. Kids love it, too.

1 6-ounce package egg pastina or alphabets
2 quarts chicken broth, preferably homemade
*   (page 240)*
1 cup finely chopped carrots
1 7-ounce can mushroom stems and pieces, drained,
*   or 3 fresh mushrooms, sliced (optional)*
1 cup fresh or frozen baby peas or shelled edamame
*   (optional)*

Cook pastina according to package directions. Drain and rinse.

Heat broth in a 3-quart saucepan. Add carrots; simmer 10 minutes, or until tender. Add mushrooms and pastina, and peas or edamame, if desired; simmer 2 to 3 minutes longer.

PER SERVING
Calories - 173
Protein - 17 g
Sodium - 400 mg
Carbohydrates - 28 g
Cholesterol - 5 mg
Total Fat - 3 g
Saturated Fat - 0 g
Dietary Fiber - 3 g

Cook's Suggestion: Serve with Roasted Garlic Bread (page 468).

Tex-Mex Chowder   8 servings

This hearty chowder is a powerhouse of protein, fiber and antioxidants—all in one bowl.

½ pound leanest ground beef

1 onion, chopped

1 28-ounce can plum tomatoes, including liquid, diced

1½ cups chicken broth, preferably homemade (page 240)

1 packet (1½ ounces) Lawry's Taco Seasoning

1 15-ounce can black beans, drained and rinsed

1 15-ounce can red kidney beans, drained and rinsed

1 4-ounce can diced green chilies (optional)

2 cups fresh or frozen corn kernels

1 cup black olives, pitted and sliced (optional)

In a nonstick skillet, sauté beef and onion until beef is no longer pink and onion is tender. Drain on paper towels; pat with additional toweling to remove excess fat. Set aside.

In a 2-quart saucepan, combine remaining ingredients and heat through. Add beef and onions and heat to serving temperature.

PER SERVING
Calories - 227
Protein - 14 g
Sodium - 876 mg
Carbohydrates - 34 g
Cholesterol - 17 mg
Total Fat - 5 g
Saturated Fat - 2 g
Dietary Fiber - 8 g

Sodium Alert: Choose low-sodium foods at other meals throughout the day to offset the higher sodium in this recipe.

Barley Mushroom Soup

Makes 3 quarts (1-cup servings)

This great-tasting soup can be ready in under an hour after soaking the barley overnight.

1 cup barley

8 cups beef broth

2 cloves garlic, minced

1 onion, coarsely chopped

3 stalks celery, sliced

½ pound leanest ground beef

½ pound fresh mushrooms, sliced

⅛ teaspoon powdered thyme

⅛ teaspoon marjoram

½ teaspoon coarse salt or to taste

½ teaspoon freshly ground black pepper

Soak barley in 3 cups of water overnight. In a medium stockpot, bring broth to a boil; add garlic, onion, celery and barley with soaking liquid and bring just to boiling (do not boil). Reduce heat and simmer uncovered, about 45 minutes, or until barley is tender.

PER SERVING
Calories - 112
Protein - 7 g
Sodium - 692 mg
Carbohydrates - 15 g
Cholesterol - 12 mg
Total Fat - 3 g
Saturated Fat - 1 g
Dietary Fiber - 3 g

Meanwhile, in a nonstick skillet, sauté ground beef. When beef is nearly cooked, add mushrooms and sauté 2 to 3 minutes. Defat beef and mushrooms by draining on paper towels. Add beef and mushrooms to soup pot; season with thyme, marjoram, salt and pepper. Heat through.

Sodium Alert: Choose low-sodium foods at other meals throughout the day to offset the higher sodium in this recipe.

Chicken and Dumpling Soup

Makes 2½ quarts (1-cup servings)

> 5 cups chicken broth, preferably homemade (page 240)
>
> 1 cup chopped onions
>
> 2 stalks celery, chopped
>
> 1 pound skinless, boneless chicken breasts
>
> 4 carrots, quartered lengthwise
>
> 2 cups sliced fresh mushrooms
>
> 2 tablespoons flour
>
> ¼ cup water
>
> 2½ cups cooked spaetzle*
>
> 1 cup peas

Combine broth, onion, celery and chicken in a medium stockpot; heat to boiling. Reduce heat and simmer 20 minutes. Add carrots and simmer 10 to 12 minutes longer, or until carrots are tender. Using tongs, remove chicken and carrots from broth and set aside.

PER SERVING
Calories - 146
Protein - 15 g
Sodium - 168 mg
Carbohydrates - 19 g
Cholesterol - 33 mg
Total Fat - 2 g
Saturated Fat - 0 g
Dietary Fiber - 2 g

Pour broth into a colander set over a bowl. Return strained broth to stockpot. Heat just to boiling; add mushrooms and simmer 5 to 7 minutes, or until mushrooms are tender.

In a small bowl, combine flour and water to make a smooth paste. Bring broth to a boil and gradually add paste, stirring constantly (you don't want lumps) until broth thickens slightly. Reduce heat to low.

Dice chicken and carrots, and put them back into broth. Stir in spaetzle; heat to serving temperature. Stir in peas.

*Look for these small dumplings in your supermarket or a specialty German market. Gemelli or other small (1½-inch-long) pasta may be substituted.

Soba Noodle Soup 4 servings

Make your own version of ramen noodle soup—it's more nutritious and has less fat and sodium.

2 cups water
6 cups chicken broth, preferably homemade
    (page 240)
1 8-ounce package soba noodles*
1¼ cups snow peas, halved lengthwise
    (optional)
1¼ cups thinly sliced cremini mushrooms
    (optional)
1 tablespoon reduced-sodium soy sauce

In a medium saucepan, bring water and 2 cups of the broth to a boil. Add noodles and cook 5 to 6 minutes, or until noodles are tender. Drain and rinse.

In a 4-quart stockpot, heat the remaining 4 cups of broth just to boiling. Add snow peas and mushrooms if desired, and cook 1 to 2 minutes. Stir in cooked noodles and soy sauce.

PER SERVING
Calories - 299
Protein - 12 g
Sodium - 377 mg
Carbohydrates - 52 g
Cholesterol - 0 mg
Total Fat - 4 g
Saturated Fat - 1 g
Dietary Fiber - 2 g

*Soba noodles are available in the Asian section of most supermarkets.

■ Monday Soup 12 servings

This is one of our favorites. We often prepare Chicken in Lettuce
Wraps on a Sunday afternoon and use the soup to start off the week.

1 recipe Chicken in Lettuce Wraps (page 456)
3 quarts chicken broth, preferably homemade
(page 240)

Prepare wraps according to recipe directions,
but omit the lettuce.

    Heat broth just to boiling. Reduce heat.
Stir wrap filling into broth. Heat to serving
temperature.

PER SERVING
Calories - 47
Protein - 5 g
Sodium - 305 mg
Carbohydrates - 3 g
Cholesterol - 5 mg
Total Fat - 1 g
Saturated Fat - 0 g
Dietary Fiber - 0 g

■

■ Tortellini Soup 4 servings

6 cups chicken broth, preferably homemade (page 240)
4 large cloves garlic, minced
1 cup diced carrots
1 cup sliced fresh cremini mushrooms
½ pound cheese tortellini, cooked al dente
4 cups fresh baby spinach

In a large saucepan, bring broth just to
boiling. Add garlic. Reduce heat and simmer
15 minutes. Add carrots and mushrooms, and
cook 5 minutes. Add tortellini and spinach;
simmer 1 minute, or just until spinach wilts.

Variation: Add 1 cup diced chicken
(½ breast), and let simmer in the broth
along with the garlic.

PER SERVING
Calories - 243
Protein - 15 g
Sodium - 644 mg
Carbohydrates - 33 g
Cholesterol - 27 mg
Total Fat - 6 g
Saturated Fat - 2 g
Dietary Fiber - 3 g

Homemade Turkey Broth

Makes 4 to 6 quarts (1-cup servings)

1 turkey carcass with meaty bones
5 to 7 quarts water or enough to cover turkey
parts by about 2 inches
3 garlic cloves, peeled
1 large yellow onion, quartered
3 carrots, peeled
3 celery stalks with leaves
3 tablespoons fresh basil leaves or
1 teaspoon dried
1 tablespoon coarse salt or to taste

Place turkey carcass in a stockpot (pull carcass apart so it will fit); add water to cover. Bring slowly to a boil, removing scum and fat that floats to the top. Add remaining ingredients and simmer 3½ hours. (Do not boil, or fat will be reabsorbed into stock, making it cloudy.) Strain stock; discard bones and vegetables. Refrigerate overnight. Skim and discard fat that rises to the top.

Return stock to stockpot. Simmer, uncovered, 1 hour, or until stock is reduced by a third. Test seasoning. Sparingly add more salt if needed. Use stock at once or store in refrigerator or freezer for later use. Freeze some stock in ice-cube trays for stir-frying or sautéing vegetables.

PER SERVING
Calories - 33
Protein - 3 g
Sodium - 240 mg
Carbohydrates - 0 g
Cholesterol - 5 mg
Total Fat - 0 g
Saturated Fat - 0 g
Dietary Fiber - 0 g

The Best Turkey Soup

Makes 4 quarts (1-cup servings)

Soup is a great comfort food. By its nature, hot soup has to be eaten slowly, giving the family time to talk. Remember, too, that leftover soups make perfect snacks.

> *3 quarts Homemade Turkey Broth*
> *   (page 253)*
> *3 carrots, peeled and diced*
> *2 celery stalks, diced*
> *1 large onion, finely chopped*
> *2 garlic cloves, minced*
> *4 cups cooked elbow macaroni*
> *½ pound fresh mushrooms, sliced*
> *   (optional)*
> *pinch coarse salt*
> *½ cup chopped fresh parsley*

Bring reduced stock just to boiling; add carrots, celery, onion and garlic. Cover; reduce heat and simmer about 30 minutes, or until vegetables are tender. Add macaroni and mushrooms, if desired; heat to serving temperature, about 2 to 3 minutes. Season. Sprinkle with parsley.

PER SERVING
Calories - 95
Protein - 4 g
Sodium - 287 mg
Carbohydrates - 13 g
Cholesterol - 0 mg
Total Fat - 2 g
Saturated Fat - 1 g
Dietary Fiber - 1 g

Homemade Bean Soup Stock

Makes 3 quarts (1-cup servings)

This soup stock is much better than the water or canned broth recommended on the packages of bean soup mixes that you buy at the market. You'll notice the superior flavor with the first sip.

>   *2 tablespoons dried parsley*
>   *1 tablespoon thyme*
>   *1 tablespoon marjoram*
>   *2 dried bay leaves*
>   *2 tablespoons celery seed*
>   *1 very meaty ham hock,*
>   *about 2½ to 3 pounds*
>   *3 quarts water*
>   *1 tablespoon salt or to taste*

Measure parsley, thyme, marjoram, bay leaves and celery seed into a square of cheesecloth; tie cloth securely at the top with string.

In a stockpot, combine seasoning pouch with ham hock, water and salt. Bring slowly to a boil, removing fat that floats to the top. Cover and simmer 2½ to 3 hours. (Do not boil, or fat will be reabsorbed into the broth, making it cloudy.)

Refrigerate overnight. Skim and discard fat that rises to the top. Cut ham off bone, reserving only very lean meat. Discard bone and seasoning pouch. Use stock at once, or store in refrigerator or freezer for later use.

PER SERVING
Calories - 33
Protein - 3 g
Sodium - 240 mg
Carbohydrates - 0 g
Cholesterol - 5 mg
Total Fat - 0 g
Saturated Fat - 0 g
Dietary Fiber - 0 g

▬ Minestrone Makes 4½ quarts (2-cup servings)

1 tablespoon extra-virgin olive oil

1 large onion, chopped

2 cloves garlic, chopped

3 stalks celery, chopped

3 carrots, peeled and chopped

6 cups chicken broth, preferably homemade (page 240)

1 28-ounce can plum tomatoes, including liquid, diced

2 Yukon Gold potatoes, cut into 1-inch cubes

1 teaspoon dried thyme

1 teaspoon coarse salt

¼ teaspoon freshly ground black pepper

8 drops Tabasco sauce

2 15-ounce cans cannellini beans, drained and rinsed

*1½ cups cut green beans (ends removed and beans
    cut into thirds)*

3 cups shredded cabbage

1 cup broccolini (little broccoli)

2 cups elbow macaroni, cooked al dente

¼ cup freshly grated Parmesan cheese

Heat oil in a nonstick frying pan. Add onion, garlic, celery and carrots. Sauté 5 to 7 minutes.

In a stockpot, combine broth and tomatoes; bring to a boil. Add sautéed vegetables, potatoes and seasonings; reduce heat to medium and cook 15 minutes. Add cannellini beans, green beans and cabbage; cook 5 minutes. Add broccolini; cook 5 minutes longer. Add pasta. Serve into bowls and sprinkle with cheese.

PER SERVING
Calories - 138
Protein - 8 g
Sodium - 490 mg
Carbohydrates - 23 g
Cholesterol - 2 mg
Total Fat - 2 g
Saturated Fat - 0 g
Dietary Fiber - 4 g

Note: This soup is a great way to use leftover vegetables or leftover grilled or roast beef, pork, chicken or turkey.

Market Vegetable Soup

Makes 5 quarts (2-cup servings)

Keep a multi-bean soup mix in your pantry, ready to be doctored up with grains, veggies and meats.

1 12-ounce package multi-bean soup mix
(3 cups dried beans)
3 quarts Homemade Bean Soup Stock (page 255)
or commercially prepared vegetable broth
1 28-ounce can plum tomatoes, including liquid,
diced
2 medium yellow onions, finely chopped
6 stalks celery, finely chopped
2 garlic cloves, minced
½ pound skinned and boned chicken breasts,
diced
½ pound thick sliced ham, diced

Thoroughly sort and wash beans. Place in a large bowl and cover with water. Soak 6 hours or overnight. Drain.

In a stockpot, heat bean soup stock or vegetable broth to almost boiling. (Do not boil, or broth will become cloudy.) Add beans, tomatoes, onions, celery and garlic. Reduce heat; cover and cook on a low boil for 3 hours, or until beans are tender. Uncover, add chicken and cook 15 minutes, or until chicken is cooked. Add ham.

PER SERVING
Calories - 197
Protein - 19 g
Sodium - 294 mg
Carbohydrates - 23 g
Cholesterol - 14 mg
Total Fat - 3 g
Saturated Fat - 1 g
Dietary Fiber - 8 g

Nutrition Note: Using homemade stock reduces the amount of sodium considerably.

Artichoke and Tomato Soup 4 servings

Soup is a great food for people who are watching their weight. Eating it slowly allows time for a message to be sent to the brain saying, "I am satisfied."

> *1 28-ounce can peeled tomatoes with basil, diced*
> *1 10-ounce jar marinated quartered artichoke hearts,*
>   *drained*
> *¼ teaspoon coarse salt or to taste*
> *½ teaspoon black pepper*
> *2 cups cooked orecchiette pasta*
> *½ cup canned chickpeas, drained and rinsed*
> *¼ teaspoon crushed red pepper (optional)*

Heat tomatoes in a medium saucepan. Add artichoke hearts and simmer 15 minutes. Season with salt and pepper. Stir in pasta and chickpeas. Heat through. Stir in red pepper, if desired.

Sodium Alert: Choose low-sodium foods at other meals to offset the higher sodium in this recipe.

PER SERVING
Calories - 181
Protein - 8 g
Sodium - 1,015 mg
Carbohydrates - 36 g
Cholesterol - 0 mg
Total Fat - 1 g
Saturated Fat - 0 g
Dietary Fiber - 5 g

Corn Chowder   Makes 4 cups

Frozen corn works well in this recipe, so there's no need to wait till summer to enjoy it!

> 2 tablespoons olive oil
> 1 cup chopped onion
> ½ cup minced celery
> 1 red pepper, minced
> 4 cups fresh corn kernels (4 or 5 cobs) or frozen
> ½ teaspoon coarse salt
> ¼ teaspoon black pepper or to taste
> 1 teaspoon chopped fresh thyme, or ¼ teaspoon dried
> 2 tablespoons chopped fresh basil, or ½ teaspoon dried
> 1 cup chicken broth, preferably homemade (page 240)
> 1 cup fat-free evaporated milk

Heat olive oil in a nonstick skillet over medium heat. Add onion and sauté 3 to 5 minutes. Add celery and sauté 5 minutes longer. Add red pepper, corn and seasonings; stir well. Reduce heat. Cover and cook 5 minutes on low heat. Add broth, cover and cook 10 minutes.

PER SERVING
Calories - 276 g
Protein - 12 g
Sodium - 421 mg
Carbohydrates - 43 g
Cholesterol - 3 mg
Total Fat - 9 g
Saturated Fat - 1 g
Dietary Fiber - 6 g

Pour half of the soup into a food processor and puree. Pour the other half into a stockpot and add pureed soup. Stir. Ten minutes before serving, add evaporated milk. Cook 10 minutes and serve.

Variation: Top with crab or lobster meat.

Manhattan Clam Chowder

Makes 3 quarts (1-cup servings)

Eating for heart health doesn't mean giving up your favorite clam chowder. Try this Manhattan version, and you won't miss its creamy cousin.

> *1 28-ounce can Italian-style plum tomatoes, chopped*
> *1 large white onion, chopped*
> *3 celery stalks, thinly sliced*
> *1 minced fresh thyme sprig or 1 teaspoon dried*
> *1/2 teaspoon salt*
> *2 peppercorns*
> *1/8 teaspoon ground pepper*
> *1/8 teaspoon Tabasco sauce*
> *1 bay leaf*
> *3 medium potatoes, peeled and diced*
> *2 carrots, thinly sliced*
> *3 6 1/2-ounce cans chopped clams with their liquid**

In a stockpot, combine all ingredients except potatoes, carrots and clams. Bring to a boil, reduce heat and simmer 20 minutes. Bring to a second boil; add potatoes and carrots, reduce heat and simmer 45 minutes, or until vegetables are just tender. Add clams with liquid and simmer 15 minutes longer. Remove bay leaf.

PER SERVING
Calories - 115
Protein - 12 g
Sodium - 262 mg
Carbohydrates - 15 g
Cholesterol - 27 mg
Total Fat - 1 g
Saturated Fat - 0 g
Dietary Fiber - 2 g

*Two pounds steamed fresh clams plus 1 1/2 cups liquid may be used in place of canned clams.

Variation: Just before serving, stir in 1 cup Dungeness or lump crabmeat.

Escarole and Rice Soup

Makes 1½ quarts (1-cup servings)

3 tablespoons olive oil

2 tablespoons minced onions

1 tablespoon minced garlic

leaves of 1 head escarole, washed and separated

dash coarse salt

5 cups chicken broth, preferably homemade
   (page 240)

3 cups cooked rice, preferably arborio

¾ teaspoon coarse salt

¼ teaspoon coarsely ground black pepper

3 tablespoons freshly grated Parmesan cheese

Heat olive oil in a nonstick skillet over medium heat. Add onion and garlic and sauté 2 to 3 minutes. Add escarole; sprinkle with a dash of coarse salt and cook one minute. Add 1 cup of the broth; cook 10 to 15 minutes to wilt the escarole.

In a medium stockpot, heat remaining 4 cups of broth. Add rice and heat to serving temperature. Add escarole mixture. Season with salt and pepper. Ladle into soup bowls. Sprinkle with cheese.

PER SERVING
Calories - 233
Protein - 8 g
Sodium - 575 mg
Carbohydrates - 30 g
Cholesterol - 4 mg
Total Fat - 9 g
Saturated Fat - 1 g
Dietary Fiber - 3 g

Side Salads

Greek Salad 6 2-cup servings

Chopping veggies the night before makes assembling this salad quick and easy the next morning. You'll have a great lunch all set to take to work.

> *2 cups hearts of romaine*
> *2 cups Bibb lettuce*
> *¾ cup small diced red onion*
> *1 cup diced English cucumber*
> *1 cup diced red pepper*
> *3 pear or plum tomatoes, halved*
> *½ cup sliced kalamata olives*
> *½ cup chopped peperoncini*
> *¼ cup Lemon Vinaigrette (page 304)*
> *3 tablespoons crumbled feta cheese*

Roll romaine and Bibb lettuce leaves into cigar-like lengths and chop into a chiffonade. Place in a salad bowl. Add onion, cucumber, red pepper, tomatoes, olives and peperoncini. Toss with vinaigrette. Sprinkle with cheese.

Variation: Add cooked chicken or shrimp to turn this salad into a one-dish meal.

PER SERVING
Calories - 112
Protein - 2 g
Sodium - 799 mg
Carbohydrates - 9 g
Cholesterol - 4 mg
Total Fat - 8 g
Saturated Fat - 1 g
Dietary Fiber - 2 g

Tuscan Bean Salad 8 servings

A tasty, satisfying way to fill about a third of your daily fiber quota.

3 15-ounce cans cannellini beans, drained and rinsed
7 tablespoons Lemon Vinaigrette (page 304)
1½ cups coarsely chopped red onion
2 large ripe tomatoes, coarsely chopped
½ cup chopped celery
¾ cup coarsely chopped fresh flat-leaf parsley

Arrange beans in a shallow salad bowl and
toss with 2 tablespoons of the lemon vinaigrette.
Chill. Just before serving, toss beans with
onion, tomatoes, celery, parsley and remaining
5 tablespoons of the vinaigrette.

PER SERVING
Calories - 245
Protein - 12 g
Sodium - 167 mg
Carbohydrates - 34 g
Cholesterol - 0 mg
Total Fat - 8 g
Saturated Fat - 1 g
Dietary Fiber - 9 g

BCT Salad 6 servings

6 cups shredded Napa cabbage
5 tablespoons Dijon Vinaigrette (page 303)
2 ripe tomatoes (preferably heirloom), coarsely chopped
1 ripe avocado, peeled, seeded and diced
4 thick slices leanest bacon, cooked and crumbled

Place cabbage in a large salad bowl. Toss with
vinaigrette. Add tomatoes. Toss again. Sprinkle
with avocado and crumbled bacon.

Fat Alert: Choose low-fat accompaniments to
offset the higher fat in this recipe.

PER SERVING
Calories - 172
Protein - 3 g
Sodium - 302 mg
Carbohydrates - 7 g
Cholesterol - 8 mg
Total Fat - 15 g
Saturated Fat - 2 g
Dietary Fiber - 3 g

▬ Classic Pasta Salad   Makes 5 quarts (1-cup servings)

DRESSING
9 tablespoons extra-virgin olive oil
3 tablespoons red wine vinegar
¾ teaspoon coarse salt
¼ teaspoon freshly ground black pepper

1 pound pennette (little penne), small shells
   or rotini
1 6½-ounce jar artichoke hearts marinated
   in olive oil*
1 15-ounce can water-packed artichoke hearts,
   drained and quartered
1 cup finely chopped red pepper (1 medium pepper)
1 cup finely chopped green pepper (1 medium pepper)
1 15-ounce can whole spears baby corn on the cob,
   drained
1 7-ounce can mushroom stems and pieces,
   drained
4 cups tiny broccoli florets or broccolini
   (little broccoli)
4 cups cherry tomatoes, halved
½ cup pitted and halved kalamata olives, for garnish
1 cup fresh basil leaves for garnish

Measure dressing ingredients into a small bowl; mix with a wire whisk or a fork until well blended.

Cook pasta according to package directions; rinse, drain and transfer to a large salad bowl. Add artichoke hearts with the marinade while pasta is still warm. Toss until pasta is coated.

PER SERVING
Calories - 164
Protein - 5 g
Sodium - 220 mg
Carbohydrates - 21 g
Cholesterol - 0 mg
Total Fat - 7 g
Saturated Fat - 1 g
Dietary Fiber - 2 g

Let cool to room temperature. Layer remaining vegetables over pasta. Chill. Just before serving, toss with dressing. Garnish with olives and basil leaves.

The most heart-healthy brands of marinated artichoke hearts are those that use olive oil or a nonhydrogenated soybean oil.

Variation: For an excellent main-meal salad, add ¾ pound diced smoked turkey breast.

■

Olive Bread Salad 12 servings

1 loaf (10 cups) olive bread, cut into ½-inch cubes
½ cup olive oil
¼ cup red wine vinegar
3 large garlic cloves, minced
2 large ripe tomatoes, diced
2 tablespoons capers
¼ cup roasted red peppers, chopped
¼ cup seeded and minced peperoncini
½ cup pitted and chopped kalamata olives
¼ cup chopped green onions
¼ cup chopped fresh flat-leaf parsley

Place the cubed olive bread in a large salad bowl. Cover and set aside.

Combine olive oil, vinegar and garlic in a jar with lid. Shake until blended. Set aside.

Combine remaining ingredients. Thirty minutes before serving, lightly toss mixture with bread. Add dressing and toss again.

PER SERVING
Calories - 218
Protein - 4 g
Sodium - 607 mg
Carbohydrates - 25 g
Cholesterol - 0 mg
Total Fat - 11 g
Saturated Fat - 1 g
Dietary Fiber - 1 g

Couscous Salad 5 servings

If you're looking for another grain to incorporate into your healthy lifestyle, try this easy-to-prepare couscous salad. The best news is that couscous (or bulgar wheat) cooks in 5 minutes.

1⅓ cups chicken broth, preferably homemade
   (page 240)
1 cup dry whole wheat couscous
1 large red bell pepper, seeded and diced
   (1½ cups)
3 green onions, sliced on the diagonal
½ English cucumber with skin on,
   diced
¼ cup pitted and halved kalamata olives
¼ cup Lemon Vinaigrette (page 304)

Bring broth to a boil. Add couscous; stir and allow to sit, covered, for 5 minutes. Remove lid and fluff lightly with a spoon.

Toss pepper, onions, cucumber and olives with 2 tablespoons of the vinaigrette. Add to couscous and toss again. Serve into bowls. Pass the remaining dressing in a pitcher on the side.

PER SERVING
Calories - 306
Protein - 10 g
Sodium - 612 mg
Carbohydrates - 51 g
Cholesterol - 1 mg
Total Fat - 7 g
Saturated Fat - 1 g
Dietary Fiber - 14 g

Mediterranean Salad 6 servings

*1 medium red onion, peeled and coarsely
    chopped*
1 English cucumber, coarsely chopped
*1 red bell pepper, seeded and coarsely
    chopped*
*1 yellow bell pepper, seeded and coarsely
    chopped*
½ cup pitted and sliced kalamata olives
2 tablespoons fresh lemon juice
2 tablespoons olive oil
¼ teaspoon coarse salt
dash freshly ground pepper
2 tablespoons crumbled feta cheese

In a shallow salad bowl, combine onion,
cucumber, bell peppers and olives.

In a cup, combine lemon juice and olive
oil. Pour over vegetables. Season with salt and
pepper. Sprinkle with cheese.

Variation: Add 1½ cups cooked baby shrimp.

PER SERVING
Calories - 125
Protein - 2 g
Sodium - 406 mg
Carbohydrates - 10 g
Cholesterol - 4 mg
Total Fat - 10 g
Saturated Fat - 2 g
Dietary Fiber - 2 g

Prawns on Endive with Avocado

6 servings

4 heads Belgian endive
2 tomatoes (preferably heirloom), diced
1 14.1-ounce can hearts of palm, drained
*   and sliced into rounds*
12 medium prawns, cooked
1 Hass avocado, peeled, seeded and diced
¼ cup Red Wine Vinaigrette (page 306)

Remove and discard endive stems. Set aside leaves of one head for garnish.

Cut leaves of remaining heads into 1-inch pieces and place in a salad bowl. Add tomatoes, hearts of palm and prawns; layer avocado slices on top. Toss with vinaigrette.

Tuck reserved endive leaves like flower petals around edges of bowl.

PER SERVING
Calories - 197
Protein - 9 g
Sodium - 439 mg
Carbohydrates - 18 g
Cholesterol - 21 mg
Total Fat - 12 g
Saturated Fat - 2 g
Dietary Fiber - 14 g

Christmas Salad   8 servings

Enjoy this colorful, heart-healthy salad all year long. The recipe was given to us by Mary Lou O'Grady, whose family named it for its festive red-and-green holiday look.

6 cups mixed greens

1 English cucumber, diced

2 cups halved cherry or pear tomatoes

2 cups diced red peppers

*3 tablespoons Balsamic Vinaigrette
     (page 301)*

½ cup diced part-skim mozzarella cheese

¼ cup sliced black olives

¼ cup thinly sliced almonds

½ cup dried cranberries

Combine mixed greens, cucumber, tomatoes and peppers in a large salad bowl. Toss with vinaigrette. Add remaining ingredients and toss again.

PER SERVING

Calories - 136

Protein - 4 g

Sodium - 94 mg

Carbohydrates - 15 g

Cholesterol - 3 mg

Total Fat - 8 g

Saturated Fat - 1 g

Dietary Fiber - 3 g

Big Veggie Salad   6 servings

Practice your lean-cooking skills with this salad. Buy the leanest
bacon and cook it until it's crisp. Then drain it on paper towels and
pat off any remaining grease. Here, the bacon is just a garnish—
not a main player.

½ head cabbage, shredded
½ head lettuce, shredded
½ zucchini, sliced
½ Bermuda or Walla Walla onion, chopped
15 fresh mushrooms, sliced
5 stalks celery, chopped
4 slices apple smoked bacon, cooked,
*   drained and crumbled*
1 bunch broccolini (little broccoli) florets
1 8-ounce can sliced water chestnuts,
*   drained*
2 cups fresh baby peas
¾ cup light mayonnaise
¾ cup nonfat sour cream
¼ cup reduced-fat cheddar cheese
¼ cup Spanish peanuts

In a large, shallow salad bowl, layer all
ingredients except mayonnaise, sour cream,
cheese and peanuts, in order given. Cover
and chill.

Combine mayonnaise with sour cream.
Chill. Just before serving, spread dressing over
salad to edges of bowl. Sprinkle with cheese.
Top with peanuts.

PER SERVING
Calories - 281
Protein - 15 g
Sodium - 566 mg
Carbohydrates - 33 g
Cholesterol - 21 mg
Total Fat - 12 g
Saturated Fat - 2 g
Dietary Fiber - 10 g

Caprese Salad on Rustic Bread

4 servings

2 tablespoons olive oil

1 clove garlic, minced

1 large beefsteak tomato, sliced into 8 slices

1 medium Walla Walla or Vidalia sweet onion,
    cut into ⅛-inch slices

½ pound fresh mozzarella cheese, sliced into
    ¼-inch-thick rounds

12 basil leaves

pinch coarse salt

pinch freshly ground black pepper

½ loaf rustic olive bread

Place olive oil and garlic in a small covered container; let sit.

On a long, rectangular platter, assemble tomato, onion, mozzarella and basil in a fan-like arrangement. Drizzle olive oil mixture over ingredients. Season with salt and pepper.

Serve open-faced on olive bread. Eat with a knife and fork.

PER SERVING

Calories - 262

Protein - 12 g

Sodium - 178 mg

Carbohydrates - 15 g

Cholesterol - 20 mg

Total Fat - 17 g

Saturated Fat - 5 g

Dietary Fiber - 1 g

Tomato, Fresh Mozzarella and Basil Salad 6 servings

Choose heirloom tomatoes whenever they're available—the old-time real tomato flavor is so much better than the taste of today's hothouse varieties.

2 cups fresh basil leaves
4 large ripe tomatoes, sliced ¼ inch thick
½ pound fresh mozzarella cheese,
  sliced ¼-inch thick
1 tablespoon extra-virgin olive oil
pinch coarse salt
pinch freshly ground black pepper

Wash and trim the basil leaves and spread them on an oval platter. Arrange alternating slices of tomatoes and mozzarella over basil. Drizzle with olive oil. Season with salt and pepper.

Variation: Garnish with 12 pitted and halved kalamata olives.

PER SERVING
Calories - 143
Protein - 8 g
Sodium - 78 mg
Carbohydrates - 6 g
Cholesterol - 13 mg
Total Fat - 11 g
Saturated Fat - 3 g
Dietary Fiber - 2 g

New Year's Eve Salad   6 servings

The dressing for this salad is made with champagne vinegar. Coincidentally, I first made it on New Year's Eve. The sun-dried tomatoes were a godsend in a winter when a good tomato was not to be found.

½ cup dry-packed sun-dried tomato halves
2 cups water
10 cups mixed baby romaine and spinach
    greens
6 tablespoons Champagne Vinaigrette
    (page 305)
1 ounce fresh Parmesan cheese

Slice each tomato in half lengthwise into strips (about 6 strips per half). Place strips in a bowl.

Bring 2 cups water just to boiling. Pour over tomatoes. Let sit 5 minutes to plump. Drain and pat dry with paper towels. Chill.

Just before serving, divide romaine and spinach greens among 6 plates. Cluster tomatoes in center of greens. Drizzle 1 tablespoon of vinaigrette over each salad. Using a carrot peeler, slice the cheese into long, thin strips; arrange 4 or 5 shavings over top of each salad.

PER SERVING
Calories - 135
Protein - 4 g
Sodium - 386 mg
Carbohydrates - 5 g
Cholesterol - 4 mg
Total Fat - 11 g
Saturated Fat - 2 g
Dietary Fiber - 2 g

Warm Pear Salad with Blue Cheese and Pecans 8 servings

Cranberries give this salad crunch and a healthy dose of vitamin C. The pecans are a rich source of monounsaturated fat.

CRANBERRY VINAIGRETTE
1/3 cup olive oil
1/4 cup cranberry juice (a variety without added sugar)
1 tablespoon raspberry vinegar
1/4 teaspoon coarse salt
1/8 teaspoon black pepper
1 1/2 teaspoons superfine sugar

1 tablespoon safflower margarine
1 teaspoon brown sugar
3 ripe pears sliced into thin wedges
8 cups baby lettuce leaves
1/2 cup dried cranberries
1/2 cup Roasted Pecans (page 275)
8 teaspoons Maytag blue cheese

Combine vinaigrette ingredients in a jar with lid. Shake well. Set aside.

Melt margarine in a nonstick skillet. Stir in sugar. Add pears. Cook over medium heat 6 to 8 minutes.

Divide lettuce leaves among 8 individual salad plates. Layer pears over lettuce. Sprinkle with cranberries and pecans. Drizzle with vinaigrette. Crumble blue cheese over top. Serve warm.

PER SERVING
Calories - 232
Protein - 8 g
Sodium - 137 mg
Carbohydrates - 21 g
Cholesterol - 2 mg
Total Fat - 17 g
Saturated Fat - 2 g
Dietary Fiber - 3 g

ROASTED PECANS
1 cup pecan halves
olive oil cooking spray
½ teaspoon olive oil
¼ teaspoon cayenne pepper
⅛ teaspoon paprika
⅛ teaspoon coarse salt

Preheat oven to 300°F. Arrange pecans on a nonstick baking sheet. Roast in oven for 5 minutes; remove. Leave oven on.

Place pecans in a shallow pie plate and spray lightly with olive oil. Toss with ½ teaspoon olive oil. Combine cayenne, paprika and salt in a small bowl. Sprinkle over pecans. Toss to cool.

Return pecans to baking sheet and put back in oven; cook 5 to 10 minutes or until slightly dark. Remove from oven and allow to cool. Use at once or store in an airtight container.

PER SERVING
Calories - 40
Protein - Tr
Sodium - 13 mg
Carbohydrates - 1 g
Cholesterol - 0 mg
Total Fat - 4 g
Saturated Fat - 0 g
Dietary Fiber - 1 g

Citrus Salad   4 servings

1 medium red grapefruit
2 medium oranges
Boston, Bibb or other lettuce leaves
¼ cup pomegranate seeds*
fresh mint leaves, for garnish

Cut off tops and bottoms of the grapefruit and oranges. Stand the fruit upright and cut off the peel in sections down to the flesh. Working over a bowl to catch the juice, hold the fruit in one hand and cut between the membranes. Rotate the fruit and let the sections fall into the bowl. Discard any seeds.

PER SERVING
Calories - 65
Protein - 1 g
Sodium - 2 mg
Carbohydrates - 16 g
Cholesterol - 0 mg
Total Fat - 0 g
Saturated Fat - 0 g
Dietary Fiber - 2 g

To serve, line 4 salad bowls with lettuce leaves. Using a slotted spoon, transfer the fruit mixture to the lettuce-lined bowls. Garnish each bowl with pomegranate seeds and mint.

*Pomegranates, one of nature's most powerful antioxidants, help guard your body against free radicals.

Romaine, Edamame and Feta Cheese   4 servings

Highlighted in this recipe, edamame are high in soy protein, vitamin C, fiber and cardioprotective isoflavones.

*4 cups hearts of romaine, rolled and
    cut into ribbons*
2 cups shelled edamame
1 cup diced tomato
1 cup diced red pepper
*3 tablespoons Italian Vinaigrette
    (page 302)*
¼ teaspoon coarse salt
*¼ teaspoon coarsely ground
    black pepper*
*3 tablespoons feta cheese,
    crumbled*

Toss romaine, edamame, tomato, red pepper and vinaigrette in a salad bowl. Season with salt and pepper. Sprinkle with cheese.

PER SERVING
Calories - 234
Protein - 13 g
Sodium - 285 mg
Carbohydrates - 15 g
Cholesterol - 6 mg
Total Fat - 14 g
Saturated Fat - 2 g
Dietary Fiber - 6 g

Avocado, Tomato and Cucumber Salad 6 servings

2 large ripe tomatoes, coarsely chopped
1 English cucumber, peeled and coarsely chopped
2 tablespoons Italian Vinaigrette (page 302)
1 Hass avocado, peeled, seeded and diced
pinch coarse salt
pinch freshly ground black pepper
6 pitted and halved kalamata olives

Toss tomatoes and cucumber with vinaigrette. Add avocado and toss gently. Season with salt and pepper. Sprinkle with olives.

Nutrition Note: Avocados can definitely fit into a heart-healthy diet because of their monounsaturated fat; pound for pound, they have less fat than butter or margarine.

PER SERVING
Calories - 110
Protein - 1 g
Sodium - 235 mg
Carbohydrates - 7 g
Cholesterol - 0 mg
Total Fat - 9 g
Saturated Fat - 1 g
Dietary Fiber - 3 g

Watercress and Radicchio Salad 4 servings

2 bunches watercress, trimmed
1 head radicchio, torn into bite-size pieces
¼ cup Very Lemon Vinaigrette
(page 304)

Just before serving, arrange watercress and radicchio in a medium salad bowl. Toss with vinaigrette.

PER SERVING
Calories - 68
Protein - 1 g
Sodium - 156 mg
Carbohydrates - 2 g
Cholesterol - 0 mg
Total Fat - 7 g
Saturated Fat - 1 g
Dietary Fiber - 0 g

Field Greens with Chickpeas and Tomatoes 4 servings

Salad is your opportunity to make a real dent in your nine-a-day goal.

2 cups mixed field greens

1 red tomato, diced

1 yellow tomato, diced

1 orange tomato, diced

½ red onion, cut into rings and then halved

4 spears fresh asparagus, cooked until crisp-tender,
*   chilled and cut into thirds*

1 cup canned chickpeas, drained and rinsed

2 tablespoons Italian Vinaigrette (page 302)

pinch coarse salt

pinch freshly ground black pepper

In a medium salad bowl, toss mixed field greens, tomatoes, onion, asparagus and chickpeas with vinaigrette. Season with salt and pepper.

PER SERVING

Calories - 148

Protein - 5 g

Sodium - 295 mg

Carbohydrates - 20 g

Cholesterol - 0 mg

Total Fat - 6 g

Saturated Fat - 1 g

Dietary Fiber - 5 g

Antipasto 12 servings

1 15-ounce jar pickled green beans

1 15-ounce jar pickled asparagus

1 15-ounce jar pickled snap peas

1 15-ounce can water-packed artichoke hearts,
   drained

1 15-ounce jar peperoncini (optional)

1 15-ounce can garbanzo beans, drained

1 15-ounce can whole black olives

2 bunches carrots

2 bunches radishes

1 red pepper, julienned

1 yellow, orange or green pepper, julienned

2 cups ripe cherry tomatoes

1 bunch red-leaf lettuce

Chill beans, asparagus, snap peas, artichoke hearts, pepperoncini, garbanzo beans and olives in their individual jars or cans. Wash carrots; trim, peel and slice on the diagonal. Trim and wash radishes. Place carrots and radishes in a bowl of ice water and refrigerate to crisp.

PER SERVING
Calories - 154
Protein - 6 g
Sodium - 837 mg
Carbohydrates - 26 g
Cholesterol - 0 mg
Total Fat - 2 g
Saturated Fat - 0 g
Dietary Fiber - 5 g

Just before serving, thoroughly drain all vegetables. Pat dry with paper towels. Arrange all ingredients except olives in mounds in a lettuce-lined basket. Tuck olives in among mounds. Accompany with Guacamole (page 314) or Artichoke Dip (page 312).

Sodium Alert: Choose low-sodium foods at other meals throughout the day to offset the high sodium in this recipe.

Tomato, Cucumber and Onion Salad 6 servings

Presentation can make eating so much more fun. Jazz up this quick-to-prepare salad by serving it in individual lettuce-leaf cups.

1 medium Bermuda or Walla Walla onion,
*   coarsely chopped*
2 large ripe tomatoes, coarsely chopped
1 medium cucumber with skin, sliced
3 tablespoons Italian Vinaigrette
*   (page 302)*
pinch coarse salt
pinch freshly ground pepper
6 Bibb lettuce-leaf cups

Toss onion, tomatoes and cucumber with vinaigrette. Season with salt and pepper. Serve in lettuce-leaf cups.

PER SERVING
Calories - 71
Protein - 1 g
Sodium - 132 mg
Carbohydrates - 6 g
Cholesterol - 0 mg
Total Fat - 5 g
Saturated Fat - 1 g
Dietary Fiber - 1 g

Field Greens with Balsamic Vinaigrette

4 servings

> 6 cups mixed greens
>> (including at least 2 cups spinach)
> 1 cup broccoli florets
> 1 cup cauliflower florets
> 4 large carrots, julienned
> 1 small red onion, chopped
> 1 large cucumber, peeled and diced
> 1 large ripe tomato, coarsely chopped
> 1/2 cup Balsamic Vinaigrette (page 301)

Layer the mixed greens in individual salad bowls. Layer broccoli, cauliflower, carrots, onion, cucumber and tomato over lettuce. Pass vinaigrette in a bowl on the side.

Note: Vinaigrette is not included in the nutritional information here. Add 81 calories and 9 grams of fat per tablespoon.

PER SERVING
Calories - 78
Protein - 4 g
Sodium - 49 mg
Carbohydrates - 17 g
Cholesterol - 0 mg
Total Fat - 1 g
Saturated Fat - 0 g
Dietary Fiber - 6 g

Make Your Own   1 serving

> 1 to 2 cups mixed green salad (dark, leafy green lettuce,
>> spinach, escarole, shredded cabbage, radicchio)
> 3/4 cup broccoli florets, carrots or cauliflower florets
> 1/2 cup canned garbanzo, pinto or soy beans,
>> drained and rinsed
> 1 tablespoon nuts or seeds or 1/8 avocado
> 1 to 2 tablespoons Italian Vinaigrette (page 302)
>> or Balsamic Vinaigrette (page 301)

Layer ingredients in a bowl in the order given, and drizzle with vinaigrette. Serve with a cluster of red grapes or fresh fruit in season.

Note: Add 90 calories, 10 grams of fat and 90 milligrams of sodium for each tablespoon of dressing.

PER SERVING
WITHOUT DRESSING
Calories - 192
Protein - 11 g
Sodium - 48 mg
Carbohydrates - 29 g
Cholesterol - 0 mg
Total Fat - 5 g
Saturated Fat - 1 g
Dietary Fiber - 11 g

■

Spinach and Tangerine Salad   4 servings

If you've never tried ugli fruit, this is a great way to sample its delicate tangerine-grapefruit flavor.

> *4 cups baby spinach leaves*
> *2 cups shredded radicchio or red-leaf lettuce*
> *4 Roma tomatoes, diced*
> *½ cup chopped red onion*
> *¼ cup Briana Blush Wine Vinaigrette**
> *2 tangerines, satsumas or ugli fruit,*
> *peeled and divided into sections*
> *and each section cut in half*
> *3 tablespoons pine nuts*

Toss spinach, radicchio, tomatoes and onion with vinaigrette. Top with fruit. Sprinkle pine nuts over top.

*Available in most supermarkets.

Variation: Add ¼ cup crumbled feta cheese.

PER SERVING
Calories - 137
Protein - 4 g
Sodium - 220 mg
Carbohydrates - 18 g
Cholesterol - 0 mg
Total Fat - 7 g
Saturated Fat - 1 g
Dietary Fiber - 3 g

Spinach, Strawberry and Walnut Salad   4 servings

4 cups fresh baby spinach leaves
*¼ cup Briana Blush Wine Vinaigrette**
1 cup thickly sliced strawberries
½ cup blueberries
¼ cup walnut halves, chopped

Toss spinach with vinaigrette. Add berries and walnuts. Toss again.

*Available in most supermarkets.

Nutrition Note: The antioxidants in the berries and the omega-3 fatty acids in the walnuts help to keep artery walls healthy.

PER SERVING
Calories - 119
Protein - 2 g
Sodium - 210 mg
Carbohydrates - 13 g
Cholesterol - 0 mg
Total Fat - 7 g
Saturated Fat - 0 g
Dietary Fiber - 3 g

■

Spinach Salad with Pine Nuts   4 servings

You'll need only a small amount of the dressing for this salad because its flavor is so intense.

DRESSING
3 tablespoons extra-virgin olive oil
1 tablespoon fresh lemon juice
¼ teaspoon coarse salt (or to taste)
⅛ teaspoon freshly ground pepper

8 cups fresh baby spinach leaves
3 tablespoons pine nuts

Combine dressing ingredients in a jar with lid.
Cover and shake until well blended.

    Place spinach in a medium salad bowl.
Toss with dressing. Sprinkle with pine nuts.

Variation: Omit the pine nuts and add thinly
sliced fresh mushrooms and purple onion cut
crosswise into $1/8$-inch slices and separated
into rings.

PER SERVING
Calories - 153
Protein - 5 g
Sodium - 221 mg
Carbohydrates - 5 g
Cholesterol - 0 mg
Total Fat - 14 g
Saturated Fat - 1 g
Dietary Fiber - 3 g

■

Spinach with Tomatoes, Blue Cheese and Pecans   4 servings

6 cups baby spinach, torn into bite-size pieces
3 Roma tomatoes, sliced
3 tablespoons Balsamic Vinaigrette (page 301)
1 ounce blue cheese, crumbled
12 pecan halves

Toss spinach and tomatoes with vinaigrette.
Sprinkle with blue cheese. Garnish with
pecans.

PER SERVING
Calories - 134
Protein - 4 g
Sodium - 223 mg
Carbohydrates - 4 g
Cholesterol - 5 g
Total Fat - 12 g
Saturated Fat - 2 g
Dietary Fiber - 2 g

Four-Bean Salad   Makes 3 quarts (1-cup servings)

1 15-ounce can chickpeas,
  drained and rinsed
1 15-ounce can black beans,
  drained and rinsed
1 15-ounce can red kidney beans,
  drained and rinsed
1 pound fresh green beans,
  steamed until just crisp-tender
2 ripe tomatoes, diced
1 small red onion, diced
1 yellow pepper, diced
1 red pepper, diced
2 tablespoons olive oil and vinegar
  dressing

Combine chickpeas, beans, tomatoes, onion and peppers in a large salad bowl. Chill. Just before serving, toss with dressing.

PER SERVING
Calories - 72
Protein - 4 g
Sodium - 11 mg
Carbohydrates - 12 g
Cholesterol - 0 mg
Total Fat - 1 g
Saturated Fat - 0 g
Dietary Fiber - 4 g

Mexicali Corn Salad   Makes 2 quarts (1-cup servings)

3½ cups fresh or frozen corn kernels
(16-ounce package)
1 15-ounce can kidney beans,
drained and rinsed
2 ripe tomatoes, diced
1 red pepper, diced
1 yellow pepper, diced
½ cup diced celery
3 scallions, diced
1 cup chopped fresh cilantro
1 tablespoon olive oil
¼ cup fresh tomato salsa
½ teaspoon chili powder

Combine all ingredients in a large salad bowl. Chill before serving.

PER SERVING
Calories - 153
Protein - 5 g
Sodium - 221 mg
Carbohydrates - 5 g
Cholesterol - 0 mg
Total Fat - 14 g
Saturated Fat - 1 g
Dietary Fiber - 3 g

Main-Meal Salads

■ All-in-One Pasta Salad 8 servings

Veggies rich in vitamins C and A add color to this pasta-based salad.
Turkey adds lean protein for balance and staying power.

1 pound fusilli or rotini, cooked al dente
1 pound smoked turkey breast, diced
1 pound fresh broccolini (baby broccoli)
*   or broccoli florets, cooked al dente*
1 6-ounce jar roasted red bell peppers,
*   drained and diced*
½ cup pitted and chopped kalamata olives
8 plum tomatoes, quartered
6 tablespoons extra-virgin olive oil
2 tablespoons cider vinegar
½ teaspoon coarse salt
¼ teaspoon freshly ground pepper
½ cup freshly grated Parmesan cheese
6 sprigs fresh basil

In a large pasta bowl, layer pasta, turkey, broccolini or broccoli florets, peppers, olives and tomatoes. Chill.

Combine olive oil, vinegar, salt and pepper. Just before serving, pour dressing over pasta and vegetables. Toss. Sprinkle with cheese. Garnish with basil leaves.

PER SERVING
Calories - 488
Protein - 29 g
Sodium - 777 mg
Carbohydrates - 54 g
Cholesterol - 44 mg
Total Fat - 18 g
Saturated Fat - 3 g
Dietary Fiber - 5 g

Warm Tortellini Salad   8 1-cup servings

By the time the tortellini is cooked, you can have the rest of this salad chopped and ready to go.

1 pound cheese tortellini

2 tablespoons olive oil

2 cloves minced garlic

1 cup cubed part-skim mozzarella

2 cups fresh baby spinach leaves,
rolled like a cigar and cut into ribbons

2 cups halved cherry tomatoes

1 tablespoon chopped fresh basil

¾ teaspoon coarse salt

¼ teaspoon freshly ground black pepper

Cook tortellini until al dente; drain, rinse and return to pot. Drizzle with olive oil and garlic. Toss gently to coat tortellini with oil. Add spinach and toss. The warmth of the tortellini will begin to wilt the spinach. Add remaining ingredients and toss thoroughly.

PER SERVING
Calories - 255
Protein - 13 g
Sodium - 529 mg
Carbohydrates - 29 g
Cholesterol - 30 mg
Total Fat - 10 g
Saturated Fat - 4 g
Dietary Fiber - 2 g

Soba Noodle Salad 6 servings

This salad goes well with grilled salmon or chicken. The dressing is so tasty you won't believe it has no added fat.

DRESSING
½ cup reduced-sodium soy sauce
⅓ cup mirin (rice wine)
3 tablespoons rice vinegar
1 tablespoon finely grated fresh ginger

1 14-ounce can chicken broth
2 cups water
1 6-ounce package dried soba (Japanese buckwheat)
  noodles, dried wheat chow-mein noodles or
  angel-hair pasta
4 cups shredded Napa cabbage
1 cup julienned daikon radishes
2 cups julienned carrots
2 cups firm tofu (½ of 14-ounce package), drained,
  patted dry and cut into squares

Combine dressing ingredients in a small bowl. Set aside.

Bring broth and water to a boil in a medium saucepan. Add noodles and cook 6 to 8 minutes, or until al dente. Drain, rinse and chill.

Just before serving, combine cabbage, radishes and carrots. Toss noodles with ¼ cup of the dressing and divide into 4 salad bowls. Arrange vegetables on top of noodles. Pour another ¼ cup of dressing over tofu and place on top of vegetables. Drizzle with remaining dressing.

PER SERVING
Calories - 241
Protein - 19 g
Sodium - 636 mg
Carbohydrates - 28 g
Cholesterol - 2 mg
Total Fat - 8 g
Saturated Fat - 1 g
Dietary Fiber - 3 g

◼ French Lentil Salad   Makes 11 1-cup servings

1 cup dry French lentils (4 cups cooked)
¼ yellow onion
4 cups water
⅓ cup Red Wine Vinaigrette (page 306)
3 cups hearts of romaine
3 cups radicchio
1½ cups diced English cucumber
1½ cups diced red onion
1½ cups diced red pepper
1 large tomato, diced
½ cup sliced kalamata olives
½ cup chopped peperoncini
3 tablespoons crumbled feta cheese

Wash and sort lentils. Place in a large saucepan. Add onion and water. Bring to a boil. Lower heat, cover and simmer 20 to 30 minutes, or until lentils are tender. (Do not overcook. Lentils should be just tender and still chewy, not soft and mushy.) Drain. While lentils are still warm, toss with 3 tablespoons of the vinaigrette. When cool, cover and chill.

Just before serving, roll romaine and radicchio leaves like a cigar and slice into ribbons. Place in a large, shallow salad bowl. Add chilled lentils, cucumber, onion, pepper, tomato, olives and peperoncini. Toss with remaining vinaigrette. Sprinkle with cheese.

PER SERVING
Calories - 153
Protein - 6 g
Sodium - 402 mg
Carbohydrates - 17 g
Cholesterol - 2 mg
Total Fat - 7 g
Saturated Fat - 1 g
Dietary Fiber - 7 g

Cook's Suggestion: For a heartier meal, accompany with Roast Chicken (page 424) and, for dessert, Rhubarb Cobbler (page 507).

■ Asian Chicken Salad   8 servings

4 cups chicken broth, preferably homemade (page 240)
4 cups water
2 skinless, boneless chicken breasts
1 8-ounce package soba noodles
1 pound fresh asparagus, ends removed,
  cut into thirds
1 medium head Napa cabbage, coarsely chopped
2 red peppers, cored, seeded and julienned
¾ cup Spicy Peanut Dressing (page 307)
4 green onions, julienned
2 tablespoons chopped peanuts

In a pan, combine 2 cups of the broth with 2 cups of the water and bring to a boil; add chicken and bring to a second boil. Reduce heat to medium; cook 20 minutes, or until chicken is done. Drain chicken and set aside to cool.

PER SERVING
Calories - 360
Protein - 18 g
Sodium - 846 mg
Carbohydrates - 32 g
Cholesterol - 22 mg
Total Fat - 20 g
Saturated Fat - 3 g
Dietary Fiber - 4 g

Fill pan with remaining 2 cups of broth and remaining 2 cups of water; bring to a boil. Add noodles and cook 3 to 5 minutes, or until noodles are tender; pour into a colander, rinse and drain. Place noodles in a bowl. Using a sharp knife, cut pile of noodles in half, then into bite-size quarters. Set aside.

Steam or microwave asparagus 3 to 5 minutes, or just until crisp-tender. Cut into thirds.

Layer cabbage in a large, shallow salad bowl. Top with noodles.

In a separate bowl, toss chicken, asparagus and peppers with dressing. Spread over cabbage and noodles. Toss lightly. Sprinkle with onion. Top with peanuts.

Sodium Alert: Choose low-sodium foods at other meals throughout the day to offset the higher sodium in this recipe.

Grilled Chicken Salad 4 servings

After a hard day, this salad is easy to do outdoors on the grill.
It's delicious served plain or drizzled lightly with a vinaigrette.

2 red peppers, seeded and julienned

1 yellow pepper, seeded and julienned

1 yellow onion, cut into ¼-inch rounds

1 tablespoon extra-virgin olive oil

1½ teaspoon coarse salt

1 teaspoon freshly ground black pepper

1 pound skinned and boned chicken breasts

12 ounces spinach leaves or mixed field greens

Toss red and yellow peppers and onion in olive oil; season with salt and pepper. Place in a nonstick grill basket. Grill 8 minutes, tossing vegetables three or four times, until onions become translucent and peppers are slightly blackened.

PER SERVING
Calories - 214
Protein - 30 g
Sodium - 864 mg
Carbohydrates - 12 g
Cholesterol - 66 mg
Total Fat - 5 g
Saturated Fat - 1 g
Dietary Fiber - 5 g

Cut chicken breasts lengthwise into slices about ½ inch thick. This will allow chicken to grill evenly and retain moisture. Grill about 4 to 5 minutes on each side, or until chicken is cooked. Cut into strips.

Arrange spinach or field greens on dinner plates. Layer with onion and peppers. Top with chicken.

Cook's Suggestions: For variety, add tomatoes or other vegetables to the grill basket. To make a fajita salad, top with shredded cheddar cheese and fresh tomato salsa.

Warm Seafood Salad   3 servings

1 tablespoon olive oil
½ pound scallops
1 cup stemmed and thinly sliced fresh
   shiitake mushrooms
⅓ pound cooked medium shrimp
2 ripe tomatoes, sliced into 2-inch strips
½ pound fresh asparagus, trimmed
4 cups mixed field greens
2 tablespoons oil-and-vinegar dressing
1 ripe Hass avocado, sliced
dash coarse salt
dash freshly ground black pepper
1 lemon, cut into wedges

Heat olive oil over medium-high heat in a nonstick grill pan or skillet. Add scallops and cook 3 minutes, turning once or twice. Add mushrooms; cook 2 minutes. Add shrimp; cook 2 minutes. Add tomatoes; cook 1 to 2 minutes.

Meanwhile, microwave or steam asparagus 2 to 3 minutes, or just until crisp-tender. Drain and cut into thirds.

Toss mixed greens with dressing and layer on dinner plates. Top with seafood, mushrooms, tomatoes and asparagus. Sprinkle with avocado. Season with salt and pepper, and garnish with lemon. Serve at once.

Cook's Suggestion: Serve with Fresh Pineapple, Papaya and Berries (page 488).

PER SERVING
Calories - 383
Protein - 29 g
Sodium - 401 mg
Carbohydrates - 21 g
Cholesterol - 123 mg
Total Fat - 23 g
Saturated Fat - 3 g
Dietary Fiber - 9 g

Crab and Shrimp Louis Salad 6 servings

DRESSING
½ cup light mayonnaise
2 tablespoons freshly squeezed lemon juice
2 tablespoons grated Bermuda or
   Walla Walla onion

1 pound fresh asparagus, tough ends removed
4 cups shredded red-leaf lettuce
2 cups shredded radicchio
¼ pound cooked Dungeness crabmeat
¼ pound cooked baby shrimp meat
2 large ripe tomatoes, coarsely chopped
¼ cup pitted and halved kalamata olives
3 hard-boiled eggs, quartered
1 lemon, cut into wedges

Combine dressing ingredients with a wire whisk. Chill.

   In a pot of boiling water, blanch asparagus 2 to 3 minutes; plunge into ice water for 2 to 3 minutes. Drain and chill. Just before serving, toss lettuce with dressing. Add crab and shrimp, and toss again. Garnish with asparagus, tomatoes, olives, eggs and lemon wedges.

PER SERVING
Calories - 249
Protein - 15 g
Sodium - 624 mg
Carbohydrates - 14 g
Cholesterol - 156 mg
Total Fat - 17 g
Saturated Fat - 2 g
Dietary Fiber - 4 g

Nutrition Note: Using light mayonnaise allows us to enjoy a marvelous salad while not undoing a good thing with a high-fat dressing.

Grilled Steak and Onion Salad

4 servings

We practiced our balancing skills on this salad. Note that we offset the sirloin steak and blue cheese with a fat-free balsamic vinegar.

1 large red onion
1 pound top sirloin steak
8 cups chopped hearts of romaine
4 Roma tomatoes, sliced into ¼-inch rounds
¼ cup balsamic vinegar or to taste
dash freshly ground pepper
2 tablespoons crumbled blue cheese

Slice onion into 1-inch chunks and arrange on wood or metal skewers. Grill over hot coals 4 minutes on each side; set aside.

Grill steak 4 to 6 minutes on each side, or to desired doneness (150° to 160°F for medium); slice into thin strips.

Divide hearts of romaine among four dinner plates. Arrange tomatoes and steak over lettuce. Top with grilled onion. Drizzle with balsamic vinegar (the steak will provide the oil). Sprinkle with pepper and cheese.

PER SERVING
Calories - 292
Protein - 39 g
Sodium - 155 mg
Carbohydrates - 12 g
Cholesterol - 104 mg
Total Fat - 10 g
Saturated Fat - 4 g
Dietary Fiber - 4 g

Caesar Salad 6 servings

No need to give up Caesar salad when it can taste this good and still be so lean.

2 large heads romaine lettuce, torn into bite-size pieces
juice of ½ large lemon
⅓ cup olive oil, preferably Garlic Olive Oil (page 306)
2½ tablespoons red wine vinegar
1 coddled egg,* chilled
¾ teaspoon coarse salt
¼ teaspoon freshly ground pepper
½ teaspoon Worcestershire sauce
¾ cup unseasoned croutons
⅓ cup freshly grated Parmesan cheese
6 anchovy fillets, finely chopped (optional)

Fill a large salad bowl with romaine. Drizzle with lemon juice, olive oil and vinegar; toss. Add coddled egg and toss again. Season with salt, pepper and Worcestershire sauce; toss. Mix in croutons. Sprinkle with cheese. Garnish with anchovies, if desired.

PER SERVING
Calories - 174
Protein - 15 g
Sodium - 465 mg
Carbohydrates - 6 g
Cholesterol - 39 mg
Total Fat - 15 g
Saturated Fat - 3 g
Dietary Fiber - 1 g

*To make a coddled egg, place a cold whole egg in a saucepan with enough warm water to completely cover. Meanwhile, in a separate saucepan, bring an equal amount of water to a boil. Immerse egg in boiling water; remove pan from heat and let stand 1 minute. Place egg in cold water to prevent further cooking. Cool in refrigerator.

Cook's Suggestion: This salad is also good topped with grilled chicken or grilled prawns or just sprinkled with cooked baby shrimp meat or Dungeness crab.

Salade Niçoise   6 servings

This classic French salad has it all: colorful vegetables, heart-healthy tuna and terrific flavor. Presenting it on a platter allows for individual preferences when dishing up a serving.

3 large red potatoes
¾ pound fresh green beans, trimmed
Niçoise Dressing (page 308)
12 cups fresh baby spinach leaves
2 6½-ounce cans water-packed tuna,
*   drained*
6 water-packed artichoke hearts,
*   cut into quarters*
½ red bell pepper, julienned
½ yellow bell pepper, julienned
½ white onion, thinly sliced
6 ripe plum tomatoes, quartered
12 niçoise or kalamata olives
2 hard-boiled eggs, peeled and quartered
fresh lemon wedges

Cook potatoes in boiling salted water for 20 to 30 minutes, or until just tender. Set aside to cool.

Meanwhile, in a pot of boiling water, blanch beans 8 to 10 minutes. Drain and immerse in ice water for 5 minutes. Drain again.

Cut potatoes into quarters. Toss potatoes and beans with 2 tablespoons of dressing. Set aside.

Arrange spinach leaves on a large, flat platter. Top with tuna, potatoes, beans, artichoke hearts and peppers. Tuck in onion slices, tomatoes and olives. Chill. Just before serving, garnish

PER SERVING
Calories - 263
Protein - 24 g
Sodium - 749 mg
Carbohydrates - 23 g
Cholesterol - 79 mg
Total Fat - 10 g
Saturated Fat - 1 g
Dietary Fiber - 9 g

with hard-boiled eggs and lemon wedges. Pass remaining dressing in a pitcher on the side.

Variation: Try serving this salad warm with Grilled Tuna Steaks (page 390).

·

Save-the-Day Fresh Fruit Salad

4 servings

A perfect lunch or light supper after a day or two of overeating. Double the recipe, and you'll have fruit already cut up for the rest of the week.

> *½ grapefruit, cut into sections*
> *½ cup 2-inch cubes watermelon*
> *½ cup 2-inch cubes cantaloupe*
> *½ cup 2-inch cubes honeydew*
> *½ cup 2-inch cubes fresh papaya*
> *½ cup 2-inch cubes fresh pineapple*
> *1 cup raspberries, strawberries or blueberries*
> *2 cups nonfat plain yogurt or fruit-sweetened*
> *   peach or raspberry yogurt*

Make sure all membranes and seeds have been removed from pieces of fruit. Arrange fruit in uniform rows on individual salad plates. Serve with yogurt.

Variation: Serve with sorbet instead of yogurt.

Nutrition Note: This fruit salad is especially high in antioxidants, vitamins A and C and folic acid.

PER SERVING
Calories - 125
Protein - 5 g
Sodium - 56 mg
Carbohydrates - 26 g
Cholesterol - 6 mg
Total Fat - 1 g
Saturated Fat - 0 g
Dietary Fiber - 3 g

Taco Salad   6 servings

1 pound leanest ground beef
2 onions, coarsely chopped
½ teaspoon Adobo All-Purpose Seasoning*
      or coarse salt
1 head romaine lettuce
1 head red-leaf lettuce, chopped
2 large tomatoes, chopped
½ cup grated reduced-fat cheddar cheese
1 Hass avocado, peeled, seeded and sliced
½ cup nonfat sour cream
1 cup fresh tomato salsa
6 warm corn tortillas

In a nonstick skillet, brown beef with half the chopped onions and add seasoning. Drain on paper towels to remove any excess grease. Line salad bowls with outside leaves of romaine lettuce. Shred remaining romaine and mix with chopped red-leaf lettuce. Top with beef, tomatoes, remaining onion, cheese and avocado. Accompany with sour cream, salsa and warm tortillas.

PER SERVING
Calories - 267
Protein - 21 g
Sodium - 294 mg
Carbohydrates - 17 g
Cholesterol - 52 mg
Total Fat - 14 g
Saturated Fat - 4 g
Dietary Fiber - 5 g

*Adobo All-Purpose Seasoning is found in the ethnic section at supermarkets. If it's unavailable where you shop, just leave it out. The recipe is delicious either way.

Salad Dressings, Sauces and Dips

Balsamic Vinaigrette Makes 1 cup

You'll never want to buy another bottled dressing once you learn to make your own!

2/3 cup extra-virgin olive oil
1/4 cup balsamic vinegar
1 tablespoon Dijon mustard
3/4 teaspoon coarse salt
1/4 teaspoon freshly ground black pepper
pinch sugar

Combine all ingredients in a jar with lid. Shake until well blended.

PER TABLESPOON
Calories - 81
Protein - 0 g
Sodium - 113 mg
Carbohydrates - 0 g
Cholesterol - 0 mg
Total Fat - 9 g
Saturated Fat - 1 g
Dietary Fiber - 0 g

A NOTE ABOUT SALAD DRESSINGS

Low in fat and calories, salads provide a tasty, attractive way to add nutrients and fiber to your diet. Salad dressings, however, are a different matter altogether. Too much dressing can turn a low-fat salad into a high-fat food. Always be sure to check the labels of store-bought dressings. Many brands simply trade fat for high-fructose corn syrup.

Most of our dressings are made with olive oil, considered by many the most healthful of all oils. But beware. Olive oil may be good for your heart, but it's still rich in fat and calories and must be used sparingly. Virgin and extra-virgin olive oils have a more powerful taste than multipurpose or "light" olive oil, so the amount can be reduced, but they provide no additional health benefit. Also, be aware that light olive oil has no less fat and no fewer calories than regular olive oil.

Italian Vinaigrette Makes 1 cup

This tried-and-true recipe was passed down from Joe's mother, who learned it from her mother, who learned it from . . .

> *¾ cup extra-virgin olive oil*
> *¼ cup cider vinegar*
> *¾ teaspoon coarse salt*
> *¼ teaspoon freshly ground black pepper*

Combine all ingredients in a jar with lid.
Shake until well blended.

PER TABLESPOON
Calories - 90
Protein - 0 g
Sodium - 90 mg
Carbohydrates - 0 g
Cholesterol - 0 mg
Total Fat - 10 g
Saturated Fat - 1 g
Dietary Fiber - 0 g

Dijon Vinaigrette Makes 1 cup

A great dressing for sparking up green beans, red potatoes, fish and shellfish.

1/4 cup Dijon mustard

1/4 cup red wine vinegar

2 cloves garlic

1 tablespoon minced white onion

1/2 teaspoon coarse salt

1/4 teaspoon coarsely ground
  black pepper

5 drops Tabasco sauce

3/4 cup extra-virgin olive oil

Combine mustard, vinegar, garlic, onion, salt, pepper and Tabasco sauce in a food processor. With machine running, add olive oil 1 tablespoon at a time. Chill.

PER TABLESPOON

Calories - 97

Protein - 0 g

Sodium - 152 mg

Carbohydrates - 1 g

Cholesterol - 0 mg

Total Fat - 10 g

Saturated Fat - 1 g

Dietary Fiber - 0 g

Lemon Vinaigrette   Makes 7 tablespoons

Try this dressing in place of butter. We like it on steamed broccoli, cauliflower, green beans and red potatoes. It's also great for shellfish.

2 garlic cloves, minced
3 tablespoons fresh lemon juice
¼ cup extra-virgin olive oil
¾ teaspoon coarse salt
¼ teaspoon freshly ground
*   black pepper*

Combine all ingredients in a jar with lid. Shake until well blended.

PER TABLESPOON
Calories - 71
Protein - Tr
Sodium - 206 mg
Carbohydrates - 1 g
Cholesterol - 0 mg
Total Fat - 8 g
Saturated Fat - 1 g
Dietary Fiber - 0 g

Very Lemon Vinaigrette   Makes 1 cup

¼ cup olive oil
¼ cup freshly squeezed lemon juice
½ teaspoon coarse salt
¼ teaspoon coarsely ground black pepper

Combine all ingredients in a jar with lid. Shake well.

PER TABLESPOON
Calories - 62
Protein - Tr
Sodium - 145 mg
Carbohydrates - 1 g
Cholesterol - 0 mg
Total Fat - 7 g
Saturated Fat - 1 g
Dietary Fiber - 0 g

Champagne Vinaigrette Makes ½ cup

⅓ cup olive oil

1 tablespoon light mayonnaise

½ teaspoon Dijon mustard

3 tablespoons champagne vinegar

1 teaspoon fresh minced garlic

¾ teaspoon coarse salt

½ teaspoon coarsely ground black pepper

Combine all ingredients in a small bowl. Stir with a fork or wire whisk until smooth and creamy.

PER TABLESPOON
Calories - 89
Protein - 0 g
Sodium - 197 mg
Carbohydrates - 1 g
Cholesterol - 0 mg
Total Fat - 10 g
Saturated Fat - 1 g
Dietary Fiber - 0 g

Red Wine Vinaigrette   Makes 1 cup

Adding a pinch of sugar mellows the tartness of the red wine vinegar.

> *¾ cup extra-virgin olive oil*
> *¼ cup red wine vinegar*
> *1 tablespoon Dijon mustard*
> *¾ teaspoon coarse salt*
> *¼ teaspoon freshly ground black pepper*
> *pinch sugar*

Combine all ingredients in a jar with lid.
Shake until well blended.

PER TABLESPOON
Calories - 93
Protein - 0 g
Sodium - 113 mg
Carbohydrates - 0 g
Cholesterol - 0 mg
Total Fat - 10 g
Saturated Fat - 1 g
Dietary Fiber - 0 g

Garlic Olive Oil   Makes 1½ cups

This flavorful oil works well in salad dressings, especially Caesar,
in marinades for grilled vegetables and over toasted breads such as
garlic bread, bruschetta and focaccia.

> *1½ cups olive oil*
> *1 head garlic, separated into cloves and peeled*

Pour olive oil into a pint-size jar; add garlic.
Cover tightly and let mellow 2 to 3 days;
remove garlic. Store in a dark place. Keeps
3 to 4 weeks.

PER TABLESPOON
Calories - 121
Protein - 0 g
Sodium - 0 mg
Carbohydrates - 0 g
Cholesterol - 0 mg
Total Fat - 14 g
Saturated Fat - 2 g
Dietary Fiber - 0 g

Spicy Peanut Dressing   Makes 1 cup

This one is high in fat, so moderation is the key.

> *10 tablespoons extra-virgin olive oil*
> *¼ cup chunky peanut butter*
> *2 tablespoons apple cider vinegar*
> *2½ tablespoons reduced-sodium soy sauce*
> *1½ tablespoons dark sesame oil*
> *1½ teaspoons honey*
> *2 cloves garlic, minced*
> *1 teaspoon peeled and grated fresh*
>   *ginger*
> *2 teaspoons coarse salt*
> *½ teaspoon freshly ground black pepper*
> *¼ teaspoon hot chili oil*

Combine all ingredients in a medium bowl. Using a wire whisk, beat until smooth and creamy.

PER TABLESPOON
Calories - 115
Protein - 1 g
Sodium - 353 mg
Carbohydrates - 2 g
Cholesterol - 0 mg
Total Fat - 12 g
Saturated Fat - 2 g
Dietary Fiber - 0 g

Niçoise Dressing   Makes ¾ cup

½ cup olive oil

2 tablespoons tarragon-flavored vinegar

2 tablespoons fresh lemon juice

2 garlic cloves, chopped

1½ teaspoons dry mustard

¼ teaspoon coarse salt

½ teaspoon freshly ground pepper

Combine all ingredients in a jar with lid. Shake well.

PER TABLESPOON
Calories - 82
Protein - 0 g
Sodium - 127 mg
Carbohydrates - 0 g
Cholesterol - 0 mg
Total Fat - 9 g
Saturated Fat - 1 g
Dietary Fiber - 0 g

Creamy Horseradish Sauce   Makes 1 cup

1 cup light mayonnaise

1 heaping tablespoon horseradish

1 teaspoon Worcestershire sauce

juice of 1 lemon

1 tablespoon minced fresh flat-leaf parsley

1 clove garlic, minced

1 tablespoon minced onion

¼ teaspoon coarse salt

Combine all ingredients in a jar. Cover; chill.

Serve with roast beef, veal, steamed vegetables, roasted peppers or onion wraps (see page 454).

PER TABLESPOON
Calories - 52
Protein - Tr
Sodium - 157 mg
Carbohydrates - 2 g
Cholesterol - 5 mg
Total Fat - 5 g
Saturated Fat - 1 g
Dietary Fiber - 0 g

Pesto   Makes 2½ cups

Delicious on pasta, chicken, seafood, vegetables and potatoes, pesto is also good for spreading on sandwiches in place of mayonnaise. Make it in the summer, when basil is at its peak. Prepare several batches and store in jars and/or ice-cube trays in the freezer for quick-to-fix dinners.

5 cups loosely packed fresh basil
8 cloves garlic
1 teaspoon coarse salt
½ cup pine nuts
¾ cup extra-virgin olive oil

Combine basil, garlic, salt and pine nuts in a blender or food processor and puree. With machine running, add olive oil 1 tablespoon at a time. Blend until smooth and oil is absorbed.

Note: Never double the pesto recipe. The oil will not absorb properly.

PER TABLESPOON
Calories - 48
Protein - 1 g
Sodium - 48 mg
Carbohydrates - 1 g
Cholesterol - 0 mg
Total Fat - 5 g
Saturated Fat - 1 g
Dietary Fiber - 0 g

Stir-Fry Sauce   Makes 9 tablespoons

This sauce tastes better than the commercial kind. It's also cheaper!

> ¼ cup reduced-sodium soy sauce
> 1 tablespoon olive oil
> 2 tablespoons oyster-flavored sauce*
> 2 tablespoons unseasoned rice vinegar
> ¼ teaspoon hot chili sauce, hot chile oil or Tabasco sauce

Combine all ingredients in a jar or small bowl.

*Oyster-flavored sauce is available in the Asian section of most supermarkets.

PER TABLESPOON
Calories - 10
Protein - 0 g
Sodium - 147 mg
Carbohydrates - 1 g
Cholesterol - 0 mg
Total Fat - 0 g
Saturated Fat - 0 g
Dietary Fiber - 0 g

■

Black Bean Dip   Makes 1 cup

> 1 15-ounce can black beans, drained and rinsed
> 1 tablespoon chili powder
> ½ teaspoon cumin
> ¼ teaspoon salt
> ¼ teaspoon Adobo All-Purpose Seasoning (optional)

Combine all ingredients in a food processor; process 2 to 3 minutes, or until smooth. Taste. Add salt if needed.

Serve with cut-up celery, carrots, cucumber, bell peppers and jicama sticks, Homemade Tortilla Chips (page 371) or warm whole wheat tortillas.

PER TABLESPOON
Calories - 24
Protein - 2 g
Sodium - 126 mg
Carbohydrates - 4 g
Cholesterol - 0 mg
Total Fat - 0 g
Saturated Fat - 0 g
Dietary Fiber - 2 g

Variation: Substitute red kidney beans for black beans.

Tuscan Bean Dip   Makes 1½ cups

1 15-ounce can cannellini beans, drained and rinsed
2 to 3 large garlic cloves, minced
1 tablespoon fresh lemon juice
4 to 6 drops Tabasco sauce
1 tablespoon extra-virgin olive oil
½ teaspoon coarse salt
¼ teaspoon freshly ground black pepper

Combine all ingredients in a food processor. Process 2 to 3 minutes, or until smooth.

Serve with cut-up celery and carrot sticks, radishes, broccoli and cauliflower florets, warm breadsticks or whole wheat pita bread or sliced and toasted whole wheat bagels.

PER TABLESPOON
Calories - 19
Protein - 1 g
Sodium - 95 mg
Carbohydrates - 3 g
Cholesterol - 0 mg
Total Fat - 1 g
Saturated Fat - 0 g
Dietary Fiber - 1 g

Layered Shrimp Dip   10 servings

1 8-ounce container whipped light cream cheese
⅓ cup cocktail sauce
½ pound shelled small cooked shrimp or crabmeat
Raw Veggies in a Basket (page 347)

Place cream cheese in the center of a 10-inch serving tray. With the back of a serving spoon, spread cheese to cover the surface of the tray. Pour cocktail sauce over cheese and spread it evenly. Sprinkle shrimp or crabmeat over top. Chill until ready to serve. Accompany with raw veggies.

PER SERVING
Calories - 77
Protein - 8 g
Sodium - 218 mg
Carbohydrates - 4 g
Cholesterol - 38 mg
Total Fat - 1 g
Saturated Fat - 0 g
Dietary Fiber - 0 g

Layered Bean Dip 10 servings

1 15-ounce can red kidney beans
1 tablespoon chili powder
½ teaspoon ground cumin
⅓ cup nonfat sour cream
¾ cup chopped dark leafy lettuce
⅓ cup white onion, chopped
1 ripe tomato, diced
¼ cup grated cheddar cheese
1½ cups tomato salsa or Pico de Gallo (page 315)
Raw Veggies in a Basket (page 347)

Puree beans in a food processor. Add chili powder and cumin, and whirl 1 minute longer. Chill at least 1 hour. Spread onto a 10-inch serving tray. Top with sour cream. Layer with lettuce, onion, tomato and cheddar cheese. Accompany with salsa or pico de gallo and raw veggies or Homemade Tortilla Chips (page 371).

PER SERVING
Calories - 138
Protein - 8 g
Sodium - 97 mg
Carbohydrates - 21 g
Cholesterol - 4 mg
Total Fat - 3 g
Saturated Fat - 1 g
Dietary Fiber - 8 g

■

Artichoke Dip Makes 1 cup

1 15-ounce can artichoke bottoms, drained
¼ cup extra-virgin olive oil
1 teaspoon fresh lemon juice
3 large garlic cloves, peeled
2 tablespoons freshly grated Parmesan cheese
½ teaspoon coarse salt
¼ teaspoon pepper

Combine artichoke bottoms, olive oil, lemon juice and garlic in a food processor; process until smooth. Add cheese, salt and pepper; process until combined (about 30 seconds).

Serve with raw vegetables or as a spread on grilled or toasted French or Tuscan bread.

PER TABLESPOON
Calories - 33
Protein - 1 g
Sodium - 174 mg
Carbohydrates - 1 g
Cholesterol - 1 mg
Total Fat - 3 g
Saturated Fat - 0 g
Dietary Fiber - 1 g

■

Avocado Spread   Makes 1 cup

1 ripe Hass avocado, peeled and seeded
1 tablespoon fresh lime juice
1 tablespoon grated onion
¼ teaspoon coarse salt
3 to 4 drops hot chili sauce or Tabasco sauce

Place avocado in a small bowl and mash with a fork. Add lime juice, onion, salt and chili sauce or Tabasco. Stir with a fork until avocado is smooth.

Variation: Add ½ cup cooked baby shrimp to ingredients.

PER TABLESPOON
Calories - 20
Protein - 0 g
Sodium - 32 mg
Carbohydrates - 1 g
Cholesterol - 0 mg
Total Fat - 2 g
Saturated Fat - 0 g
Dietary Fiber - 1 g

Cook's Suggestion: For a shrimp wrap, spread mixture on a tortilla and top with diced tomato and chopped mixed greens. Roll and slice.

313

Guacamole Makes 3 cups

Use this as a dip in moderation with fresh carrots and radishes or as a complement to Mexican food.

> *4 ripe avocados, peeled and seeded*
> *juice of 1 lemon*
> *¼ teaspoon Tabasco sauce*
> *1 small red onion, diced*
> *1 medium tomato, diced*
> *2 cloves garlic, minced*
> *1 teaspoon coarse salt*
> *¾ teaspoon freshly ground pepper*

Place avocado in a medium bowl; cover with lemon juice to seal and sprinkle with Tabasco. Layer onion, tomato and garlic over top. Cover with plastic wrap and chill for 2 hours.

Just before serving, slice through the mixture with a sharp knife to dice the avocado and mix the ingredients. Add salt and pepper, and stir gently with a fork.

PER TABLESPOON
Calories - 27
Protein - 0 g
Sodium - 42 mg
Carbohydrates - 1 g
Cholesterol - 0 mg
Total Fat - 3 g
Saturated Fat - 0 g
Dietary Fiber - 1 g

Variation: Add 1½ cups of cooked shrimp to the mixture.

Pico de Gallo Makes 2 cups

Whenever we ate the salsa served at our favorite Mexican restaurant, I'd go home and try to duplicate the taste. At long last, I not only succeeded but topped it!

1¼ cups finely chopped ripe tomatoes
½ cup finely chopped white onion
1 jalapeño pepper, seeded and finely
*   chopped*
⅓ cup finely chopped cilantro
2 tablespoons fresh lime juice
½ teaspoon coarse salt

Just before serving, combine tomatoes, onion, jalapeño, cilantro and lime juice. Season with salt.

PER ½ CUP
Calories - 24
Protein - 1 g
Sodium - 246 mg
Carbohydrates - 6 g
Cholesterol - 0 g
Total Fat - 0 g
Saturated Fat - 0 g
Dietary Fiber - 1 g

Vegetables

Artichokes and Garlic 4 servings

8 fresh baby artichokes
½ lemon, in wedges,
   plus juice of 1 whole lemon
3 tablespoons chopped onion
3 garlic cloves, minced
1½ cups dry white wine
dash of salt
Roasted Garlic (page 327)

Wash artichokes. Slice off stems to form a flat base. Snap off tough outer leaves closest to base. Trim ½ inch off pointed tops, then use scissors to snip off tips of outer leaves. Rub all cut edges with the lemon wedges.

In a small saucepan, combine lemon juice, onion, garlic, wine and salt; bring to a boil. Place artichokes upright in mixture; cover and simmer 15 to 20 minutes, or until bottom leaves pull off easily and bottoms can be pierced with a knife tip.

Serve warm with roasted garlic. After dipping individual leaves into the paste, cut away the prickly choke and dip the tender base into the garlic.

Variation: Instead of garlic paste, serve with light mayonnaise mixed with a touch of fresh lemon juice and some grated onion.

PER SERVING
Calories - 292
Protein - 6 g
Sodium - 250 mg
Carbohydrates - 26 g
Cholesterol - 0 mg
Total Fat - 14 g
Saturated Fat - 2 g
Dietary Fiber - 8 g

Artichokes and String Beans   6 servings

Steaming is an easy, low-calorie way to prepare all sorts of vegetables. Even better, steamed vegetables keep their color and nutrients— and taste delicious!

1 pound fresh string beans
1 15-ounce can water-packed artichoke hearts,
drained and quartered
¼ cup fresh lemon juice
2 tablespoons extra-virgin olive oil
½ teaspoon coarse salt
¼ teaspoon freshly ground pepper

Wash beans; remove ends and strings. Place a metal vegetable steamer basket in a medium saucepan filled with 2 inches of water. Bring water to a boil. Add beans; cover and steam 10 to 20 minutes, or until beans are just tender (do not overcook).

Transfer beans from steamer to serving bowl; add artichokes. Combine lemon juice, olive oil, salt and pepper. Pour over beans and artichokes. Serve hot or cold.

PER SERVING
Calories - 57
Protein - 2 g
Sodium - 437 mg
Carbohydrates - 9 g
Cholesterol - 0 mg
Total Fat - 2 g
Saturated Fat - 0 g
Dietary Fiber - 3 g

Pan-Steamed Asparagus 4 servings

Getting your vitamins and iron has never been easier!

1 pound fresh asparagus
2 tablespoons water
1 lemon, cut into wedges

Wash and trim asparagus. Bring water to a boil in a nonstick skillet and add asparagus. Cover tightly and steam over medium-high heat 3 to 5 minutes, or until asparagus is crisp-tender. Shake pan occasionally during cooking. Serve with lemon wedges.

PER SERVING
Calories - 25
Protein - 3 g
Sodium - 2 mg
Carbohydrates - 4 g
Cholesterol - 0 g
Total Fat - 0 g
Saturated Fat - 0 g
Dietary Fiber - 2 g

Roasted Asparagus with Garlic 4 servings

2 bunches fresh asparagus, trimmed
(thick stalks work best)
1 tablespoon olive oil
6 cloves garlic, chopped
¼ teaspoon coarse salt
pinch coarsely ground black pepper
½ lemon

In a bowl, toss asparagus with oil and garlic. Arrange asparagus and garlic on a nonstick baking sheet; roast in a preheated 400°F oven 8 to 10 minutes. Turn and roast 5 to 6 minutes longer or until crisp-tender. Remove to serving platter. Sprinkle with salt and pepper. Squeeze lemon juice over top.

PER SERVING
Calories - 56
Protein - 2 g
Sodium - 122 mg
Carbohydrates - 5 g
Cholesterol - 0 mg
Total Fat - 4 g
Saturated Fat - 0 g
Dietary Fiber - 2 g

Roasted Asparagus with Parmesan 4 servings

1 pound fresh asparagus, trimmed
1 teaspoon olive oil
pinch coarse salt
pinch freshly ground black pepper
1 tablespoon freshly grated Parmesan
  cheese

Place asparagus in a pie plate and toss with olive oil. Arrange stalks in a single layer on a nonstick baking sheet. Roast in 400°F oven, 7 to 10 minutes for thin stalks, 15 to 20 for thicker stalks or until al dente. Season with salt and pepper. Sprinkle with cheese.

PER SERVING
Calories - 42
Protein - 3 g
Sodium - 146 mg
Carbohydrates - 5 g
Cholesterol - 1 mg
Total Fat - 2 g
Saturated Fat - 0 g
Dietary Fiber - 2 g

Sautéed Baby Broccoli 4 servings

Broccolini, a cross between broccoli and Chinese kale, has a wonderfully sweet flavor and crunchy texture.

1 tablespoon olive oil
2 bunches broccolini (baby broccoli), sliced
6 cloves garlic, chopped
½ lemon
pinch coarse salt

Heat olive oil in a nonstick skillet over medium-high heat. Add broccolini and garlic. Stir-fry 4 to 5 minutes, or until broccolini is crisp-tender. Remove to serving platter. Squeeze lemon over top. Sprinkle with salt.

PER SERVING
Calories - 69
Protein - 4 g
Sodium - 32 mg
Carbohydrates - 8 g
Cholesterol - 0 mg
Total Fat - 4 g
Saturated Fat - 1 g
Dietary Fiber - 0 g

Stir-Fried Broccoli and Cauliflower with Red Peppers 4 servings

2 teaspoons sesame oil
2 cups broccoli florets
2 cups cauliflower florets
¼ cup chicken broth, preferably homemade
    (page 240)
1 cup ¼-inch strips seeded red pepper

Preheat a nonstick wok or skillet over high heat. When wok is hot, add sesame oil. When oil is hot, add broccoli and cauliflower; stir-fry, uncovered, for 1 minute. Add chicken broth. Cover and cook 2 minutes. Add red peppers. Cover and cook 1 minute longer, or until vegetables are crisp-tender.

PER SERVING
Calories - 52
Protein - 3 g
Sodium - 82 mg
Carbohydrates - 6 g
Cholesterol - 0 mg
Total Fat - 3 g
Saturated Fat - 0 g
Dietary Fiber - 3 g

Chinese Snow Peas 4 servings

2 teaspoons extra-virgin olive oil
1 teaspoon finely minced garlic
¼ teaspoon crushed red pepper
¾ pound snow peas, ends and strings removed

Preheat a nonstick wok or skillet over high heat. When wok is hot, add olive oil, garlic and red pepper. When oil is hot, add snow peas; stir-fry, uncovered, 2 to 3 minutes, until crisp-tender.

PER SERVING
Calories - 56
Protein - 2 g
Sodium - 4 mg
Carbohydrates - 7 g
Cholesterol - 0 mg
Total Fat - 2 g
Saturated Fat - 0 g
Dietary Fiber - 2 g

Roasted Carrots 4 servings

Roasting in high heat brings out the sweetness in veggies by caramelizing their sugars.

> *12 carrots, sliced diagonally into thirds*
> *1½ tablespoons extra-virgin olive oil*
> *pinch coarse salt*
> *pinch freshly ground black pepper*

Place carrots in a pie plate and toss with olive oil. Arrange carrots in a single layer on a nonstick baking sheet. Roast in 400°F oven for 10 to 20 minutes, until tender. Sprinkle with salt and pepper.

Note: When selecting carrots, look for ones that are firm and have no cracks.

PER SERVING
Calories - 123
Protein - 2 g
Sodium - 184 mg
Carbohydrates - 19 g
Cholesterol - 0 mg
Total Fat - 5 g
Saturated Fat - 1 g
Dietary Fiber - 5 g

ROASTED BABY VEGETABLES. Select a combination of baby eggplants, baby zucchini, pattypan squash, red, green or yellow peppers cut into squares and small white cremini or portobello mushrooms. Toss with enough olive oil to coat. Roast 20 to 30 minutes, or until vegetables are tender.

Green Beans with Artichokes and Red Pepper 6 servings

2 pounds fresh string beans, trimmed
2 15-ounce cans water-packed artichoke hearts, drained
1 red bell pepper, seeded
dash coarse salt
dash freshly ground black pepper

Blanch beans 3 minutes in a large pot of boiling water. Plunge immediately into ice water to set color and flavor. Drain.

Cut each artichoke heart lengthwise into eighths. Dice red pepper.

In a large serving bowl, toss beans with artichokes and red pepper. Season.

PER SERVING
Calories - 69
Protein - 5 g
Sodium - 409 mg
Carbohydrates - 15 g
Cholesterol - 0 mg
Total Fat - 0 g
Saturated Fat - 0 g
Dietary Fiber - 6 g

Green Beans with Shallots 6 servings

2 pounds string beans, ends removed
1 tablespoon olive oil
3 large shallots, diced
dash coarse salt
dash freshly ground black pepper

Blanch beans 3 minutes in a large pot of boiling water. Plunge immediately into ice water to set color and flavor. Drain.

Heat oil in a nonstick skillet over medium heat. Add shallots and sauté 8 to 10 minutes, stirring frequently, until lightly browned. Add beans and heat to serving temperature. Season.

PER SERVING
Calories - 70
Protein - 3 g
Sodium - 50 mg
Carbohydrates - 12 g
Cholesterol - 0 mg
Total Fat - 2 g
Saturated Fat - 0 g
Dietary Fiber - 5 g

Sautéed Spinach with Garlic 4 servings

1 tablespoon olive oil
5 cloves garlic, peeled and minced
1 pound baby spinach leaves, trimmed and washed
1 tablespoon water
½ lemon
pinch coarse salt
pinch fresh ground black pepper

Preheat a nonstick skillet over medium heat. Add olive oil; when hot, add garlic and sauté about 1 minute until golden. Add spinach and water. Cover and cook over medium heat 2 to 3 minutes, or until spinach is wilted. Remove spinach, shaking off excess water, and place on a serving platter. Drizzle with lemon juice. Season with salt and pepper.

PER SERVING
Calories - 61
Protein - 3 g
Sodium - 210 mg
Carbohydrates - 6 g
Cholesterol - 0 mg
Total Fat - 4 g
Saturated Fat - 1 g
Dietary Fiber - 3 g

Nutrition Note: The vitamin C in the lemon juice helps your body absorb iron from the spinach.

Sautéed Spinach with Pine Nuts 4 servings

1 teaspoon extra-virgin olive oil
2 pounds fresh spinach, trimmed
2 tablespoons pine nuts
pinch coarse salt
pinch freshly ground black pepper

Heat olive oil in a nonstick skillet. Add spinach and cook over medium-high heat about 3 to 5 minutes, or just until wilted. Sprinkle with pine nuts. Season with salt and pepper.

Note: When selecting spinach, look for crisp, dark green leaves that *smell* like spinach.

PER SERVING
Calories - 94
Protein - 8 g
Sodium - 176 mg
Carbohydrates - 9 g
Cholesterol - 0 mg
Total Fat - 6 g
Saturated Fat - 1 g
Dietary Fiber - 6 g

Edamame 2 ½-cup servings

These Japanese soybeans are rich in isoflavones and contain all the essential amino acids. They make a delicious snack or hors d'oeuvre.

1 pound fresh or frozen edamame
1 teaspoon coarse salt

Bring 6 cups of water to a boil in a large saucepan. Add edamame; boil 2 minutes for fresh or 4 to 5 minutes for frozen. Drain and rinse. Sprinkle with salt. Serve hot or cold. To eat, push beans out of pods directly into your mouth.

PER SERVING
Calories - 120
Protein - 10 g
Sodium - 10 mg
Carbohydrates - 9 g
Cholesterol - 0 mg
Total Fat - 5 g
Saturated Fat - 1 g
Dietary Fiber - 4 g

Roasted Balsamic Red Onions 8 servings

4 small red onions, peeled and halved
olive oil cooking spray
1 tablespoon olive oil
1½ teaspoons balsamic vinegar
¼ teaspoon coarse salt
pinch coarsely ground black pepper

Arrange onions, cut side down, in a baking dish coated with cooking spray.

In a small bowl, whisk together oil, vinegar, salt and pepper. Drizzle over onions. Bake at 400°F for 1 hour, or until onions are tender.

Serve with roast chicken, turkey or beef.

PER SERVING
Calories - 29
Protein - 0 g
Sodium - 61 mg
Carbohydrates - 3 g
Cholesterol - 0 mg
Total Fat - 2 g
Saturated Fat - 0 g
Dietary Fiber - 1 g

Portobello Mushrooms 6 servings

Try portobellos grilled or in sandwiches, salads and stir-fries.

> *1 recipe Stir-Fry Sauce (page 310)*
> *½ pound portobello mushrooms, thinly sliced*
> *1 tablespoon olive oil*

Pour stir-fry sauce over mushrooms.
Marinate 10 to 15 minutes. Pour off marinade.

Heat olive oil in a nonstick skillet over medium-high heat. Add mushrooms. Stir fry 8 to 10 minutes, or until mushrooms are cooked.

PER SERVING
Calories - 36
Protein - 1 g
Sodium - 80 mg
Carbohydrates - 2 g
Cholesterol - 0 mg
Total Fat - 3 g
Saturated Fat - 0 g
Dietary Fiber - 1 g

Stir-Fried Wild Mushrooms 4 servings

> *2 teaspoons extra-virgin olive oil*
> *½ pound shiitake mushrooms, sliced ¼ inch thick**
> *3 garlic cloves, minced*
> *2 tablespoons reduced-sodium soy sauce*
> *2 tablespoons mirin (rice wine)*
> *2 tablespoons finely chopped fresh flat-leaf parsley*

Heat olive oil in a nonstick wok or skillet over medium-high heat. Add mushrooms and stir-fry 1 to 2 minutes. Add garlic and soy sauce, and cook 1 minute longer. Add wine and cook 1 to 2 minutes, or until sauce thickens slightly. Sprinkle with parsley.

PER SERVING
Calories - 61
Protein - 2 g
Sodium - 348 mg
Carbohydrates - 8 g
Cholesterol - 0 g
Total Fat - 3 g
Saturated Fat - 0 g
Dietary Fiber - 1 g

If fresh shiitake mushroom are not available, substitute one 2-ounce package dried shiitake mushrooms. To reconstitute, place mushrooms in a bowl and cover with boiling water. Let stand 30 to 35 minutes to soften. Remove stems. Drain, rinse and pat dry with paper towels.

■

Roasted Garlic   4 servings

4 whole heads garlic
4 tablespoons olive oil
dash coarse salt

Lay each head of garlic on its side and cut off ½ inch across the top. Place each head in an individual 5-inch ovenproof pie plate or ramekin. Drizzle with olive oil and cover with foil. Bake at 350°F for 45 to 60 minutes, or until garlic is tender when tested with a fork.

PER SERVING
Calories - 164
Protein - 2 g
Sodium - 65 mg
Carbohydrates - 10 g
Cholesterol - 0 mg
Total Fat - 14 g
Saturated Fat - 2 g
Dietary Fiber - 1 g

Using a fork, make a spread by releasing garlic from skins right onto baking dish. Stir into oil. Sprinkle with coarse salt. Spread onto bread, potatoes or vegetables.

Stir-Fried Peppers and Onion 4 servings

3 cloves garlic
1 medium white onion
1 large red bell pepper
1 large yellow bell pepper
1 large green bell pepper
1 tablespoon extra-virgin olive oil

Chop garlic. Cut onion in half, then slice again into ⅛-inch-thick half-rounds. Cut each pepper in half, then into julienne strips. Heat olive oil in a nonstick grill pan or skillet over medium heat. Add garlic and onions; sauté 10 minutes until onions are just tender. Add peppers; sauté 2 to 3 minutes longer, or until peppers are crisp-tender.

PER SERVING
Calories - 77
Protein - 2 g
Sodium - 4 mg
Carbohydrates - 11 g
Cholesterol - 0 mg
Total Fat - 4 g
Saturated Fat - 0 g
Dietary Fiber - 3 g

■

Grilled Parmesan Zucchini 4 servings

2 small zucchini
juice of ½ lemon
pinch coarse salt
pinch freshly ground pepper
1 tablespoon freshly grated Parmesan cheese

Cut zucchini lengthwise into quarters. Sprinkle with lemon juice, salt and pepper. Wrap in foil. Grill 10 to 15 minutes, or until hot and crisp-tender. Sprinkle with cheese.

PER SERVING
Calories - 15
Protein - 1 g
Sodium - 145 mg
Carbohydrates - 2 g
Cholesterol - 1 mg
Total Fat - 0 g
Saturated Fat - 0 g
Dietary Fiber - 1 g

Baked Stuffed Zucchini 5 servings

5 medium zucchini (about 8 inches long),
    halved lengthwise*
2 teaspoons olive oil
1 yellow onion, chopped
1 pound extra-lean ground beef
1 cup cooked Sticky Rice (page 378)
¾ teaspoon Lawry's seasoning salt
¼ teaspoon freshly ground black pepper
3 tablespoons freshly grated Parmesan cheese

Using a spoon, scoop out a trough down the center of each zucchini half. Arrange halves in an ovenproof casserole.

Heat olive oil in a nonstick skillet over medium-high heat. Add onion and sauté 6 to 8 minutes. Add ground beef and sauté 10 to 15 minutes longer, or until meat is cooked. Drain meat on paper toweling to remove excess fat.

Mix beef with cooked rice. Season with salt and pepper. Spoon mixture into zucchini boats. Cover with foil. Bake 60 minutes at 375°F. Remove foil for last 10 minutes. Sprinkle with cheese.

PER SERVING
Calories - 290
Protein - 22 g
Sodium - 110 mg
Carbohydrates - 19 g
Cholesterol - 59 mg
Total Fat - 14 g
Saturated Fat - 5 g
Dietary Fiber - 3 g

*The 8-inch zucchini are usually younger and have softer skins than the larger ones.

Nutrition Note: Zucchini is high in vitamins A and C, folic acid, niacin, magnesium and potassium.

Variation: Add 1 cup 20-Minute Marinara (page 350) to beef-and-rice mixture.

Grilled Parmesan Tomatoes 4 servings

For best flavor, always store tomatoes at room temperature.

> *2 ripe tomatoes, halved*
> *½ teaspoon extra-virgin olive oil*
> *pinch coarse salt*
> *pinch freshly ground pepper*
> *2 tablespoons chopped fresh basil*
> *2 teaspoons freshly grated Parmesan cheese*
> *or 1 teaspoon bread crumbs*

Brush tomatoes lightly with olive oil. Cook, cut side down, 3 to 5 minutes on a hot grill, rotating tomatoes for crisscross grill marks. Turn cut side up. Sprinkle with salt, pepper and basil. Top with cheese or bread crumbs. Grill 2 to 3 minutes longer.

PER SERVING
Calories - 22
Protein - 1 g
Sodium - 141 mg
Carbohydrates - 3 g
Cholesterol - 1 mg
Total Fat - 1 g
Saturated Fat - 0 g
Dietary Fiber - 1 g

Nutrition Note: Tomatoes are a rich source of vitamin C. They also contain vitamins A and B, iron, phosphorus and fiber.

Grill Basket Tomatoes   4 servings

2 cups red cherry or pear-shaped tomatoes
2 cups yellow or orange cherry or pear-shaped tomatoes
2 teaspoons extra-virgin olive oil
pinch coarse salt
pinch freshly ground black pepper
¼ cup chopped fresh basil leaves

Toss tomatoes in olive oil. Grill in a nonstick grill basket over hot coals 8 to 10 minutes, or until tomatoes are soft. Season with salt and pepper. Sprinkle with basil leaves.

PER SERVING
Calories - 57
Protein - 2 g
Sodium - 135 mg
Carbohydrates - 8 g
Cholesterol - 0 mg
Total Fat - 3 g
Saturated Fat - 0 g
Dietary Fiber - 2 g

Spinach-Stuffed Tomatoes   4 servings

¼ cup chopped onion
2 teaspoons olive oil
6 cups baby spinach leaves, chopped
½ cup nonfat sour cream
dash Tabasco sauce
4 medium tomatoes
3 tablespoons grated part-skim mozzarella cheese

Sauté onion in olive oil until tender; add spinach and cook 3 to 4 minutes. Cool; drain, squeezing excess water from spinach. Add sour cream and Tabasco sauce.

Cut tops off tomatoes and remove centers. Fill shells with spinach mixture. Bake at 375°F for 20 to 25 minutes. Sprinkle with cheese.

PER SERVING
Calories - 103
Protein - 5 g
Sodium - 99 mg
Carbohydrates - 13 g
Cholesterol - 6 mg
Total Fat - 4 g
Saturated Fat - 1 g
Dietary Fiber - 3 g

Tomato and Basil Skewers Makes 8 skewers

This is a filling late-afternoon snack. Try it with a spicy tomato drink.

8 6-inch wooden skewers
½ cup fresh small basil leaves
16 pear or grape tomatoes
8 bocconcini (small mozzarella balls), halved
16 pitted kalamata olives

On each skewer, thread a basil leaf, a tomato, another basil leaf, a mozzarella ball, a basil leaf, 2 olives, a basil leaf and a tomato.

Variation: Add diced red or yellow peppers, quartered artichoke hearts, cubed cucumbers or peperoncini.

PER SERVING
Calories - 58
Protein - 3 g
Sodium - 243 mg
Carbohydrates - 3 g
Cholesterol - 5 mg
Total Fat - 5 g
Saturated Fat - 1 g
Dietary Fiber - 0 g

■

Roast Fingerling Potatoes 6 servings

1½ pounds fingerling potatoes with skins
2 whole heads garlic
3 tablespoons olive oil

Scrub potatoes. Cut in half lengthwise.
Lay each head of garlic on its side and cut off about ½ inch straight across the top. Separate the cloves but do not peel.
Toss potatoes and garlic with olive oil; arrange in a single layer in a nonstick roasting pan. Bake at 425°F for 45 to 50 minutes, turning once.

PER SERVING
Calories - 106
Protein - 3 g
Sodium - 7 mg
Carbohydrates - 10 g
Cholesterol - 0 mg
Total Fat - 7 g
Saturated Fat - 1 g
Dietary Fiber - 3 g

Roast Red Potatoes   6 servings

It's a shame that potatoes have gotten such a bad rap! Tucked inside their jackets are all sorts of good things, including potassium and vitamins B_6 and C.

1 pound tiny red potatoes with skins, halved
2 tablespoons extra-virgin olive oil
1 head garlic cloves, peeled
½ teaspoon coarse salt
¼ teaspoon freshly ground black pepper

Move oven rack to second-highest position. Preheat oven to 425°F. Place potatoes in a nonstick roasting pan. Toss with olive oil. Turn each potato cut side up. Bake for 15 minutes. Remove pan from oven. Using a fork, gently turn potatoes cut side down. Tuck garlic cloves among potatoes. Put back in oven and bake 40 minutes longer, or until potatoes are golden brown. Season with salt and pepper.

PER SERVING
Calories - 67
Protein - 2 g
Sodium - 166 mg
Carbohydrates - 6 g
Cholesterol - 0 mg
Total Fat - 5 g
Saturated Fat - 1 g
Dietary Fiber - 2 g

Variation: Add 2 tablespoons of fresh rosemary sprigs just before baking.

Jalapeño-Stuffed Potatoes 4 servings

2 large baking potatoes

1½ teaspoons extra-virgin olive oil

8 sprigs fresh rosemary

1 small white onion, finely chopped

*2 tablespoons finely chopped pickled jalapeño
    nacho rings*

¼ cup low-fat (1%) buttermilk

½ cup nonfat sour cream

2 tablespoons chopped green onions

¼ cup shredded reduced-fat cheddar cheese

¼ cup shredded part-skim mozzarella cheese

Scrub potatoes; cut in half lengthwise. Lay each potato half, cut side down, on a piece of aluminum foil. Drizzle with ½ teaspoon of the olive oil and rub each half on all sides with the oil. Tuck 2 sprigs of rosemary under each half and wrap in aluminum foil. Bake at 325°F for 30 to 40 minutes, or until tender.

PER SERVING
Calories - 140
Protein - 7 g
Sodium - 162 mg
Carbohydrates - 23 g
Cholesterol - 3 mg
Total Fat - 2 g
Saturated Fat - 0 g
Dietary Fiber - 2 g

In a nonstick skillet, heat remaining teaspoon of olive oil. Add onion and sauté 3 to 5 minutes. Toss with jalapeño rings in a bowl and set aside.

Carefully scoop the insides of each potato half into a large bowl, leaving a thin shell.* Using a potato masher or electric mixer, mash hot potatoes thoroughly until no lumps remain. Gradually beat in buttermilk until potatoes are smooth and fluffy. Gently stir in sour cream, green onions, sautéed onions and jalapeños. Divide potato mixture among 4 potato shells. Top with cheddar and mozzarella. Rebake potatoes at 350°F for about 10 minutes, or until the cheese melts.

*If potato shells fall apart when you scoop out the insides, just piece them together as best you can before placing the mashed potatoes on top. Once the cheese melts, they'll look perfect.

■

Herbed Dijon Potatoes   6 servings

5 tablespoons Dijon mustard
3 tablespoons olive oil
1 teaspoon minced garlic
½ teaspoon Italian seasoning
6 medium red potatoes with skins,
    cut into chunks
olive oil cooking spray

Combine mustard, olive oil, garlic and Italian seasoning. Pour over potatoes and toss.

Spray an ovenproof casserole dish with olive oil. Arrange potatoes in dish. Bake at 375°F for 40 to 50 minutes, or until potatoes are tender.

PER SERVING
Calories - 124
Protein - 5 g
Sodium - 155 mg
Carbohydrates - 12 g
Cholesterol - 0 mg
Total Fat - 7 g
Saturated Fat - 1 g
Dietary Fiber - 5 g

Potatoes with Sour Cream and Cottage Cheese 4 servings

You won't miss the butter when you discover how much flavor the fresh rosemary adds. You'll also be surprised by the satisfying taste of a topping made with sour cream and cottage cheese.

2 large russet potatoes with skins
1 teaspoon extra-virgin olive oil
8 sprigs fresh rosemary
pinch coarse salt
pinch freshly ground black pepper
¼ cup chopped fresh chives
¼ cup nonfat sour cream
¼ cup nonfat cottage cheese

Scrub potatoes; cut in half lengthwise. Lay each half, cut side down, on a piece of aluminum foil; rub on all sides with olive oil. Tuck 2 sprigs of rosemary under each potato half and wrap in foil. Bake at 425°F for 30 to 40 minutes, or until tender. Season with salt and pepper.

Place chives in a small ramekin. Combine sour cream and cottage cheese in a small bowl. Pass ramekin and bowl with potatoes.

PER SERVING
Calories - 102
Protein - 7 g
Sodium - 118 mg
Carbohydrates - 17 g
Cholesterol - 1 mg
Total Fat - 1 g
Saturated Fat - 0 g
Dietary Fiber - 1 g

Jumbo Oven Fries 4 servings

Our fries have less than a quarter the fat of regular fries and more real food flavor. Keeping the skins on ensures vitamin C and other nutrients.

> *3 large russet potatoes with skins,*
> > *quartered*
> *2 tablespoons extra-virgin olive oil*
> *pinch coarse salt*

Preheat oven to 400°F. Move oven rack to highest position. Cut each potato quarter lengthwise into ¼-inch strips. Place in a pie plate and toss with olive oil.

Arrange potatoes, on a nonstick baking sheet. Roast 20 minutes, or until brown. Using a metal spatula, turn potatoes and bake 10 to 15 minutes longer, until tender and evenly brown on all sides. Sprinkle with salt.

PER SERVING
Calories - 119
Protein - 5 g
Sodium - 16 mg
Carbohydrates - 12 g
Cholesterol - 0 mg
Total Fat - 7 g
Saturated Fat - 1 g
Dietary Fiber - 5 g

Variation: Prepare as directed above. After tossing with olive oil, sprinkle with 2 to 3 tablespoons fresh rosemary sprigs and salt and pepper to taste.

Country Fried Potatoes with Garlic 4 servings

1¹/₂ tablespoons extra-virgin olive oil
1¹/₂ tablespoons minced garlic
4 medium red potatoes with skins
    (about 1 pound), very thinly sliced

In a nonstick skillet, heat olive oil over medium-high heat. Add garlic and potatoes; sauté 4 to 5 minutes, turning frequently. Reduce heat to medium and partially cover with lid so steam can escape; cook 8 to 10 minutes longer, turning frequently. When potatoes are tender, remove lid and reduce heat to low; sauté 2 to 3 minutes longer, or until nicely browned.

PER SERVING
Calories - 124
Protein - 2 g
Sodium - 6 mg
Carbohydrates - 16 g
Cholesterol - 0 mg
Total Fat - 6 g
Saturated Fat - 1 g
Dietary Fiber - 1 g

Yukon Gold Smashed Potatoes

4 servings

Yukon Golds are excellent boiling potatoes with a smooth texture.

*4 pounds Yukon Gold potatoes
    with skins
2 tablespoons olive oil
1/3 cup warm nonfat milk
1/2 teaspoon coarse salt or to taste
1/4 teaspoon freshly ground
    black pepper*

Scrub and rinse potatoes; place in a large saucepan and cover with water. Bring to a boil, reduce heat and simmer, uncovered, 15 to 20 minutes until just tender.

    Drain potatoes in a colander; cover with a dish towel and let sit for 5 minutes. Cut potatoes into quarters and place in a medium bowl; toss with olive oil. Smash with a potato masher. Add warm milk; beat with a fork until creamy. Season with salt and pepper. Reheat quickly, if necessary, and pile lightly in a hot dish.

PER SERVING
Calories - 122
Protein - 5 g
Sodium - 266 mg
Carbohydrates - 12 g
Cholesterol - 0 mg
Total Fat - 7 g
Saturated Fat - 1 g
Dietary Fiber - 5 g

Turnip Fries 4 servings

2 whole turnips with skins
2 tablespoons olive oil
¼ teaspoon coarse salt
pinch freshly ground black pepper

Preheat oven to broil. Arrange oven rack in position between center and top of oven.

Cut turnips into thick wedges; place in a pie plate and toss in oil until lightly coated. Arrange turnips in a single layer on a nonstick baking sheet and broil 20 minutes, turning two or three times until tender. Remove to serving plate. Season with salt and pepper.

Cook's Suggestion: Serve turnip fries with ketchup or dip in coarse salt and apple cider vinegar.

Variation: Use parsnips instead of turnips. Depending on the thickness, you may need to shorten the cooking time by a few minutes.

PER SERVING
Calories - 76
Protein - 5 g
Sodium - 161 mg
Carbohydrates - 4 g
Cholesterol - 0 mg
Total Fat - 7 g
Saturated Fat - 1 g
Dietary Fiber - 1 g

Roasted Root Vegetables 6 servings

These vitamin-rich vegetables always look so beautiful in the
supermarket during the fall and winter. Take them home and cook
them according to this simple recipe.

1 cup 1-inch cubes carrots
1 cup 1-inch cubes parsnips
1 cup 1-inch cubes turnips
1 cup 1-inch cubes sweet potato
1 cup 1-inch cubes butternut squash
1½ tablespoons olive oil
¼ teaspoon coarse salt
¼ teaspoon freshly ground black pepper
½ cup finely chopped basil

Place vegetables in a bowl; add olive oil and
toss to coat.

Arrange vegetables in a single layer on
a nonstick baking sheet. Roast in a 425°F
oven for 30 minutes, or until tender. Remove
to a warm serving plate. Season with salt and
pepper. Sprinkle with basil.

PER SERVING
Calories - 96
Protein - 1 g
Sodium - 108 mg
Carbohydrates - 16 g
Cholesterol - 0 mg
Total Fat - 4 g
Saturated Fat - 0 g
Dietary Fiber - 3 g

Cook's Suggestion: For roasted vegetable soup, heat the leftovers
in 2 cups of chicken broth for every 2 cups of vegetables.

Asian Stir-Fry with Noodles   4 servings

Stir-fries are the perfect way to incorporate high-protein soy into your eating plan. The tofu in this recipe soaks up the sauce and flavors it.

NOODLES

1 10-ounce package firm tofu

1 15-ounce can chicken broth

2 cups water

1 8-ounce package soba noodles

1 tablespoon sesame oil

SAUCE

1 cup chicken broth

1 tablespoon plus 1 teaspoon cornstarch

2 tablespoons reduced-sodium soy sauce

1 teaspoon spicy Thai chili sauce

  (2 teaspoons for extra-spicy flavor)

VEGETABLES

1 tablespoon extra-virgin olive oil

1 tablespoon peeled and minced fresh ginger

2 cups broccoli or broccolini florets and stems, chopped

1 cup chopped red pepper

2 cups snow peas, ends and strings removed

6 white mushrooms sliced

½ cup chopped green onions

Cut tofu in half lengthwise and place halves on a dinner plate. Cover with multiple layers of paper towel, then place a heavy object on top to force water out of tofu. Let sit 15 to 20 minutes.

   In a medium saucepan, bring broth and water to a boil. Add noodles and cook

PER SERVING
Calories - 259
Protein - 13 g
Sodium - 716 mg
Carbohydrates - 40 g
Cholesterol - 0 mg
Total Fat - 7 g
Saturated Fat - 1 g
Dietary Fiber - 4 g

6 to 8 minutes, or until just tender. Drain. Transfer to a serving bowl. Toss with sesame oil. Set aside.

To make the sauce, combine one cup chicken broth with cornstarch in a small saucepan; stir until smooth and no lumps remain. Stir in soy sauce and chili sauce. Bring to a boil, stirring constantly until sauce thickens slightly. Set aside on stovetop to keep warm.

To stir-fry vegetables, preheat a nonstick wok or skillet over medium-high heat. When pan is hot, add olive oil. When oil is hot, add ginger; stir-fry 30 seconds. Add broccoli or broccolini, red pepper and snow peas; stir-fry 2 minutes. Add mushrooms and green onions; stir-fry 1 to 3 minutes. Remove tofu from covering and slice into 1-inch cubes; add to stir-fry. Stir gently 2 to 3 minutes. Pour vegetables over noodles and toss.

Variation: Replace tofu with ¾ pound cubed skinless, boneless chicken breast or ¾ pound cooked medium prawns.

Ginger Stir-Fry   4 servings

1 teaspoon extra-virgin olive oil

½ teaspoon Asian sesame oil

3 medium carrots, cut diagonally into
    ⅛-inch-thick slices

3 large garlic cloves, thinly sliced

¼ cup chicken broth, preferably homemade
    (page 240)

1 teaspoon peeled, minced fresh ginger

½ pound snow peas, ends and strings removed

1 red pepper, seeded and cut into
    ½-inch-wide strips

1 tablespoon reduced-sodium soy sauce

⅛ teaspoon crushed red pepper (optional)

Preheat a nonstick wok or skillet over high heat. When wok is hot, add olive oil and sesame oil. When oils are hot, add carrots and garlic; stir-fry, uncovered, 1 minute. Add broth, cover and cook 3 minutes. Add ginger, snow peas and red pepper; cook, covered, 1 minute longer, or until vegetables are crisp-tender. Drizzle with soy sauce. Sprinkle with crushed red pepper, if desired.

PER SERVING
Calories - 76
Protein - 3 g
Sodium - 235 mg
Carbohydrates - 3 g
Cholesterol - 0 mg
Total Fat - 2 g
Saturated Fat - 0 g
Dietary Fiber - 4 g

Grilled Vegetables 4 servings

2 red bell peppers, cut into eighths
1 yellow, orange or green bell pepper,
    cut into eighths
2 red onions sliced into 1/2-inch rings

OR

1/2 pound asparagus, tough ends removed
18 to 20 cherry tomatoes

OR

1 medium zucchini, sliced into 1/4-inch ovals
1 white onion, cut into 1/2-inch rings

1 tablespoon extra-virgin olive oil
1 1/2 teaspoons coarse salt
1 teaspoon freshly ground black pepper

Choose one of the vegetable combinations above (or try your own) and toss with the olive oil, salt and pepper. Grill in a grill basket over high heat about 15 to 20 minutes, turning every 5 minutes. Cook until vegetables are soft and slightly charred.

PER SERVING
Calories - 123
Protein - 4 g
Sodium - 494 mg
Carbohydrates - 21 g
Cholesterol - 0 g
Total Fat - 4 g
Saturated Fat - 1 g
Dietary Fiber - 6 g

Grilled Vegetable Skewers

4 servings

Add more essential antioxidants to your day with these quick-to-fix vegetable skewers.

> *juice of ½ lemon*
> *½ tablespoon olive oil*
> *6 cloves garlic, chopped*
> *¼ teaspoon coarse salt*
> *⅛ teaspoon freshly ground black pepper*
> *8 cherry tomatoes*
> *12 fresh shiitake or cremini mushrooms,*
> *   trimmed*
> *1 red pepper, seeded and cut into eighths*
> *1 orange or yellow pepper, seeded and*
> *   cut into eighths*
> *4 yellow squash or yellow sunburst squash,*
> *   cut into 2-inch cubes*

Combine lemon juice, olive oil, garlic, salt and pepper in a shallow baking dish. Add vegetables; toss lightly to coat with marinade. Let stand in marinade 30 minutes. Drain, reserving marinade. Alternate vegetables on skewers. Grill 4 inches from heat 10 to 12 minutes, turning often and basting frequently with marinade.

PER SERVING
Calories - 58
Protein - 3 g
Sodium - 127 mg
Carbohydrates - 10 g
Cholesterol - 0 mg
Total Fat - 2 g
Saturated Fat - 0 g
Dietary Fiber - 2 g

Cook's Suggestion: Serve with couscous and Grilled Lamb Skewers (page 442).

Raw Veggies in a Basket

6 servings

No matter your age, nothing's more fun than dipping food that's really good for you into something that's really tasty. And by arranging the vegetables in a pretty basket, you have a perfect party appetizer packed with health.

> *16 baby carrots or 4 larger carrots,*
> *peeled and cut into thirds*
> *4 stalks celery, trimmed and cut into thirds*
> *1 bunch green onions, trimmed*
> *1 small bunch radishes, rinsed and trimmed*
> *1 small summer squash, cut crosswise*
> *into rings*
> *1 English cucumber, cut crosswise*
> *into rings*
> *8 cherry tomatoes, halved*
> *2 cups sugar snap peas*
> *1 red pepper, julienned*
> *1 yellow pepper, julienned*
> *1 small bunch fresh spinach,*
> *rinsed and trimmed*

Chill vegetables. Arrange in a spinach-lined basket.

Variations: Other options include blanched green beans or asparagus, daikon radishes or jicama strips.

PER SERVING
Calories - 55
Protein - 2 g
Sodium - 52 mg
Carbohydrates - 10 g
Cholesterol - 0 mg
Total Fat - 0 g
Saturated Fat - 0 g
Dietary Fiber - 3 g

(continued on next page)

Serving Suggestions: Raw veggies are delicious with Guacamole (page 314), Pico de Gallo (page 315), Tuscan Bean Dip (page 311), Black Bean Dip (page 310) or Layered Shrimp Dip (page 311). They're also a great complement to saucy entrées such as Classic Lasagna (page 304) and Mac and Cheese (page 366). Encourage your family to dip the vegetables into the sauce.

Pasta and Fixings

Five-Star Marinara Sauce · Makes 2 quarts

2 tablespoons olive oil

2 cups finely chopped yellow onion

3 garlic cloves, minced

1 28-ounce can plum tomatoes, including liquid,
   diced

4 cups water

1 6-ounce can tomato paste

2 tablespoons chopped fresh basil

¾ teaspoon oregano

½ teaspoon coarse salt or to taste

¼ teaspoon coarsely ground fresh pepper

Heat olive oil in a nonstick skillet over medium heat. Add onion and cook 8 to 10 minutes, or until translucent. Add garlic and cook 2 to 3 minutes longer.

Heat tomatoes and remaining ingredients over medium-high heat in a large saucepan. Add onion and garlic. Reduce heat and simmer 1 hour.

PER 2 CUPS
Calories - 138
Protein - 4 g
Sodium - 881 mg
Carbohydrates - 18 g
Cholesterol - 0 mg
Total Fat - 7 g
Saturated Fat - 1 g
Dietary Fiber - 4 g

Sodium Alert: Be sure to eat low-sodium foods throughout the day to balance the sodium in the marinara sauce.

Cook's Suggestion: If you're lucky enough to have leftover sauce, you can make Chicken and Polenta (page 417).

A NOTE ABOUT STORE-BOUGHT CANNED TOMATO PRODUCTS

Many of our recipes call for canned Italian plum tomatoes. The better the grade, the more flavorful the sauce. For recipes that call for diced plum tomatoes, buy the whole plum tomatoes and dice them yourself.

Store-bought tomato sauce, tomato puree and tomato paste should also be of the highest grade available. Freeze any leftover paste by the tablespoonful on a sheet of waxed paper; once frozen, remove to a plastic freezer bag and store in the freezer for later use.

20-Minute Marinara   Makes 3½ cups

1 28-ounce can Italian-style peeled tomatoes
  with basil, diced
2 tablespoons extra-virgin olive oil
10 fresh basil leaves
1 teaspoon finely chopped fresh oregano or
  ½ teaspoon dried
¾ teaspoon coarse salt or to taste
½ teaspoon freshly ground black pepper

Combine all ingredients in a medium saucepan. Heat to almost boiling. Reduce heat to low and simmer 10 minutes.

Variation: While sauce is simmering, add ½ cup pitted and sliced kalamata olives and a 17-ounce can of mushroom stems and pieces, drained.

PER SERVING
Calories - 118
Protein - 2 g
Sodium - 814 mg
Carbohydrates - 14 g
Cholesterol - 0 mg
Total Fat - 7 g
Saturated Fat - 1 g
Dietary Fiber - 2 g

Chunky Meat Sauce 8 servings

This variation on the classic bolognese sauce has been passed down
in our family through several generations.

> 1 tablespoon olive oil
> 1 yellow onion, coarsely chopped
> 10 garlic cloves, minced
> 1 cup sliced fresh mushrooms
> 1 pound extra-lean ground beef, shaped into a large patty
> 1 28-ounce can plum tomatoes, including liquid,
>   diced
> 1 tablespoon dried basil or 1/4 cup chopped fresh
> 3/4 teaspoon dried oregano
> 3/4 teaspoon coarse salt
> 1/4 teaspoon coarsely ground black pepper
> 1/4 teaspoon crushed red pepper flakes

Heat olive oil in a nonstick skillet over
medium heat; add onion and sauté 8 to 10
minutes, or until translucent. Add garlic and
mushrooms; sauté 2 to 3 minutes longer.

Add whole patty of ground beef and sauté
3 to 4 minutes; turn and sauté 3 to 4 minutes
longer, keeping patty whole as long as
possible. Add diced canned tomatoes, basil,
oregano, salt, black pepper and red pepper flakes. Reduce heat
and simmer 1 hour. (The meat will start to just fall apart on its own.)
Stir gently to mix.

PER SERVING
Calories - 181
Protein - 12 g
Sodium - 371 mg
Carbohydrates - 8 g
Cholesterol - 39 mg
Total Fat - 12 g
Saturated Fat - 4 g
Dietary Fiber - 2 g

Penne with Veal Sauce   8 servings

Adding ground veal to a classic red sauce turns a lean pasta dish into a hearty supper.

> 1 pound penne
> 1 28-ounce can plum tomatoes,
>   including liquid, diced
> 1 15-ounce can tomato sauce
> 1/4 cup dry white wine
> 1 1/2 teaspoons extra-virgin olive oil
> 2 garlic cloves, minced
> 1/2 pound lean ground veal
> 1/2 cup chopped fresh basil
> pinch coarse salt
> pinch freshly ground black pepper

Cook penne according to package directions. Drain and set aside. Meanwhile, in a 4-quart saucepan, heat tomatoes, tomato sauce and wine; allow to simmer while cooking the veal.

In a nonstick skillet, heat olive oil; add garlic and ground veal. Sauté until veal is cooked. Drain excess fat; pat veal with paper towels to remove any remaining fat. Add veal to sauce. Season with basil, salt and pepper.

Divide penne into individual bowls; top with sauce.

PER SERVING
Calories - 288
Protein - 4 g
Sodium - 460 mg
Carbohydrates - 49 g
Cholesterol - 22 g
Total Fat - 4 g
Saturated Fat - 1 g
Dietary Fiber - 4 g

Pasta with Pesto and Tomatoes

8 servings

We make a lot of pesto in the summer, when basil is readily available. This is our favorite recipe for the first batch.

> *1 pound rotelle*
> *1¼ cups fresh Pesto (page 309)*
> *3 large ripe tomatoes, diced*
> *¼ cup freshly grated Parmesan cheese*

Cook rotelle 10 to 12 minutes, or until al dente. Drain in a colander and toss in a large bowl with pesto. Add tomatoes. Sprinkle with cheese.

PER SERVING
Calories - 355
Protein - 10 g
Sodium - 177 mg
Carbohydrates - 47 g
Cholesterol - 2 mg
Total Fat - 14 g
Saturated Fat - 2 g
Dietary Fiber - 3 g

Penne with Sun-Dried Tomatoes

8 servings

Make this dish in the summertime, when tomatoes and fresh basil are at their peak.

4 large ripe tomatoes, coarsely chopped
10 oil-packed sun-dried tomatoes, drained
        and coarsely chopped
6 large garlic cloves, chopped
¼ cup extra-virgin olive oil
½ teaspoon coarse salt
¼ teaspoon freshly ground pepper
1½ cups fresh basil leaves
1 pound penne
crushed red pepper (optional)

Combine ripe and sun-dried tomatoes, garlic, olive oil, salt and pepper. Let stand 1 hour at room temperature. Coarsely chop 1 cup of the basil leaves; reserve remaining leaves for garnish.

PER SERVING
Calories - 299
Protein - 10 g
Sodium - 197 mg
Carbohydrates - 46 g
Cholesterol - 0 g
Total Fat - 10 g
Saturated Fat - 1 g
Dietary Fiber - 3 g

Cook penne according to package directions; drain. While still hot, toss with tomato mixture. Add chopped basil and toss again. Just before serving, garnish with remaining basil leaves. Accompany with crushed red pepper, if desired.

Mostaccioli with Fresh Tomatoes and Basil   8 servings

6 large ripe tomatoes
1½ cups fresh basil
6 large garlic cloves, minced
⅓ cup olive oil
¾ teaspoon salt
¼ teaspoon pepper
1 pound mostaccioli or other tube-shaped pasta
1 cup freshly grated Parmesan cheese

Cut tomatoes into ½-inch chunks. Coarsely chop 1 cup of the basil leaves; reserve the remaining leaves for garnish. Combine tomatoes with chopped basil; add garlic, olive oil, salt and pepper; toss. Let stand for 1 hour at room temperature.

Cook pasta according to package directions; drain. Toss with tomatoes while still hot. Sprinkle with cheese. Garnish with remaining ½ cup basil.

PER SERVING
Calories - 373
Protein - 14 g
Sodium - 422 mg
Carbohydrates - 49 g
Cholesterol - 10 g
Total Fat - 14 g
Saturated Fat - 4 g
Dietary Fiber - 3 g

Spaghetti with Meatballs 10 servings

BASIC TOMATO SAUCE
1 28-ounce can plum tomatoes
1 28-ounce can tomato puree
1 12-ounce can tomato paste
1 8-ounce can tomato sauce
3 cups water
1½ teaspoons salt
2 tablespoons chopped fresh basil
*   or 1½ teaspoons dried*
1½ tablespoons minced fresh oregano leaves
*   or ¾ teaspoon dried*
½ pound pork loin chops, bone in

1 pound leanest ground beef
1 cup dry bread crumbs
5 cloves garlic, finely minced
1 egg
¼ cup nonfat milk
½ cup chopped fresh parsley
salt and pepper to taste
2 pounds spaghetti or corkscrew-shaped pasta
fresh basil sprigs for garnish
crushed red pepper (optional)

In a food processor, puree tomatoes until smooth; transfer to a stockpot. Add canned tomato puree, tomato paste, tomato sauce, water, salt, basil and oregano. Stir thoroughly to combine ingredients. Heat sauce just to boiling (do not allow to boil). Reduce to a simmer. Meanwhile, trim all visible fat from

PER SERVING
Calories - 584
Protein - 32 g
Sodium - 737 mg
Carbohydrates - 88 g
Cholesterol - 64 mg
Total Fat - 13 g
Saturated Fat - 3 g
Dietary Fiber - 8 g

pork chops. In a nonstick skillet, brown chops 3 to 4 minutes on each side. Remove from skillet and drain on paper towels; pat dry with additional paper toweling to remove all excess fat. Add chops to sauce as it cooks.

Place ground beef in a medium bowl. Add bread crumbs, garlic, egg, milk, parsley, salt and pepper. Knead until mixture is smooth, adding more milk if needed for moisture. Form 20 firm meatballs and add to sauce. Simmer 2 to 2½ hours longer. Remove the pork bones, breaking the meat into pieces in the sauce.

Cook pasta according to package directions. Drain and transfer to a pasta bowl. Pour one cup of the sauce over the top—just enough for color. Garnish with basil sprigs. Serve with meatballs and additional sauce. Accompany with crushed red pepper, if desired.

Sauce Variations: For a vegetarian sauce, omit pork chops and meatballs. (You'll also save 106 calories and 5 grams of fat.)

SAUSAGE AND MEATBALL SAUCE FOR SPECIAL OCCASIONS. In a nonstick skillet over medium-high heat, sauté 6 extra-lean Italian sausages 8 to 10 minutes or microwave on full power in a covered dish 8 to 10 minutes, turning once. Drain and pat with paper towels. Cut each sausage crosswise into thirds. Add to spaghetti sauce along with the meatballs. Simmer as directed above. Add 97 calories and 7 grams of fat per ⅓ sausage.

Penne alla Puttanesca   8 servings

1 tablespoon olive oil
1 cup chopped onion
5 cloves garlic, minced
1 28-ounce can Italian-style peeled tomatoes
  with basil
1 tablespoon chopped fresh basil
1 2-ounce can anchovy fillets, drained
½ teaspoon coarse salt
3 tablespoons capers, drained and rinsed
1 pound penne, cooked al dente
½ cup pitted and halved kalamata olives
¼ cup grated pecorino romano or
  Parmesan cheese
fresh basil for garnish
¼ teaspoon crushed red pepper (optional)

Heat olive oil in a nonstick skillet over medium-high heat. Add onion and garlic, and sauté 6 to 8 minutes, or until onions are tender. Spoon into food processor. Add tomatoes, basil and anchovies, and process 2 to 3 minutes until mixture is smooth. Pour into medium saucepan. Heat just to boiling; reduce heat and simmer 10 to 15 minutes.

PER SERVING
Calories - 309
Protein - 13 g
Sodium - 840 mg
Carbohydrates - 49 g
Cholesterol - 3 g
Total Fat - 8 g
Saturated Fat - 0 g
Dietary Fiber - 4 g

Season with salt. Add capers. Serve penne into pasta bowls. Ladle sauce over top; garnish with olives. Sprinkle with cheese. Garnish with basil. Season with crushed red pepper, if desired.

Sodium Alert: This dish is high in sodium. Serve it with low-sodium accompaniments or decrease the sodium by omitting the anchovies.

Shells with Olive Sauce 8 servings

*1 pound pennette (little penne), little shells
   or gemelli*
1 tablespoon olive oil
1 teaspoon crushed hot red pepper flakes
2 large garlic cloves, minced
½ cup finely chopped onion
2 cups tomato sauce
½ cup pitted and chopped kalamata olives
1 tablespoon capers, drained and rinsed
10 large basil leaves

Cook pasta according to package directions; drain. Meanwhile, heat olive oil in a nonstick skillet. Add pepper flakes and garlic; cook 2 to 3 minutes, or until garlic begins to soften. Add onion and sauté 2 to 3 minutes longer. Add tomato sauce; heat just to boiling and reduce heat; simmer 5 minutes.

   Just before serving, add olives and capers. Divide pasta among individual pasta bowls. Ladle sauce over top. Garnish with basil.

PER SERVING
Calories - 258
Protein - 10 g
Sodium - 340 mg
Carbohydrates - 46 g
Cholesterol - 0 g
Total Fat - 4 g
Saturated Fat - 0 g
Dietary Fiber - 3 g

Rotelle with Prawns, Tomatoes and Olives 8 servings

It looks like you've been cooking for hours, but this dish can be prepped and on the table in the time it takes to cook the pasta. Perfect for family or a last-minute dinner with friends.

1 pound rotelle or other tube-shaped pasta
2 teaspoons Garlic Olive Oil (page 306)
  or 2 teaspoons extra-virgin olive oil
  plus 2 minced garlic cloves
1 pound large prawns, shelled and deveined
¼ cup extra-virgin olive oil
2 tablespoons balsamic vinegar
3 large garlic cloves
1 teaspoon coarse salt
½ teaspoon freshly ground pepper
3 cups fresh basil
1½ pounds ripe tomatoes, cut into 1-inch cubes
1 cup pitted and halved kalamata olives*

Cook pasta until al dente. Keep warm in serving bowl.

In a nonstick skillet over medium-high heat, heat garlic olive oil; add prawns and cook 5 to 6 minutes, or until prawns are done. Remove from heat.

In a blender or food processor, combine olive oil, vinegar, garlic, salt, pepper and 2 cups of the basil; whirl 1 minute. Pour over warm pasta. Add tomatoes and olives; toss. Add prawns; toss again. Garnish with remaining basil.

PER SERVING
Calories - 496
Protein - 25 g
Sodium - 1013 mg
Carbohydrates - 62 g
Cholesterol - 107 mg
Total Fat - 16 g
Saturated Fat - 1 g
Dietary Fiber - 4 g

*If sodium is a concern for you, cut down on the olives.

Orecchiette with Sausage   8 servings

A good way to enjoy the taste of sausage without all the calories and fat involved in an entrée-size portion.

> *1 pound orecchiette or medium shell-shaped pasta*
> *3/4 pound extra-lean sweet Italian sausage*
> *4 medium garlic cloves, minced*
> *1 28-ounce can plum tomatoes, including liquid,*
> *   diced*
> *2 tablespoons tomato paste*
> *1 1/2 teaspoons minced fresh oregano or*
> *   1/2 teaspoon dried*
> *2 tablespoons chopped fresh basil or*
> *   1/2 teaspoon dried*
> *1/2 teaspoon salt*
> *1/4 teaspoon pepper*
> *1/8 to 1/4 teaspoon crushed red pepper (optional)*
> *fresh basil leaves for garnish*

Cook pasta according to package directions. Drain and set aside.

Slit open, remove and discard the sausage casing. In a preheated nonstick skillet over medium heat, brown sausage 6 to 8 minutes, or until cooked, breaking it apart as it browns. Drain on paper towels; pat dry with additional toweling to remove all excess fat. Set aside.

PER SERVING
Calories - 346
Protein - 17 g
Sodium - 629 mg
Carbohydrates - 45 g
Cholesterol - 33 mg
Total Fat - 9 g
Saturated Fat - 1 g
Dietary Fiber - 3 g

In a medium saucepan, combine garlic, tomatoes, tomato paste, oregano, basil, salt, pepper and crushed red pepper, if desired. Simmer 10 to 15 minutes. Stir sausage into sauce. Serve over pasta. Garnish with basil leaves.

Linguine with Clam Sauce 8 servings

Tired of the same old spaghetti sauce? Here's a quick, tasty variation on a red sauce. It's delicious even without the fresh clams.

1 pound linguine

1 28-ounce can plum tomatoes, including liquid, diced

1½ tablespoons extra-virgin olive oil

4 large garlic cloves, finely minced

1 cup dry white wine

¾ teaspoon coarse salt

¼ teaspoon freshly ground black pepper

2 6½-ounce cans chopped clams with liquid

2 pounds fresh manila, littleneck or butter clams

½ cup hot water

¼ cup chopped fresh Italian parsley

crushed red pepper (optional)

Cook linguine according to package directions; drain and set aside. Meanwhile, in a 1½-quart saucepan, combine tomatoes, olive oil, garlic, wine, salt, pepper and chopped clams. Simmer, uncovered, 15 to 20 minutes.

Scrub and wash clams (see page 406). Place in steamer with water; cover tightly and steam 5 to 10 minutes, or until clams open. Discard unopened clams.

Divide linguine among individual pasta bowls; ladle sauce over pasta. Top with steamed clams in their shells. Sprinkle with parsley. Accompany with red pepper, if desired.

Cook's Suggestion: Accompany with Roasted Garlic Bread (page 468) to sop up the sauce.

PER SERVING

Calories - 348

Protein - 22 g

Sodium - 439 mg

Carbohydrates - 50 g

Cholesterol - 36 mg

Total Fat - 4 g

Saturated Fat - 0 g

Dietary Fiber - 3 g

Linguine with Shrimp 8 servings

It's hard to believe that something this good can be on the table
in 30 minutes or less!

1 pound linguine
¼ cup olive oil
½ cup finely chopped green onion
3 cloves garlic, minced
1½ pound peeled (tails left on), deveined, cooked
  medium shrimp
¼ cup lemon juice
¼ cup chopped fresh basil
¼ cup chopped fresh Italian parsley
1 teaspoon coarse salt
½ teaspoon freshly ground black pepper
⅓ cup freshly grated Parmesan cheese (optional)

Cook pasta al dente according to package
directions. Meanwhile, heat olive oil in
a nonstick skillet over medium-high
heat. Add onion and garlic; sauté 1 to 2
minutes. Add shrimp; sauté 2 to 3 minutes
longer. Add lemon juice, basil, parsley, salt
and pepper; simmer until pasta is ready.

Arrange pasta in a large shallow bowl.
Toss with shrimp. Sprinkle with cheese, if desired.

PER SERVING
Calories - 367
Protein - 25 g
Sodium - 372 mg
Carbohydrates - 45 g
Cholesterol - 129 g
Total Fat - 9 g
Saturated Fat - 1 g
Dietary Fiber - 2 g

Classic Lasagna   12 servings

Save your fat calories for another day by making your own lasagna.
It's even better-tasting this way.

>   1 12-ounce package lasagna noodles
>   1 pound leanest Italian sausage
>   2 garlic cloves, minced
>   1 small onion, chopped
>   3 16-ounce cans plum tomatoes,
>   including liquid
>   2 tablespoons extra-virgin olive oil
>   3 8-ounce cans tomato sauce
>   ½ teaspoon dried oregano
>   1 teaspoon dried basil
>   ¾ teaspoon coarse salt or to taste
>   ¼ teaspoon freshly ground pepper
>   2 bunches fresh spinach leaves
>   2 cups nonfat ricotta cheese
>   ½ pound reduced-fat mozzarella cheese,
>   grated
>   ½ pound fat-free mozzarella cheese,
>   grated

Cook lasagna noodles according to package
directions. Drain and set aside.

Meanwhile, slit open, remove and discard
sausage casing. In a preheated nonstick
skillet, brown sausage with garlic and onion
until sausage is done and onion is tender.
Drain sausage mixture on paper towels; pat
dry with additional paper toweling to remove
all excess fat. Set aside.

PER SERVING
Calories - 346
Protein - 23 g
Sodium - 1,095 mg
Carbohydrates - 31 g
Cholesterol - 43 mg
Total Fat - 14 g
Saturated Fat - 3 g
Dietary Fiber - 6 g

In a food processor, puree tomatoes; add olive oil, tomato sauce, oregano, basil, salt and pepper. Process 2 to 3 minutes, or until smooth. Set aside.

Wash spinach; shake dry and remove any tough stems. Steam in a covered skillet 2 to 3 minutes, or until wilted; cool. Squeeze dry; chop. Combine spinach, sausage and ricotta.

Combine reduced-fat mozzarella and fat-free mozzarella.

Cover bottom of a 13- by 9-inch baking pan with about one fifth of the tomato sauce. Add a layer of lasagna noodles. Spread with sausage mixture. Add a layer of mozzarella. Cover with a little more tomato sauce. Repeat layers two or three more times. Pour remaining sauce over final layer. Top with additional cheese. Bake, covered, at 350°F for 60 minutes. (For a smaller group, use two 8-inch square pans and freeze one.)

Sodium Alert: Choose low-sodium foods at other meals throughout the day to offset the higher sodium in this recipe.

Variation: Omit the sausage to prepare an equally delicious meatless lasagna that saves 100 calories and 8 grams of fat.

Mac and Cheese 10 servings

With just a few modifications, even your favorite comfort foods can fit into a lifelong heart-healthy eating plan.

1 pound large elbow macaroni

¼ cup all-purpose flour

2½ cups nonfat milk

1 tablespoon margarine

¼ teaspoon paprika

1 teaspoon dry mustard

½ teaspoon hot sauce

1 teaspoon salt

¼ teaspoon pepper

1 pound reduced-fat cheddar cheese, shredded

1 large ripe tomato, sliced

3 tablespoons freshly grated Parmesan cheese

Cook macaroni according to package directions. Drain and set aside. In a screw-top jar, combine flour with ½ cup of the nonfat milk to form a smooth paste. Set aside.

PER SERVING
Calories - 353
Protein - 24 g
Sodium - 649 mg
Carbohydrates - 39 g
Cholesterol - 35 mg
Total Fat - 11 g
Saturated Fat - 5 g
Dietary Fiber - 2 g

In a saucepan over medium heat, melt margarine; add remaining milk, paprika, mustard, hot sauce, salt and pepper, stirring constantly. When milk is hot, gradually stir in reserved flour mixture. Cook, stirring constantly, until slightly thickened and bubbly. Add cheddar cheese; stir until melted. Stir macaroni into cheese sauce. Transfer to a 2-quart casserole. Arrange tomato slices over top, pushing edges of each slice into macaroni. Bake, uncovered, at 350°F for 45 minutes. Sprinkle with Parmesan and serve.

Nutrition Note: Substituting leaner cheese and adding the Parmesan at the end lowers the fat but maximizes the flavor.

Mac and Peas 8 servings

This recipe goes together quickly if you keep the ingredients on hand.

> *1 pound penne*
>
> *1 10-ounce package frozen tiny peas (2 cups)*
>
> *2 tablespoons water*
>
> *¼ cup olive oil*
>
> *3 tablespoons chopped shallots*
>
> *3 cloves garlic, finely chopped*
>
> *½ teaspoon coarse salt*
>
> *¼ teaspoon freshly ground black pepper*
>
> *¼ teaspoon crushed red pepper*
>
> *¼ cup freshly grated Parmesan cheese*

Cook penne al dente according to package direction; drain. Keep warm. Place peas in a saucepan with water and bring to a boil over high heat. Reduce heat to medium, cover and cook 2 to 3 minutes, or until peas are just tender. Remove peas from pan at once and set aside.

PER SERVING
Calories - 332
Protein - 12 g
Sodium - 289 mg
Carbohydrates - 49 g
Cholesterol - 5 mg
Total Fat - 10 g
Saturated Fat - 2 g
Dietary Fiber - 3 g

Heat olive oil in a nonstick skillet over medium heat. Add shallots, garlic, salt, pepper and red pepper; sauté, stirring constantly, 2 to 3 minutes until shallots are tender.

Arrange penne in a shallow pasta bowl. Add shallot mixture and toss. Add peas and toss gently. Sprinkle with cheese.

Cook's Suggestion: You can elevate the nutritional value of this dish by serving it with a side salad of mixed greens topped with chickpeas.

Tuna Casserole 8 servings

Serve this dish with broccolini (little broccoli) so you can dip the vegetables in the sauce.

1 pound elbow macaroni
2 10¾-ounce cans reduced-fat cream of chicken soup*
1 cup nonfat milk
1 6-ounce can water-packed tuna
1 8-ounce can sliced water chestnuts, drained
2 tablespoons freshly grated Parmesan cheese

Cook macaroni according to package directions. Drain and set aside.

Meanwhile, in a saucepan, heat chicken soup; gradually stir in nonfat milk and cook, stirring, until mixture is smooth and bubbly. Gently stir in tuna, water chestnuts and the cooked macaroni. Transfer to a 2-quart casserole dish. Bake at 375°F for 15 minutes. Sprinkle with cheese; bake 5 minutes longer. Serve at once.

PER SERVING
Calories - 288
Protein - 16 g
Sodium - 296 mg
Carbohydrates - 46 g
Cholesterol - 15 mg
Total Fat - 3 g
Saturated Fat - 0 g
Dietary Fiber - 0 g

*Using reduced-fat cream of chicken soup yields fat and calorie savings that allow this old favorite to fit into today's eating plan. Substitute Campbell's Healthy Request Cream of Chicken Soup for the reduced-fat soup to save an additional 2 grams of fat and 470 milligrams of sodium per serving.

Beans and Grains

Cheese-and-Bean Quesadillas

6 servings (3 slices per serving)

So easy to make, even your kids can put them together.

> *1 15½-ounce can black beans*
> *½ cup diced red onion*
> *¾ cup diced tomatoes*
> *½ teaspoon ground cumin*
> *6 8-inch tortillas*
> *1½ cups grated low-fat cheddar cheese*

Preheat cookie sheet in 400°F oven.

Drain beans, rinse and pour into a bowl. Add onion and tomatoes. Sprinkle with cumin and mix with a fork.

Place one tortilla on cookie sheet. Sprinkle with ¼ cup of the cheese and 5 heaping tablespoons of the bean mixture (about ⅓ cup). Add an additional ¼ cup of cheese and top with another tortilla. Repeat procedure with remaining tortillas.

Bake quesadillas 5 minutes. Turn over and bake 5 minutes longer. Using a pizza cutter, slice each quesadilla into 6 pieces.

PER SERVING
Calories - 286
Protein - 16 g
Sodium - 701 mg
Carbohydrates - 42 g
Cholesterol - 6 mg
Total Fat - 6 g
Saturated Fat - 2 g
Dietary Fiber - 7 g

Sodium Alert: Choose low-sodium foods at other meals throughout the day to offset the higher sodium in this recipe.

A NOTE ABOUT STORE-BOUGHT BEANS

In most cases, we use canned beans in our recipes. Home-cooked dried beans are preferable, but canned beans shorten cooking time. Some brands taste better than others, and some are more heart-healthy. Be sure to read the labels. Canned beans tend to be higher in sodium than home-cooked beans, so watch your sodium intake from other foods throughout the day. Rinsing canned beans will reduce their sodium content by half.

Veggie Chili Makes 3 quarts (1-cup servings)

3 tablespoons olive oil

1 red onion, diced

2 garlic cloves, minced

2 red peppers, diced

1 yellow pepper, diced

1 28-ounce can plum tomatoes with puree

1 14-ounce can chili-style tomatoes, including liquid

3 tablespoons chili powder

3 tablespoons cumin

1 teaspoon coarse salt

1/4 teaspoon coarsely ground black pepper

1 15-ounce can pinto beans, drained and rinsed

1 15-ounce can kidney beans, drained and rinsed

1 15-ounce can black beans, drained and rinsed

2 cups frozen corn

2 cups chopped white onions (optional)

3/4 cup grated reduced-fat cheddar cheese (optional)

3/4 cup nonfat sour cream (optional)

Homemade Tortilla Chips (optional, page 371)

Heat olive oil in a nonstick skillet over
medium-high heat. Add onion and sauté
8 to 10 minutes. Add garlic and sauté
2 to 3 minutes longer.

In a stockpot, combine red and yellow
peppers, plum tomatoes and chili-style
tomatoes; squeeze and crush tomatoes by hand
as you add them. Add chili powder, cumin,
salt and pepper. Heat just to boiling. Reduce heat to simmer and
add sautéed onions and garlic. Cook 30 minutes. Add beans and
simmer 20 minutes. Add corn and cook 15 minutes longer. Serve
into bowls. Top with onions, cheese, sour cream and tortilla chips,
if desired.

PER CUP
Calories - 267
Protein - 15 g
Sodium - 529 mg
Carbohydrates - 44 g
Cholesterol - 3 mg
Total Fat - 5 g
Saturated Fat - 1 g
Dietary Fiber - 12 g

Homemade Tortilla Chips   4 servings

4 6-inch whole wheat flour tortillas
olive oil cooking spray

Cut tortillas into wedges and arrange on a
nonstick baking sheet. Spray lightly with olive
oil. Bake at 400°F for 6 to 7 minutes or until
crisp.

Cook's Suggestion: Serve with 1 cup Pico
de Gallo (page 315) and ½ cup Guacamole
(page 314).

PER SERVING
Calories - 126
Protein - 3 g
Sodium - 407 mg
Carbohydrates - 17 g
Cholesterol - 0 mg
Total Fat - 5 g
Saturated Fat - 1 g
Dietary Fiber - 11 g

Three-Bean Chili 8 servings

1 pound leanest ground beef

1 medium onion, chopped

2 garlic cloves, minced

1½ teaspoons Lawry's Chili Seasoning (optional)

1 28-ounce can plum tomatoes, including liquid

⅛ teaspoon ground cumin (¼ teaspoon for spicy)

½ teaspoon cayenne

1 tablespoon chili powder

¾ teaspoon coarse salt

2 15-ounce cans red kidney beans, drained and rinsed

1 15-ounce can black beans, drained and rinsed

1 15-ounce can cannellini beans, drained and rinsed

In a nonstick skillet, brown beef with onion and garlic; drain excess fat and pat with paper towels to remove any additional fat. Sprinkle meat with chili seasoning, if desired.

Meanwhile, puree tomatoes in a food processor 2 to 3 minutes, or until smooth. Pour tomatoes into a 3-quart saucepan and add seasonings. Heat just to boiling; reduce heat to simmer. Add beef and beans; simmer 10 minutes.

PER SERVING

Calories - 255

Protein - 22 g

Sodium - 651 mg

Carbohydrates - 30 g

Cholesterol - 35 mg

Total Fat - 7 g

Saturated Fat - 2 g

Dietary Fiber - 11 g

Nutrition Note: Beans are jam-packed with B vitamins, minerals and fiber. They're also a plant source of protein, providing an array of phytochemicals for disease prevention.

Cook's Suggestion: Serve with warm tortillas and fresh strawberries.

Pasta e Fagioli   8 servings

Another recipe that you can make right out of your pantry and have on the table in no time at all.

¼ cup olive oil

3 tablespoons chopped shallots

3 cloves garlic, chopped

4 cups cooked orecchiette or other small
   noodle-shaped pasta

3 cups cooked cannellini beans

2 cups peas

½ teaspoon coarse salt

¼ teaspoon coarsely ground black pepper

3 tablespoons freshly grated Parmesan cheese

Heat olive oil in a nonstick skillet over medium-high heat. Add shallots and garlic; sauté, stirring constantly, 2 to 3 minutes, or until shallots are tender.

Arrange pasta and beans in a pasta bowl. Toss with olive oil and shallots. Gently stir in peas. Season with salt and pepper. Sprinkle with cheese.

PER SERVING
Calories - 299
Protein - 10 g
Sodium - 197 mg
Carbohydrates - 46 g
Cholesterol - 0 mg
Total Fat - 10 g
Saturated Fat - 1 g
Dietary Fiber - 3 g

Variation: Instead of peas, substitute sautéed zucchini, broccoli or any other suitable vegetable you have on hand. This dish is also a good way to use leftover pasta.

Chicken and Bean Burritos

6 servings

MARINADE
¼ cup freshly squeezed orange juice
1 tablespoon freshly squeezed lime juice
2 tablespoons cider vinegar
1 tablespoon extra-virgin olive oil
1 teaspoon fresh oregano or
  ½ teaspoon dried
½ teaspoon coarse salt
¼ teaspoon freshly ground black pepper

2 whole skinned and boned chicken breasts,
  cut into ½-inch strips
6 6-inch warm whole wheat or flour tortillas
1 cup Black Bean Dip (page 310)
6 cups shredded lettuce
⅓ cup tomato salsa or Pico de Gallo
  (page 315)
1 ripe avocado, peeled, seeded and chopped
½ cup nonfat sour cream (optional)

Combine marinade ingredients in a jar with lid and shake to blend. Pour over chicken strips; marinate 10 minutes. Drain chicken and set aside.

Preheat a nonstick skillet over medium-high heat. Add chicken strips and stir-fry 8 to 10 minutes, or until done. Transfer chicken to a serving platter.

PER SERVING
Calories - 370
Protein - 26 g
Sodium - 825 mg
Carbohydrates - 46 g
Cholesterol - 35 mg
Total Fat - 10 g
Saturated Fat - 2 g
Dietary Fiber - 8 g

To prepare burritos, spoon black bean dip along the center of each tortilla. Top with shredded lettuce and chicken. Add salsa, avocado and sour cream, if desired. Fold opposite sides of tortilla over filling, then fold ends over folded sides.

Cook's Suggestion: We like to serve these burritos with Sticky Rice (page 378).

Nutrition Note: This recipe decreases the chicken (animal protein) and increases the black beans (vegetable protein).

■

Fava Beans, Artichokes and Tomatoes   4 servings

1 tablespoon extra-virgin olive oil
4 garlic cloves, minced
1 19-ounce can fava beans, drained and rinsed
1 15-ounce can quartered artichoke hearts, drained
2 tablespoons chopped fresh thyme
¼ teaspoon salt or to taste
¼ to ½ teaspoon black pepper
1 tablespoon freshly squeezed lemon juice
1 cup diced ripe tomato

Heat olive oil in a nonstick skillet over medium-high heat. Add garlic and sauté 3 to 4 minutes, until tender. Add beans, artichoke hearts, thyme, salt, pepper and lemon juice, and heat to serving temperature. Stir in tomatoes.

PER SERVING
Calories - 163
Protein - 8 g
Sodium - 843 mg
Carbohydrates - 25 g
Cholesterol - 0 mg
Total Fat - 4 g
Saturated Fat - 1 g
Dietary Fiber - 7 g

Rice and Beans · 6 servings

7 cups cold water
1 pound dried cranberry beans*
2 meaty smoked ham hocks
5 cloves garlic, chopped
2 teaspoons freshly ground black pepper
1½ teaspoons coarse salt or to taste
6 cups cooked rice

Place beans in large bowl and cover with water. Soak 6 hours or overnight, or use quick-cook method below. Drain and rinse. Place water, beans, ham hocks, garlic and pepper in a stockpot and bring to a boil. Reduce heat; cover and simmer 2½ to 3 hours, or until beans are tender. Remove ham hocks. Season with salt. Serve over or alongside rice—either way is good.

PER SERVING
Calories - 500
Protein - 22 g
Sodium - 685 mg
Carbohydrates - 100 g
Cholesterol - 2 mg
Total Fat - 1 g
Saturated Fat - 0 g
Dietary Fiber - 19 g

Cook's Suggestion: Serve with sliced tomatoes and sliced jalapeño peppers on the side. Grilled salmon or chicken also goes well.

*To quick-cook dried beans: Sort and wash one 1 pound package of dried beans and put them in a stockpot with 2 quarts of water; cover and bring to a boil; boil 2 minutes. Remove from heat and let soak, covered tightly, 1 hour. Drain.

Tuscan Beans and Rigatoni

8 servings

Looking for ways to increase your fiber intake? Beans top the list for high-fiber foods.

1 pound rigatoni

2 tablespoons olive oil, preferably Garlic Olive Oil
(page 306)

4 garlic cloves, finely chopped

1½ pounds ripe plum tomatoes, coarsely chopped

1 15-ounce can cannellini beans, drained and
rinsed

½ teaspoon coarse salt

¼ teaspoon freshly ground black pepper

Cook pasta al dente according to package directions; drain. Heat olive oil in a medium saucepan; add garlic and sauté 3 to 4 minutes, or until just tender. Add tomatoes; simmer 5 minutes, or until tomatoes begin to soften. Add beans; simmer 5 minutes longer. Season with salt and pepper. Toss pasta with sauce. Transfer to a serving bowl.

PER SERVING
Calories - 338
Protein - 12 g
Sodium - 397 mg
Carbohydrates - 61 g
Cholesterol - 0 mg
Total Fat - 5 g
Saturated Fat - 1 g
Dietary Fiber - 6 g

Sticky Rice 4 servings

"Double up" on the nutrients in short-grain rice, also known as pearl or Japanese new-variety rice, by adding shelled edamame beans, slivered green onions, slivered toasted almonds and/or red bell peppers.

1 cup short-grain rice

Cover rice with cold water in a 2-quart saucepan. Stir and drain; repeat 2 to 3 times until water runs clear. Return drained rice to saucepan and add 1¼ cups cold water. Bring to a boil over high heat; reduce heat, cover and simmer 20 minutes, or until rice is tender and liquid is nearly absorbed. Remove from heat and let stand, covered, 5 to 10 minutes. Uncover; fluff with a fork.

PER SERVING
Calories - 170
Protein - 3 g
Sodium - 5 mg
Carbohydrates - 39 g
Cholesterol - 0 mg
Total Fat - 1 g
Saturated Fat - 0 g
Dietary Fiber - 0 g

Variation: Sprinkle cooked rice with dried crushed red pepper.

Note: Using a rice cooker makes cooking rice even simpler.

Wild Rice, Brown Rice and Barley

4 servings

Try this whole-grain combination. It's chock-full of fiber.

> *1 tablespoon olive oil*
> *½ cup chopped onion*
> *4 cups chicken broth, preferably homemade*
>   *(page 240)*
> *¼ cup wild rice*
> *⅓ cup Texmati or basmati long-grain*
>   *brown rice*
> *¼ cup barley*
> *2 tablespoons wheat berries*

Heat olive oil in a nonstick skillet over medium-high heat. Add onion and sauté 6 to 8 minutes, or until tender. Transfer to a medium saucepan and add broth. Bring to a boil and stir in wild rice, long-grain rice, barley, and wheat berries. Cover, reduce heat and simmer 30 to 35 minutes, or until grains are tender and moisture is absorbed.

PER SERVING
Calories - 213
Protein - 8 g
Sodium - 253 mg
Carbohydrates - 34 g
Cholesterol - 2 mg
Total Fat - 5 g
Saturated Fat - 1 g
Dietary Fiber - 4 g

Brown and Wild Rice 7 1-cup servings

The new dietary guidelines encourage adults to eat at least three servings of whole grains each day. This side dish will help you reach that goal.

1 small onion, chopped

1 tablespoon olive oil

2½ cups chicken broth, preferably homemade
  (page 240)

2¼ cups water

⅔ cup wild rice

1 cup long-grain brown rice

½ pound fresh mushrooms, sliced (optional)

2 tablespoons chopped fresh parsley

Heat olive oil in a nonstick skillet over medium-high heat; add onion and sauté 6 to 8 minutes, or until tender. Transfer to a 3-quart saucepan and add broth, water, wild rice and brown rice. Bring to a boil. Reduce heat; stir once. Cover and simmer 35 to 40 minutes, or until rice is tender and most of the moisture is absorbed. Add mushrooms, if desired, and simmer 5 minutes longer. Sprinkle with parsley.

PER SERVING
Calories - 191
Protein - 7 g
Sodium - 103 mg
Carbohydrates - 34 g
Cholesterol - 1 mg
Total Fat - 3 g
Saturated Fat - 0 g
Dietary Fiber - 2 g

Nutrition Note: Wild rice is high in protein, low in fat and contains potassium, phosphorus and B vitamins.

Wild Rice and Mushrooms   6 servings

1 cup wild rice
4 cups chicken broth, preferably homemade (page 240)
½ pound fresh shiitake, cremini or button mushrooms,
*   trimmed and thinly sliced*

Place rice in a medium bowl and fill bowl
with cold water. Stir and let sit 2 minutes.
Pour off any debris that floats to the surface.
Rinse again.

In a heavy saucepan, combine rice and
chicken broth. Bring to a boil; reduce heat and
cover. Simmer 40 to 50 minutes, or until rice
is tender and liquid is mostly absorbed. Add
mushrooms and cook 5 to 10 minutes longer.

PER SERVING
Calories - 123
Protein - 8 g
Sodium - 187 mg
Carbohydrates - 22 g
Cholesterol - 1 mg
Total Fat - 1 g
Saturated Fat - 0 g
Dietary Fiber - 2 g

■

Just Long-Grain Rice   6 ½-cup servings

1 cup chicken broth, preferably homemade (page 240)
1 cup water
1 cup long-grain Texmati or basmati rice
1 tablespoon finely chopped fresh flat-leaf parsley

In a 2-quart saucepan, bring broth and water
to a boil. Add rice; stir lightly with a fork.
Reduce heat; cover and simmer 15 to 20
minutes, or until rice is soft and moisture is
absorbed. Stir in parsley.

PER SERVING
Calories - 114
Protein - 5 g
Sodium - 41 mg
Carbohydrates - 23 g
Cholesterol - 0 mg
Total Fat - 0 g
Saturated Fat - 0 g
Dietary Fiber - 1 g

Egg Risotto   6 servings

¼ cup olive oil

½ cup finely chopped yellow onion

*1½ cups chicken broth, preferably homemade
(page 240)*

1 teaspoon coarse salt

½ teaspoon finely ground black pepper

2 eggs, scrambled

*2½ cups cooked rice, preferably arborio or
Sticky Rice (page 378)*

3 tablespoons freshly grated Parmesan cheese

1 tablespoon chopped fresh flat-leaf parsley

Heat olive oil in a nonstick skillet over medium-high heat. Add onions and sauté 6 to 8 minutes, or until translucent. Add broth, salt and pepper. Bring to a boil. Turn off the heat. Add scrambled eggs and fluff with a fork. Add cooked rice and stir gently. Sprinkle with cheese and parsley.

PER 1 CUP

Calories - 226

Protein - 6 g

Sodium - 455 mg

Carbohydrates - 24 g

Cholesterol - 65 mg

Total Fat - 12 g

Saturated Fat - 2 g

Dietary Fiber - 0 g

Cook's Suggestion: Serve with Christmas Salad (page 269).

Barley Mushroom Pilaf 8 servings

Make this dish on a weekend as an accompaniment to a beef roast. Later in the week, you can make a great barley soup by warming a can of beef broth in a saucepan and adding leftover pilaf and any leftover roast, finely diced.

1 tablespoon olive oil
1 onion, chopped
1¼ cups barley
¼ pound fresh mushrooms, sliced
4 cups beef broth

Heat olive oil in a nonstick skillet over medium-high heat. Add onion and sauté 6 to 8 minutes, or until tender. Add garlic and sauté 2 to 3 minutes. Stir in barley; cook 3 to 4 minutes, or until barley is lightly toasted. Add mushrooms; cook 2 to 3 minutes longer. Spoon into a 9 x 13 x 2-inch ovenproof casserole.

Pour broth over barley and mushrooms. Stir. Bake, covered, at 350°F for 1½ hours, or until liquid is absorbed.

PER SERVING
Calories - 194
Protein - 11 g
Sodium - 646 mg
Carbohydrates - 34 g
Cholesterol - 0 mg
Total Fat - 2 g
Saturated Fat - 0 g
Dietary Fiber - 8 g

Polenta with Parmesan 4 ¾-cup servings

We enjoy this northern Italian dish as a first course or as a side dish with chicken. It's especially good topped with our marinara sauce.

2 cups chicken broth, preferably homemade
    (page 240)
1 cup water
⅛ teaspoon coarse salt
1 teaspoon olive oil
1 cup polenta
2 tablespoons freshly grated Parmesan
    cheese
½ teaspoon finely chopped fresh thyme

Bring broth and water to a boil in a medium saucepan. Add salt and olive oil. Slowly add polenta, stirring constantly to prevent lumps, until mixture thickens. Stir in cheese and thyme.

PER SERVING
Calories - 179
Protein - 7 g
Sodium - 244 mg
Carbohydrates - 33 g
Cholesterol - 13 mg
Total Fat - 2 g
Saturated Fat - 1 g
Dietary Fiber - 1 g

A NOTE ABOUT COUSCOUS

The style of couscous common in northern Africa and many other regions of the Mediterranean has a very fine texture, traditionally produced by pressing semolina dough through a fine mesh. Israeli couscous is larger and cooked much the way standard pasta is cooked. The two types of couscous cannot be used interchangeably without modifying the recipe. Look for Israeli couscous in ethnic markets or in the ethnic section of your supermarket; if you can't find it, orzo is an acceptable substitute.

Couscous with Cranberries and Almonds 5 1-cup servings

2 teaspoons olive oil
½ red onion, small dice
1½ cup Israeli couscous
1½ cups chicken broth, preferably homemade (page 240)
¾ cup minced carrots
½ cup dried cranberries, raisins or currants
¼ cup sliced almonds
2 green onions, thinly sliced
2 tablespoons finely chopped flat-leaf parsley

Heat olive oil in a nonstick skillet; add onion and sauté over medium heat 4 to 5 minutes. Add couscous and sauté 3 to 4 minutes, or until couscous is lightly browned.

In a small saucepan, bring broth to a boil. Pour over couscous. Cover and let sit 5 to 8 minutes. Fluff with a fork. Add remaining ingredients and toss to mix.

PER SERVING
Calories - 309
Protein - 10 g
Sodium - 98 mg
Carbohydrates - 56 g
Cholesterol - 1 mg
Total Fat - 5 g
Saturated Fat - 1 g
Dietary Fiber - 5 g

Seafood

Sea Bass with Sun-Dried Tomato Crust   4 servings

The sweet tomato mixture and mild sea bass flavor in this recipe balance the tartness of the lemon and kalamata olives.

8 marinated sun-dried tomatoes, drained
3 garlic cloves
1 teaspoon olive oil
6 fresh lemon slices
1 pound sea bass fillets
1 tablespoon fresh lemon juice
8 kalamata olives, pitted and halved
lemon wedges

Place tomatoes, garlic and olive oil in a food processor. Process until tomatoes are finely chopped.

   Arrange lemon slices in an 8-inch ovenproof casserole. Layer sea bass over top. Drizzle fish with lemon juice. Using a spatula, spread tomato mixture over top of fish. Bake uncovered at 375°F for 10 to 20 minutes, or until fish flakes easily when pierced with a fork. Sprinkle with olives the last 3 minutes of cooking time. Serve with lemon wedges.

PER SERVING
Calories - 154
Protein - 21 g
Sodium - 314 mg
Carbohydrates - 7 g
Cholesterol - 91 mg
Total Fat - 5 g
Saturated Fat - 1 g
Dietary Fiber - 0 g

A NOTE ABOUT COOKING FISH

The Canadian Department of Fisheries suggests measuring fish at the thickest point and allowing 10 minutes cooking time per inch. For example, if a salmon measures 3 inches at its thickest point, the total cooking time should be 30 minutes, 15 minutes per side. A 1-inch-thick halibut fillet should require 10 minutes total cooking time, 5 minutes per side. Always test fish a few minutes early to avoid overcooking. It's done the second it loses translucency and flakes easily when tested with a fork at its thickest point.

Halibut with Two Cheeses 4 servings

1 pound halibut cheeks or steaks
3 tablespoons plain nonfat yogurt
2 teaspoons light mayonnaise
1 tablespoon chopped fresh tarragon
½ cup grated part-skim mozzarella cheese
2 tablespoons freshly grated Parmesan cheese

Arrange halibut in an ovenproof casserole dish. Combine yogurt, mayonnaise, tarragon and cheese; spread over fish. Bake at 400°F for 15 minutes, or until fish flakes easily when tested with a fork.

Cook's Suggestion: Serve with Classic Pasta Salad (page 264).

PER SERVING
Calories - 192
Protein - 29 g
Sodium - 211 mg
Carbohydrates - 2 g
Cholesterol - 47 mg
Total Fat - 7 g
Saturated Fat - 3 g
Dietary Fiber - 0 g

Snapper and Capers 4 servings

This is old-style Mediterranean cooking at its best.

> *2 tablespoons olive oil*
> *2 cups canned plum tomatoes, including liquid, diced*
> *1 cup dry white wine*
> *4 cloves garlic, minced*
> *¼ cup capers*
> *¼ cup chopped fresh flat-leaf parsley*
> *½ teaspoon coarse salt*
> *¼ teaspoon crushed red pepper*
> *¼ teaspoon coarsely ground black pepper*
> *¼ cup pitted and halved kalamata olives (optional)*
> *1 pound red snapper fillets*

Combine 1 tablespoon of the olive oil, plum tomatoes, wine, garlic and capers in a medium saucepan. Cook over low heat 30 minutes. Stir in parsley, seasonings and olives, if desired.

Heat remaining tablespoon of olive oil over medium heat in a nonstick grill pan. Add snapper fillets and cook 4 to 5 minutes. Turn and cook 2 to 3 minutes longer, or until fish flakes easily when tested with a fork. Serve onto plates. Spoon sauce over top.

PER SERVING
Calories - 247
Protein - 23 g
Sodium - 577 mg
Carbohydrates - 11 g
Cholesterol - 54 mg
Total Fat - 8 g
Saturated Fat - 1 g
Dietary Fiber - 1 g

Sodium Alert: Adding the olives increases the sodium substantially, so you'll need to watch other food selections throughout the day.

Red Snapper with Creamy Parmesan Sauce 4 servings

1 pound fresh red snapper or flounder fillets
olive oil cooking spray
1/3 cup light mayonnaise
2 tablespoons freshly grated Parmesan cheese
2 tablespoons chopped green onions
1/2 teaspoon white Worcestershire sauce
 (Worcestershire for chicken)

Divide fillets into four pieces and arrange in a shallow ovenproof casserole sprayed with olive oil cooking spray. Combine mayonnaise, cheese, onion and Worcestershire; spread mixture over fish. Bake at 450°F for 12 to 15 minutes.

PER SERVING
Calories - 183
Protein - 23 g
Sodium - 306 mg
Carbohydrates - 2 g
Cholesterol - 63 mg
Total Fat - 9 g
Saturated Fat - 2 g
Dietary Fiber - 0 g

■

Asian Grilled Fish 4 servings

The flavor of fish is enhanced by this simple rub, featuring ginger and the Japanese horseradish called wasabi. You can find wasabi at your supermarket or in specialty and Asian markets.

1 pound tuna, swordfish, monkfish
 or snapper
1 tablespoon minced garlic
2 teaspoons peeled and minced ginger
1 teaspoon wasabi powder
1 tablespoon black sesame seeds
1/4 cup reduced-sodium soy sauce

(continued on next page)

389

Arrange fish in a shallow glass bowl. Rub with garlic, ginger and wasabi powder. Sprinkle with sesame seeds. Pour soy sauce over fish. Marinate 30 minutes.

Grill fish over hot coals 6 to 8 minutes on each side for tuna or snapper; 9 to 10 minutes for swordfish or monkfish, or until done.

PER SERVING
Calories - 147
Protein - 28 g
Sodium - 575 mg
Carbohydrates - 2 g
Cholesterol - 51 mg
Total Fat - 2 g
Saturated Fat - 0 g
Dietary Fiber - 0 g

■

Grilled Tuna Steaks 4 servings

½ cup reduced-sodium soy sauce
1 tablespoon sesame oil
1 tablespoon fresh lemon juice
2 tablespoons mirin (rice wine)
3 garlic cloves
1 2-inch piece fresh ginger, peeled
1 tablespoon crushed red pepper
1 pound fresh tuna, swordfish or
    mahimahi
lemon wedges

Combine soy sauce, sesame oil, lemon juice, wine, garlic, ginger and red pepper. Pour over fish. Marinate 20 to 30 minutes. Remove fish from marinade and shake off excess.

Grill fish over hot coals 6 to 8 minutes on each side, or until done. Serve with plenty of fresh lemon.

PER SERVING
Calories - 190
Protein - 36 g
Sodium - 451 mg
Carbohydrates - 7 g
Cholesterol - 65 g
Total Fat - 3 g
Saturated Fat - 1 g
Dietary Fiber - 0 g

Nutrition Note: Tuna is another great way to eat those heart-healthy omega-3 fatty acids.

Grilled Swordfish with Olives and Capers 4 servings

Each year, seafood ranks higher on American popularity polls. Eating swordfish is a great way to increase your intake of omega-3s.

MARINADE
2 tablespoons extra-virgin olive oil
¼ cup fresh lemon juice
2 garlic cloves, minced
1 tablespoon minced fresh flat-leaf parsley
1½ tablespoons fresh rosemary sprigs

1 pound swordfish steaks, salmon or tuna
    (about 1 inch thick)
fresh rosemary and thyme sprigs for garnish
    (optional)
1 lime, cut into wedges
¼ cup pitted and chopped kalamata olives
    (optional)
2 teaspoons capers (optional)

Combine marinade ingredients. Arrange swordfish in a casserole and pour marinade over fish. Marinate 15 to 20 minutes at room temperature.

When grill is hot, brush it with oil. Cook fish on grill 9 to 10 minutes, turning once. Place on a bed of herb sprigs, if desired. Garnish with lime. Sprinkle with olives and capers, if desired.

PER SERVING
Calories - 163
Protein - 23 g
Sodium - 103 mg
Carbohydrates - 2 g
Cholesterol - 44 mg
Total Fat - 7 g
Saturated Fat - 2 g
Dietary Fiber - 0 g

Grilled Swordfish with Garlic and Ginger 4 servings

¼ cup fresh lemon juice
grated zest of 1 lemon
¼ cup rice vinegar
2 tablespoons reduced-sodium soy sauce
2 tablespoons chopped garlic cloves
1 tablespoon peeled and minced fresh ginger
¼ cup chopped cilantro
1 pound swordfish steaks
2 cups Pico de Gallo (page 315)

Combine lemon juice, lemon zest, vinegar, soy sauce, garlic, ginger and cilantro. Pour over swordfish. Marinate 30 minutes.

Grill swordfish over hot coals about 10 minutes per inch of thickness of fish. Serve with pico de gallo.

PER SERVING
Calories - 161
Protein - 23 g
Sodium - 404 mg
Carbohydrates - 4 g
Cholesterol - 44 mg
Total Fat - 5 g
Saturated Fat - 1 g
Dietary Fiber - 0 g

Grilled Salmon and Shiitake Mushrooms 4 servings

When we learned that hoisin sauce has even less sodium than reduced-sodium soy sauce, we used a combination of the two. We like it better!

MARINADE
2 tablespoons reduced-sodium soy sauce
2 tablespoons hoisin sauce
1 tablespoon Asian sesame oil

1 tablespoon mirin (rice wine)
1/2 teaspoon sugar
1 tablespoon peeled and minced fresh ginger

1 pound salmon steaks or fillets
3/4 pound fresh shiitake mushroom caps,
*   wiped clean*
1 1/2 tablespoons extra-virgin olive oil
pinch coarse salt
pinch freshly ground pepper
1 bunch fresh spinach leaves
1/2 lemon, cut into wedges
1/2 lime, cut into wedges

Combine the marinade ingredients. Place salmon in a casserole; pour marinade over top and marinate 10 minutes. Turn and marinate 10 minutes longer.

PER SERVING
Calories - 354
Protein - 28 g
Sodium - 774 mg
Carbohydrates - 14 g
Cholesterol - 75 mg
Total Fat - 21 g
Saturated Fat - 4 g
Dietary Fiber - 4 g

Slice mushrooms. Arrange in a pie plate. Drizzle with olive oil and toss to coat. Season with salt and pepper.

While fish is marinating, prepare grill. When grill is hot, brush with oil. Remove salmon from marinade and place on grill; cook 10 minutes per inch of thickness of fish. If grill has a lid and you keep it down during cooking, you won't have to turn the salmon. If not, turn salmon once.

Five minutes before salmon is done, grill mushrooms in a nonstick grill basket about 4 minutes, or until cooked. Shake basket two or three times to turn mushrooms for even cooking.

Line a serving platter with spinach leaves. Arrange salmon and grilled mushrooms on top. Garnish with lemon and lime wedges.

Poached Salmon with Summer Vegetables 4 servings

The freshness of summer vegetables makes this "one dish" meal a winner!

SAUCE
1 cup chopped white onion
2 teaspoons minced garlic
3 tablespoons olive oil
⅓ cup freshly squeezed lemon juice
2 tablespoons Dijon mustard
1 teaspoon coarse salt
¼ cup finely chopped fresh basil
¼ cup finely chopped flat-leaf parsley

1 cup dry white wine
4 cups water
½ onion
1 parsley stem
1 tablespoon Old Bay Seasoning
¾ pound salmon steak
½ pound petite red potatoes, scrubbed and
  cut into quarters
¼ pound fresh asparagus, trimmed
⅓ pound fresh green beans, ends and strings
  removed
2 teaspoons olive oil
6 cups fresh baby spinach, rolled like a cigar
  and sliced into ribbons
12 pitted kalamata olives

Combine onion, garlic, olive oil, lemon juice, mustard and salt in a small bowl. Set aside.

PER SERVING
Calories - 310
Protein - 22 g
Sodium - 713 mg
Carbohydrates - 16 g
Cholesterol - 56 mg
Total Fat - 19 g
Saturated Fat - 3 g
Dietary Fiber - 6 g

In a 4-quart saucepan, heat wine, water, onion, parsley and Old Bay Seasoning. Add salmon, cover and cook 10 minutes per inch of thickness of fish. Salmon should flake easily when tested with a fork. (Do not allow liquid to boil; this will cause the fish to toughen or break up.)

Place a metal steamer in a medium saucepan filled with 3 inches of water. Bring to a boil. Add potatoes; steam 5 to 10 minutes, or until just tender. Remove from steamer and set aside. Add more water to steamer if needed. Add asparagus and steam 2 to 3 minutes, or until just tender. Remove from steamer and set aside. Add green beans to steamer and steam 5 to 7 minutes, or until just tender. Remove from steamer and set aside. While vegetables are still warm, toss with olive oil.

Just before serving, line a shallow salad bowl with baby spinach. Position salmon in center. Arrange vegetables in piles around salmon. Stir basil and parsley into the sauce; drizzle half the sauce over salmon and vegetables. (Reserve remaining sauce for another meal.) Garnish with olives.

Baked Salmon 6 servings

When starting up the grill seems like too much work, don't forget the simple, old-fashioned method of baking fish.

1 ½ pounds salmon fillets
1 teaspoon extra-virgin olive oil
2 heaping teaspoons finely minced garlic
1 teaspoon fresh oregano or ¼ teaspoon dried
1 tablespoon finely minced fresh basil
¼ teaspoon black pepper
pinch coarse salt
1 bunch fresh watercress or parsley
2 fresh lemons, cut into wedges

Cover a shallow baking dish or jelly-roll pan with foil. Position salmon skin side down on top of foil. Rub with olive oil; season with garlic, oregano, basil and pepper. Bake at 325°F for 25 to 35 minutes, or until salmon is barely opaque throughout and flakes easily when tested with a fork. Do not overcook. (The salmon will continue cooking for a few minutes once removed from the oven.) Season with salt.

PER SERVING
Calories - 218
Protein - 23 g
Sodium - 143 mg
Carbohydrates - 1 g
Cholesterol - 75 g
Total Fat - 13 g
Saturated Fat - 2 g
Dietary Fiber - 0 g

Transfer to a serving platter. Garnish with watercress or parsley and fresh lemon.

Just Grilled Salmon   4 servings

Here's a great way to get your daily dose of omega-3s. The same recipe can be used for tuna, swordfish, mahimahi or any other fish of this kind.

> 1 pound fresh salmon fillets
> 2 teaspoons extra-virgin olive oil
> pinch coarse salt
> pinch freshly ground black pepper
> 1 lemon, cut into wedges

Brush grill rack with oil or line with a piece of aluminum foil to prevent fish from sticking.

Rub salmon fillets with olive oil; sprinkle with salt and pepper. Cook fillets on a hot grill 5 to 7 minutes on each side, or until fish flakes evenly when tested with a fork at its thickest point.

Serve with plenty of fresh lemon.

PER SERVING
Calories - 275
Protein - 32 g
Sodium - 76 mg
Carbohydrates - 6 g
Cholesterol - 99 mg
Total Fat - 15 g
Saturated Fat - 2 g
Dietary Fiber - 0 g

Grilled Fish Tacos   4 servings

> MARINADE
> 2 tablespoons olive oil
> ¼ cup fresh lime juice
> 4 large heads of garlic, minced
> 1 teaspoon ground cumin
> ½ cup chopped cilantro

(continued on next page)

1 pound halibut fillets

2 tablespoons olive oil

1 large onion, cut into half-rings

1 yellow bell pepper, julienned

1 red bell pepper, julienned

4 whole wheat or flour tortillas,* warmed

1 ripe avocado, peeled and sliced

Combine marinade ingredients. Cut halibut into thin strips; place in marinade and turn to coat. Marinate halibut for 15 minutes, turning two or three times.

Prepare coals. When coals are ready, place a piece of tin foil over the grill. Grill halibut strips 6 to 8 minutes, or until cooked. Remove to hot serving platter.

4-SERVING TOTAL
Calories - 470
Protein - 30 g
Sodium - 303 mg
Carbohydrates - 39 g
Cholesterol - 36 g
Total Fat - 22 g
Saturated Fat - 4 g
Dietary Fiber - 6 g

Meanwhile, heat 2 tablespoons of olive oil in nonstick skillet. Add onions and cook over medium heat 4 to 5 minutes. Add peppers and cook 2 to 3 minutes longer, or until peppers are crisp-tender. Remove to serving plate alongside halibut. Pass with warm tortillas and sliced avocado.

*Whole wheat tortillas have a third fewer calories than flour tortillas and no fat. They also have 9 grams of fiber, compared to 1.5 grams for flour tortillas.

Pan-Seared Tuna 4 servings

How easy is this? Five or six minutes from start to finish!

1 bunch fresh cilantro
juice of 2 limes
1 pound tuna steaks
2 teaspoons extra-virgin olive oil
½ teaspoon salt
¼ teaspoon pepper
1 lemon, cut into wedges

Shred ½ cup of cilantro leaves and combine with lime juice; set aside.

Rub tuna steaks on both sides with 1 teaspoon of the olive oil; season with salt and pepper. Heat remaining teaspoon of olive oil in a nonstick skillet or grill pan until very hot but not smoking. Add tuna steaks and cook over high heat 2 to 3 minutes on each side, or until fish flakes easily. (Reduce heat a notch if pan begins to smoke during cooking.) Serve on a bed of cilantro. Spoon cilantro-lime sauce over top of tuna. Garnish with lemon wedges.

PER SERVING
Calories - 146
Protein - 21 g
Sodium - 325 mg
Carbohydrates - 3 g
Cholesterol - 29 g
Total Fat - 6 g
Saturated Fat - 0 g
Dietary Fiber - 0 g

Variation: Grill tuna over hot coals about 5 minutes, turning only once.

Maryland Crab Cakes   Makes 18 appetizer-size crab cakes

1 pound blackfin/lump blue crab
1½ tablespoons light mayonnaise
2 egg whites
½ red bell pepper, seeded and finely chopped
1 teaspoon Dijon mustard
1½ tablespoons dried parsley
2 teaspoons dried oregano
¼ teaspoon coarse salt
½ teaspoon coarsely ground black pepper
⅛ teaspoon garlic powder
½ teaspoon cayenne pepper (optional for spicy)
olive oil cooking spray

In a large mixing bowl, combine crabmeat with mayonnaise, egg whites, red pepper, mustard, parsley, oregano, salt, pepper, garlic powder and cayenne pepper, if desired. Gently mix with a spoon to combine ingredients (try to keep crabmeat intact).

Spray a large nonstick skillet with olive oil. Heat skillet over high heat. Shape about ¼ cup of the crab mixture into a ball (about the size of a silver dollar) and place in skillet; flatten with a spatula to ensure even cooking. Repeat with remaining mixture.

Cook crab cakes 2 to 3 minutes, or until golden brown. Flip cakes, reduce heat to medium-low and continue cooking 5 to 6 minutes, until no liquid comes out the sides when cakes are pressed lightly with a spatula. Cakes are done when they're firm and golden brown on both sides.

PER APPETIZER
Calories - 33
Protein - 5 g
Sodium - 117 mg
Carbohydrates - 1 g
Cholesterol - 20 mg
Total Fat - 1 g
Saturated Fat - Tr
Dietary Fiber - Tr

PER ENTRÉE
Calories - 99
Protein - 15 g
Sodium - 352 mg
Carbohydrates - 2 g
Cholesterol - 60 mg
Total Fat - 3 g
Saturated Fat - 0 g
Dietary Fiber - 1 g

Variation: For entrée-size crab cakes, shape into baseball-size balls and flatten to 3-inch diameter. Makes 6 cakes.

Cook's Suggestion: For added taste and a bit more of a Maryland tradition, sprinkle some Old Bay Seasoning on top of crab cakes before cooking.

■

Sautéed Shrimp   4 servings

2 teaspoons extra-virgin olive oil
3 large cloves garlic, finely minced
1 pound large shrimp, peeled and deveined,
    tails left on
2 tablespoons finely chopped fresh
    flat-leaf parsley
2 whole lemons, cut into quarters

In a nonstick skillet, heat olive oil. Add garlic and cook 1 minute over medium-high heat. Add shrimp and cook 3 to 4 minutes. Turn; sprinkle with parsley and cook 3 minutes longer, or until opaque. Serve with fresh lemons.

PER SERVING
Calories - 143
Protein - 23 g
Sodium - 169 mg
Carbohydrates - 2 g
Cholesterol - 172 g
Total Fat - 4 g
Saturated Fat - 1 g
Dietary Fiber - 0 g

Grilled Shrimp Kebabs 4 servings

1 large red pepper

1 large yellow pepper

1 large green pepper

1 medium white onion

1 medium red onion

1 pound large shrimp

¼ cup extra-virgin olive oil

1½ teaspoons balsamic vinegar

2 tablespoons fresh lemon juice

4 garlic cloves, chopped

2 tablespoons chopped fresh basil leaves

12 cherry tomatoes

1 cup fresh or canned pineapple chunks, drained

Wash peppers and remove seeds; cut into 2-inch chunks. Peel onions; cut into 2-inch cubes. Shell and devein shrimp; pat dry.

In a shallow bowl, combine olive oil, vinegar, lemon juice, garlic and basil. Add peppers, onions and shrimp; marinate 20 to 30 minutes, turning two or three times to coat with sauce.

Thread shrimp, vegetables, tomatoes and pineapple onto metal skewers. Grill over hot coals 8 to 10 minutes, turning frequently, until shrimp turn pink and are cooked through.

PER SERVING

Calories - 231

Protein - 25 g

Sodium - 180 mg

Carbohydrates - 16 g

Cholesterol - 172 mg

Total Fat - 8 g

Saturated Fat - 1 g

Dietary Fiber - 3 g

Grilled Prawns   4 servings

1 pound large prawns (about 16)
¼ cup extra-virgin olive oil
1½ teaspoons balsamic vinegar
2 tablespoons fresh lemon juice
4 garlic cloves, chopped
2 tablespoons chopped fresh basil
1½ teaspoons minced fresh oregano
pinch coarse salt
¾ teaspoon pepper
2 tablespoons chopped fresh flat-leaf
*   parsley*

Peel prawns, leaving tails on; devein. Combine olive oil, vinegar, lemon juice, garlic, basil, oregano, salt, pepper and parsley. Pour over prawns. Marinate 20 to 30 minutes, turning prawns two or three times to coat. Remove from marinade and shake off excess.

Thread prawns onto metal skewers. Grill over hot coals 4 to 5 minutes, turning frequently, until prawns turn pink and are cooked through.

PER SERVING
Calories - 108
Protein - 6 g
Sodium - 115 mg
Carbohydrates - 0 g
Cholesterol - 12 mg
Total Fat - 9 g
Saturated Fat - 1 g
Dietary Fiber - 0 g

Cook's Suggestion: Prawns are low in total fat, but moderately high in cholesterol. Include prawns on a day that emphasizes low-cholesterol food choices, such as our Grilled Vegetable Skewers (page 346).

Stir-Fried Scallops and Prawns

4 servings

Peel and devein the prawns early in the day (or start out with precooked prawns), and you can prepare this dish in under 10 minutes.

½ pound medium prawns
1 tablespoon extra-virgin olive oil
2 garlic cloves, minced
½ pound sea scallops
1 bunch fresh flat-leaf parsley
2 fresh lemons, cut into wedges

Peel prawns, leaving tails on; devein. In a nonstick skillet, heat olive oil over medium-high heat. Add garlic and scallops, and sauté 2 to 3 minutes on each side; add prawns and cook 2 to 3 minutes longer, or until both scallops and prawns are cooked. Serve on a parsley-lined platter. Garnish with lemon wedges.

PER SERVING
Calories - 147
Protein - 22 g
Sodium - 184 mg
Carbohydrates - 3 g
Cholesterol - 105 mg
Total Fat - 5 g
Saturated Fat - 1 g
Dietary Fiber - 0 g

Cook's Suggestion: This is a great company meal that goes well with Pasta with Pesto and Tomatoes (page 353) or Penne with Sun-Dried Tomatoes (page 354).

Basic Steamed Clams   4 servings

3 pounds fresh manila, littleneck or butter clams, washed
½ cup chopped fresh flat-leaf parsley
5 fresh lemons, cut into wedges

Arrange clams on a rack in a steamer; add
2 cups hot water. Cover tightly and steam
over medium-high heat 5 to 10 minutes, or
just until shells open. (Discard any unopened
shells. Reserve nectar for chowder.)

Remove clams to a serving platter. Sprinkle
with parsley. Accompany with lemon wedges.

PER SERVING
Calories - 82
Protein - 11 g
Sodium - 47 mg
Carbohydrates - 17 g
Cholesterol - 23 mg
Total Fat - 1 g
Saturated Fat - 0 g
Dietary Fiber - 0 g

Steamers in Wine and Garlic   4 servings

2 pounds manila, littleneck or butter clams, washed
2 tablespoons olive oil
¼ cup dry white wine
1 small onion, chopped
5 garlic cloves, minced
1 celery stalk, chopped
½ cup chopped fresh flat-leaf parsley
3 fresh lemons, cut into wedges

Wash clams (see page 406) and place in a
large pot. Add olive oil, wine, onion, garlic
and celery. Cover and bring to a boil. Reduce
heat to medium; simmer 10 minutes, or just
until shells open. Transfer clams and broth to
shallow dish. Sprinkle with parsley. Squeeze
½ lemon over clams. Accompany with
remaining lemons.

PER SERVING
Calories - 92
Protein - 14 g
Sodium - 64 mg
Carbohydrates - 8 g
Cholesterol - 36 mg
Total Fat - 2 g
Saturated Fat - 0 g
Dietary Fiber - 2 g

A NOTE ABOUT WASHING CLAMS

Scrub clams to remove sand and grit. Place in a large glass bowl and cover with salt water or a solution of ⅓ cup salt to 1 gallon of water. Soak 15 to 20 minutes; drain and rinse. Repeat procedure twice. Discard any clams that are not tightly closed.

Steamers with Garlic and Tomatoes

4 servings

You don't have to wait for summer to enjoy this indoor clambake!

2 pounds manila, littleneck or butter clams, washed
1 tablespoon olive oil
1 onion, chopped
2 celery stalks, chopped
3 minced garlic cloves
1 28-ounce can Italian-style peeled tomatoes with basil, diced
½ teaspoon coarse salt
¼ teaspoon freshly ground black pepper
⅛ teaspoon crushed red pepper
¼ cup chopped fresh flat-leaf parsley

PER SERVING
Calories - 129
Protein - 11 g
Sodium - 686 mg
Carbohydrates - 15 g
Cholesterol - 23 mg
Total Fat - 4 g
Saturated Fat - 0 g
Dietary Fiber - 3 g

Arrange clams on a rack in a steamer or Dutch oven. Add 2 cups hot water, cover tightly and steam over medium heat 5 to 10 minutes, or just until shells open. Discard unopened clams.

Heat olive oil in a nonstick skillet over medium-high heat. Add onion and celery; sauté 6 to 8 minutes. Add garlic; sauté 2 to 3 minutes. Add tomatoes; reduce heat and simmer 30 minutes. Add seasonings. Place clams in large soup bowls. Spoon tomato sauce over clams. Sprinkle with parsley.

Mussels with Tomatoes   4 servings

5 dozen mussels
1 leek with greens, chopped
1 medium onion, thinly sliced
3 cloves garlic, minced
1½ cups dry vermouth
¾ cup water
½ teaspoon coarse salt
1 14½-ounce can Italian-style peeled tomatoes
    with basil
2 tablespoons olive oil
¼ cup chopped fresh flat-leaf parsley

Scrub mussel shells with a wire brush; remove and discard beards. Rinse mussels in cold water; discard those with broken or open shells.

Place mussels on a rack in a steamer or Dutch oven; add leek, onion, garlic, vermouth, water and salt. Cover tightly and steam over medium-high heat for 6 to 8 minutes, or just until shells open. Remove mussels to a serving dish and cover tightly to keep warm.

Boil cooking liquid for 2 to 3 minutes to reduce. Add tomatoes and olive oil. Heat to serving temperature. Pour over mussels. Sprinkle with parsley.

Cook's Suggestion: Serve with rustic bread for dipping in sauce.

Variation: Prepare as above but use a 28-ounce can of tomatoes and increase salt to 1 teaspoon. Serve over linguine.

PER SERVING
Calories - 306
Protein - 23 g
Sodium - 744 mg
Carbohydrates - 16 g
Cholesterol - 51 mg
Total Fat - 10 g
Saturated Fat - 2 g
Dietary Fiber - 2 g

Steamed Mussels in Wine and Garlic

8 servings

Enjoy these mussels as an appetizer, a first course or an entrée.

4 pounds fresh mussels
¾ cup dry white wine
3 garlic cloves, peeled

Scrub mussel shells with a wire brush; remove and discard beards. Rinse mussels in cold water; discard those with broken or open shells.

Place mussels in a steamer; add wine and garlic. Cover tightly; steam 6 to 8 minutes, or just until shells open. Drain.

Mussels can be served hot or cold.

PER SERVING
Calories - 140
Protein - 19 g
Sodium - 295 mg
Carbohydrates - 6 g
Cholesterol - 45 mg
Total Fat - 4 g
Saturated Fat - 1 g
Dietary Fiber - 0 g

Seafood Risotto   4 servings

Save this recipe for an occasion when you have time to linger at the table and enjoy good food with family or friends.

> 5 cups chicken broth, preferably homemade
>   (page 240)
> ¼ teaspoon saffron threads
> ¼ pound lean Italian chicken sausage
> 12 manila or littleneck clams
> 1 tablespoon olive oil
> 1 small yellow onion, finely chopped
> 2 carrots, finely chopped
> 1 cup portobello mushrooms, finely chopped
> 1½ cups arborio rice
> ¾ cup dry white wine
> ½ cup frozen peas
> 12 medium precooked prawns, deveined
> pinch cayenne pepper
> ¼ teaspoon Parmesan cheese
> 2 tablespoons chopped flat-leaf parsley

Warm broth in a medium saucepan. Crush saffron threads between your fingers into the broth. Keep broth warm over low heat.

Heat a nonstick skillet over medium-high heat. Squeeze sausage from its casing into skillet and fry 4 to 5 minutes, or until cooked. Drain on paper towels and pat with additional toweling to remove any excess fat. Crumble sausage into tiny pieces. Set aside.

PER SERVING
Calories - 480
Protein - 25 g
Sodium - 576 mg
Carbohydrates - 67 g
Cholesterol - 66 mg
Total Fat - 9 g
Saturated Fat - 1 g
Dietary Fiber - 4 g

(continued on next page)

Steam clams and set aside.

Heat olive oil in nonstick skillet over medium-high heat. Add onion, carrots and mushrooms; sauté 5 minutes. Add rice; sauté 2 minutes longer. Add wine. Stir with a wooden spoon until liquid is absorbed. Add peas and one cup of warm broth; stir continuously until broth is absorbed. Add another cup of broth; stir until absorbed. Keep adding broth, one cup at a time, stirring continuously. Repeat for 20 minutes, or until all broth is used. Add prawns during last 3 minutes of cooking.

Remove to shallow serving bowl. Top with clams and sausage. Sprinkle with cayenne pepper, cheese and parsley.

■

South of the Border Stew 6 servings

1 pound mussels

1 pound clams

3 tablespoons olive oil

1 medium yellow onion, diced

5 cloves garlic, minced

1 red pepper, diced

1 yellow pepper, diced

1 orange pepper, diced

1 jalapeño pepper, diced

1 28-ounce can plum tomatoes, including liquid,
   diced

1 cup dry white wine

juice of 1 lime

¼ pound red snapper, cut into 3-inch cubes

¼ pound cod, cut into 3-inch cubes

¼ pound scallops

½ pound medium shrimp, peeled and deveined
1 cup chopped cilantro
3 greens onions, chopped
pinch coarse salt
pinch freshly ground black pepper

Scrub mussel shells with a wire brush; remove and discard beards.
Rinse mussels in cold water; discard those
with broken or open shells. Scrub clams.

PER SERVING
Calories - 337
Protein - 36 g
Sodium - 612 mg
Carbohydrates - 19 g
Cholesterol - 115 mg
Total Fat - 10 g
Saturated Fat - 2 g
Dietary Fiber - 3 g

Arrange mussels and clams on a rack in a
steamer with a lid filled with 2 cups hot water.
Steam covered 6 to 8 minutes, or just until
shells open. Set aside. Reserve ½ cup nectar
(liquid from steaming mussels and clams).

Heat olive oil in a nonstick skillet, add
onions and sauté 8 to 10 minutes; add garlic and peppers and cook
3 to 4 minutes longer.

Meanwhile, combine tomatoes, wine, lime juice and reserved
nectar. Heat just to boiling. Add snapper, cod and scallops. Cook
4 to 6 minutes. Add shrimp. Cook 2 to 3 minutes. Add sautéed
onions and peppers. Sprinkle with cilantro and green onions. Season
with salt and pepper. Serve into bowls. Top with clams and mussels.

Poultry

Chicken Parmesan 4 servings

1 cup oyster crackers or saltines
¼ cup freshly grated Parmesan cheese
2 tablespoons finely chopped fresh parsley
½ teaspoon ground thyme
½ teaspoon dried oregano
½ teaspoon dried basil
½ teaspoon paprika
½ teaspoon coarse salt
½ teaspoon freshly ground black pepper
2 whole skinned and boned chicken breasts,
*   halved*
2 teaspoons olive oil
½ cup low-fat (1%) buttermilk

Place crackers in a gallon- or jumbo-size zip-lock plastic bag and crush them with your hands or a rolling pin. Add cheese, herbs and seasonings. Shake bag to combine ingredients.

Brush chicken with olive oil and dip in buttermilk. Place in the plastic bag; shake bag until chicken pieces are evenly coated with seasonings. In a nonstick pan, bake chicken at 400°F for 30 minutes. Reduce heat to 350°F and bake 10 minutes longer, or until chicken is tender.

PER SERVING
Calories - 240
Protein - 31 g
Sodium - 645 mg
Carbohydrates - 11 g
Cholesterol - 78 mg
Total Fat - 7 g
Saturated Fat - 2 g
Dietary Fiber - 0 g

A NOTE ABOUT POULTRY

The most healthful poultry is skinless white breast (white meat is leaner than dark). The skin should always be removed from poultry, since that's where the fat is. Three ounces of chicken breast without skin contains just 3 grams of fat; with skin, it contains twice that amount. Similarly, 3 ounces of turkey breast without skin has just 2.7 grams of fat; with skin, it has 8.7 grams of fat. Watch out for ground turkey and ground chicken—both can be higher in fat than ground round.

Quick Chicken   4 servings

Double the recipe and you'll have the makings for salad or lunch-box sandwiches the following day.*

> *1 15-ounce can chicken broth or 2 cups homemade
>   (page 240)*
> *2 cups water*
> *1 pound skinned and boned chicken breasts*
> *pinch coarse salt*

In a 1½-quart saucepan, bring broth and water to a boil. Add chicken and bring to a second boil; reduce heat to medium and cook 20 minutes, or until chicken is done. Remove chicken and reserve stock for later use. Sprinkle with salt.

PER SERVING
Calories - 157
Protein - 28 g
Sodium - 178 mg
Carbohydrates - 0 g
Cholesterol - 73 g
Total Fat - 4 g
Saturated Fat - 1 g
Dietary Fiber - 0 g

*If chicken is to be used for sandwiches, cool
10 minutes and tear into strings or slice diagonally across top.*

Chicken Fajitas   6 servings

Fajitas are the perfect way to get everything you need in proper balance. The tortillas and vegetables offer an abundance of carbohydrates, while the chicken provides moderate amounts of protein.

2 garlic cloves, minced

3 tablespoons freshly squeezed lime juice

1/4 cup loosely packed cilantro plus additional
    cilantro for garnish

1 tablespoon plus 1 teaspoon extra-virgin olive oil

2 whole skinned and boned chicken breasts,
    cut into 1/4-inch strips

2 white onions, halved and sliced lengthwise
    into 1/3-inch-thick slices

1 yellow bell pepper, cut into 1/3-inch strips

1 red bell pepper, cut into 1/3-inch strips

1 green bell pepper, cut into 1/3-inch strips

1 recipe Pico de Gallo (page 315)

1/2 cup nonfat sour cream

6 warm flour or corn tortillas (see page 415)

In a medium bowl, combine garlic, lime juice and cilantro with 1 tablespoon olive oil. Add chicken and toss to coat. Let sit 30 minutes.

Preheat a nonstick skillet over medium-high heat. Add chicken and stir-fry 8 to 10 minutes; remove and set aside. In the same skillet, heat remaining teaspoon of olive oil over medium-high heat. Add onions and stir-fry 2 minutes. Add peppers and stir-fry 3 to 4 minutes until crisp-tender.

Arrange chicken with onions and peppers on a platter or in a shallow serving bowl. Accompany with pico de gallo, sour cream and warm tortillas. Serve with steamed long-grain rice.

PER SERVING
Calories - 280
Protein - 19 g
Sodium - 369 mg
Carbohydrates - 33 g
Cholesterol - 29 mg
Total Fat - 8 g
Saturated Fat - 2 g
Dietary Fiber - 4 g

To Warm Tortillas:

Easiest Method. Invest in an inexpensive terra-cotta tortilla warmer available at your local kitchen store or by mail order.

Oven Method. Wrap tortillas in aluminum foil and heat in a 325°F oven, about 15 minutes.

Microwave Method. Place tortillas between 2 slightly dampened paper towels. Microwave on high for 1 to 2 minutes, or until warm. Keep wrapped until ready to serve.

Variation: For a spicier chicken dish, mince a canned chipotle chili and add it to the marinade.

■

Asian Chicken 4 servings

1 recipe Quick Chicken (page 413)
3 tablespoons rice wine vinegar
1 tablespoon extra-virgin olive oil
1 tablespoon reduced-sodium soy sauce
1 tablespoon hoisin sauce
2 garlic cloves, finely minced
2 to 3 drops Tabasco sauce or hot chili oil

Prepare chicken as directed in recipe. Combine remaining ingredients in a small bowl. Pass with chicken.

Cook's Suggestion: Serve with Sticky Rice (page 378) and stir-fried vegetables.

PER SERVING
Calories - 202
Protein - 27 g
Sodium - 362 mg
Carbohydrates - 6 g
Cholesterol - 73 mg
Total Fat - 6 g
Saturated Fat - 1 g
Dietary Fiber - 0 g

A NOTE ABOUT NONSTICK PANS

Investing in a set of high-quality nonstick frying pans allows you to fry with ease and yet use only a minimum amount of fat or, in many cases, no fat at all. Heavier pans work best. Although you can stir-fry in the frying pans, a good nonstick wok is a wonderful addition, as are nonstick cake pans and cookie sheets.

Chicken Cutlets 4 servings

1 pound skinned and boned chicken breasts
¼ cup egg substitute
¼ cup bread crumbs
¼ cup flour
2 tablespoons freshly grated Parmesan cheese
pinch coarse salt
pinch coarsely ground black pepper
olive oil cooking spray

Place chicken breasts in freezer for 20 to 30 minutes, or until just barely frozen. Slice chicken thin. (Partial freezing makes it easier to slice.)

Put egg substitute in a shallow casserole. In another casserole, combine bread crumbs, flour, cheese, salt and pepper.

Spray an ovenproof casserole with olive oil. Dip chicken in egg, then into bread crumb mixture. Arrange in a single layer in casserole; spray with olive oil and bake 10 minutes in 350°F oven. Flip chicken, spray with oil and bake 10 minutes longer, or until chicken is cooked.

PER SERVING
Calories - 186
Protein - 30 g
Sodium - 224 mg
Carbohydrates - 8 g
Cholesterol - 68 mg
Total Fat - 3 g
Saturated Fat - 1 g
Dietary Fiber - 0 g

Chicken Cordon Bleu   4 servings

Once you've mastered our chicken cutlet recipe, try this for a more
upscale presentation.

1 recipe Chicken Cutlets (page 416)
¼ pound thinly sliced prosciutto
1 ounce (8 very thin slices) part-skim mozzarella cheese

Prepare cutlets as directed in recipe except for
the last step. Instead, after flipping chicken,
cook 5 to 6 minutes, or until chicken is almost
cooked. Top each cutlet first with a slice of
prosciutto and then with a slice of cheese.
Cook 5 minutes longer, or until chicken is
cooked and cheese is melted.

PER SERVING
Calories - 297
Protein - 37 g
Sodium - 257 mg
Carbohydrates - 8 g
Cholesterol - 87 mg
Total Fat - 11 g
Saturated Fat - 2 g
Dietary Fiber - 0 g

Chicken and Polenta   4 servings

1 pound Chicken Cutlets (page 416)
2½ cups warm 20-Minute Marinara (page 350)
½ cup grated part-skim mozzarella cheese
3 cups Polenta with Parmesan (page 384)

Prepare cutlets as directed in recipe except
for last step. Instead, 5 minutes after chicken
is flipped, pour ½ cup sauce over chicken
and sprinkle with cheese. Cook 5 to 7 minutes
longer, until chicken is cooked and cheese
is melted.

Arrange chicken and polenta on dinner
plates. Pass remaining sauce on the side.

PER SERVING
Calories - 265
Protein - 37 g
Sodium - 574 mg
Carbohydrates - 9 g
Cholesterol - 79 mg
Total Fat - 8 g
Saturated Fat - 3 g
Dietary Fiber - 0 g

Southern Fried Chicken 4 servings

Imagine not having to give up fried chicken! Follow the braising technique in this recipe to enjoy an old favorite.

> *1 cup low-fat (1%) buttermilk*
> *2 whole skinned and boned chicken breasts,*
> *   halved*
> *1 cup all-purpose flour*
> *1½ teaspoons salt*
> *½ teaspoon pepper*
> *2 teaspoons paprika*
> *2 teaspoons extra-virgin olive oil*

Pour buttermilk into a casserole. Dip chicken in buttermilk, turning once to coat.

Combine flour and seasonings in a paper bag. Add chicken and shake to coat.

In a nonstick skillet, heat olive oil over medium-high heat. Add chicken and cook 10 to 15 minutes, turning often to brown evenly. Add 3 tablespoons of water and cover. Reduce heat and cook chicken 25 minutes; uncover and cook 5 to 10 minutes longer, or until chicken is tender. Remove to a serving platter.

PER SERVING
Calories - 304
Protein - 32 g
Sodium - 392 mg
Carbohydrates - 28 g
Cholesterol - 75 mg
Total Fat - 6 g
Saturated Fat - 2 g
Dietary Fiber - 1 g

Chicken Curry   8 servings

1 tablespoon extra-virgin olive oil

½ cup chopped onion

*2 cups chicken broth, preferably homemade
    (page 240)*

2 cups nonfat milk

½ cup all-purpose flour

½ teaspoon salt

1 tablespoon curry powder, preferably Madras

¼ teaspoon ground ginger

1 tablespoon lemon juice

4 cups cubed cooked chicken breast

1 8-ounce can sliced water chestnuts

6 cups Sticky Rice (page 378)

2 tablespoons slivered almonds

¼ cup raisins or dried cranberries

⅔ cup pineapple chunks

Heat olive oil in a nonstick skillet. Add onions and sauté until tender. Stir in broth; bring to a boil. Combine milk and flour to form a smooth paste; gradually add to boiling broth, stirring constantly until thick. Add seasonings. Pour lemon juice over chicken; add chicken to broth. Stir in water chestnuts. Heat. Serve over steamed rice. Garnish with almonds, raisins or dried cranberries and pineapple chunks.

PER SERVING
Calories - 435
Protein - 30 g
Sodium - 473 mg
Carbohydrates - 64 g
Cholesterol - 62 mg
Total Fat - 6 g
Saturated Fat - 1 g
Dietary Fiber - 2 g

Grilled Herbed Chicken Breasts

4 servings

Cooking with fresh herbs makes all the difference. Try this recipe for your family and enjoy the compliments!

3 tablespoons extra-virgin olive oil
2 tablespoon fresh lemon juice
1 tablespoon minced fresh thyme
½ tablespoon minced fresh rosemary
¾ teaspoon coarse salt
½ teaspoon freshly ground pepper
2 whole skinned and boned chicken breasts, halved

Combine first six ingredients in a casserole. Add chicken and turn so both sides are coated. Marinate 10 minutes.

Cook chicken on a hot grill about 5 minutes on each side, or until cooked. When chicken is done, it will feel firm to the touch but not hard.

PER SERVING
Calories - 184
Protein - 27 g
Sodium - 327 mg
Carbohydrates - 1 g
Cholesterol - 73 mg
Total Fat - 8 g
Saturated Fat - 1 g
Dietary Fiber - 0 g

Note: This chicken can also be cooked on the stove in a nonstick skillet or grill pan.

Grilled Lemon Chicken   4 servings

1 freshly squeezed lemon
2 tablespoons extra-virgin olive oil
½ teaspoon coarse salt
¼ teaspoon freshly ground black pepper
2 skinless, boneless chicken breasts, halved

Combine lemon juice, olive oil, salt and pepper. Place chicken in a casserole. Pour marinade over chicken. Marinate 10 minutes.

Heat a grill pan and cook chicken 10 to 12 minutes on each side, until done. Cut diagonally into ½-inch-thick slices.

PER SERVING
Calories - 171
Protein - 23 g
Sodium - 305 mg
Carbohydrates - 1 g
Cholesterol - 58 mg
Total Fat - 8 g
Saturated Fat - 1 g
Dietary Fiber - 0 g

■

Grilled Chicken Burgers 4 servings

1 recipe Grilled Herbed Chicken Breasts
*   (page 420)*
4 whole wheat hamburger buns, split
mustard to taste
4 teaspoons light mayonnaise (optional)
2 tablespoons sweet pickle relish (optional)
1 large tomato, sliced
4 dark green lettuce leaves
4 slices red or white onion (optional)
sliced dill pickle (optional)
sliced English cucumber (optional)

Prepare chicken breasts according to recipe. Toast buns, cut side down, on grill during last 1 minute of cooking.

Spread mustard and, if desired, mayonnaise and relish on half of each bun. Add chicken, tomato, lettuce and onion; top with other bun half. Accompany with pickle and cucumber, if desired.

PER SERVING
Calories - 335
Protein - 31 g
Sodium - 671 mg
Carbohydrates - 25 g
Cholesterol - 75 mg
Total Fat - 12 g
Saturated Fat - 2 g
Dietary Fiber - 1 g

40 Cloves of Garlic Chicken   6 servings

Double the recipe and keep on enjoying the special flavor of this dish for days to come.

1½ teaspoons extra-virgin olive oil
3 whole skinned and boned chicken breasts,
　　halved
40 garlic cloves (about 4 heads), unpeeled
1¼ cups dry white wine
1 tablespoon chopped fresh rosemary
1 tablespoon chopped fresh thyme
¼ cup fresh chopped flat-leaf parsley
pinch coarse salt
pinch freshly ground black pepper
6 ¼-inch slices Tuscan-style bread

Heat oil in a nonstick skillet. Add chicken and cook over medium-high heat 4 to 5 minutes. Turn chicken, add garlic and cook 4 to 5 minutes longer, or until garlic begins to brown. Transfer chicken and garlic to an ovenproof baking dish and set aside.

PER SERVING
Calories - 223
Protein - 23 g
Sodium - 236 mg
Carbohydrates - 18 g
Cholesterol - 49 mg
Total Fat - 3 g
Saturated Fat - 1 g
Dietary Fiber - 1 g

Pour wine into skillet to deglaze the pan; add rosemary and thyme and pour mixture over chicken. Cover tightly with foil. Bake at 350°F for 30 to 45 minutes, or until chicken is done. Sprinkle with parsley. Season with salt and pepper. Set aside.

In a preheated broiler, toast Tuscan bread slices until golden brown on each side. Pass bread for dipping with chicken and garlic sauce.

Citrus Marinated Chicken   6 servings

MARINADE

¼ cup freshly squeezed orange juice

1 tablespoon freshly squeezed lime juice

2 tablespoons cider vinegar

1 tablespoon extra-virgin olive oil

1 teaspoon fresh oregano or ½ teaspoon dried

½ teaspoon coarse salt

¼ teaspoon freshly ground black pepper

*3 whole skinned and boned chicken breasts,
    halved*

Combine marinade ingredients in a jar with lid; shake to blend. Arrange chicken in casserole dish. Pour marinade over chicken. Marinate 20 minutes.

Grill chicken over medium-hot coals about 5 to 7 minutes, depending on thickness of chicken. Turn and grill 10 minutes longer, or until chicken is cooked.

PER SERVING
Calories - 137
Protein - 23 g
Sodium - 225 mg
Carbohydrates - 2 g
Cholesterol - 58 mg
Total Fat - 4 g
Saturated Fat - 1 g
Dietary Fiber - 0 g

Nutrition Note: Remember, you can cut over 50% of the fat simply by choosing a skinless chicken breast.

Roast Chicken   4 3½-ounce servings

3-to-4-pound chicken
pinch fresh chopped or ground sage
pinch fresh chopped or powdered rosemary
pinch coarse salt
pinch coarsely ground black pepper
2 celery ribs with leaves, chopped
2 carrots, chopped
1 large onion, quartered
3 garlic cloves, peeled

Wash outside of chicken with cold water and rub with sage, rosemary, salt and pepper. Wipe inside of chicken with a damp paper towel; place celery, carrots, onion and garlic inside cavity. Skewer neck skin to back; tuck wing tips behind shoulder joints.

Place chicken breast side up in a shallow roasting pan. Roast at 350°F for 60 to 75 minutes, or until juices have no trace of pink. Meat thermometer should register 180°F. Let stand 10 minutes before slicing.

PER SERVING
Calories - 205
Protein - 30 g
Sodium - 104 mg
Carbohydrates - 4 g
Cholesterol - 89 mg
Total Fat - 7 g
Saturated Fat - 2 g
Dietary Fiber - 5 g

Roast Breast of Turkey 12 servings

Buy the biggest turkey breast available and serve this dish as an entrée. Use any leftover turkey for sandwiches the rest of the week.

4 pounds fresh turkey breast
½ teaspoon extra-virgin olive oil
2 heaping tablespoons chopped fresh rosemary leaves
2 heaping tablespoons chopped fresh sage
pinch coarse salt
pinch freshly ground black pepper
pinch paprika

Rub turkey breast on both sides with olive oil. Sprinkle with rosemary, sage, salt, pepper and paprika. Position turkey breast on a rack in a roasting pan. Roast at 325°F for 1½ hours, or until juices have no trace of pink. A meat thermometer should register 170°F.

PER 4.8 OUNCES
Calories - 149
Protein - 33 g
Sodium - 71 mg
Carbohydrates - 0 g
Cholesterol - 90 g
Total Fat - 1 g
Saturated Fat - 0 g
Dietary Fiber - 0 g

■

Roast Turkey with Bread Stuffing

15 3-ounce servings

You can save fat and calories by choosing to eat the white meat without skin. (Save the dark meat and skin for the soup pot.)

8-to-10-pound fresh turkey
pinch fresh or ground sage to taste
pinch coarse salt
pinch freshly ground black pepper
3 celery stalks, cut into 2-inch pieces
2 onions, quartered

(continued on next page)

Rinse inside and outside of turkey with cold water. Rub outside with seasonings. Place celery and onions inside cavity. Skewer neck skin to back; tuck wing tips behind shoulder joints.

In a roasting pan, place turkey breast side up on a rack; roast at 325°F. Turkey is done when drumsticks move easily or twist out of joint. A meat thermometer should register 185°F. If turkey browns too quickly, cover it with a cap of aluminum foil. Remove skin before slicing.

Roasting Chart:

6–8 pounds: 2¾ to 3½ hours

8–12 pounds: 3¼ to 4 hours

12–16 pounds: 3¾ to 5 hours

16–20 pounds: 4¾ to 6½ hours

20–24 pounds: 6¼ to 8 hours

Bread Stuffing:

1 tablespoon virgin olive oil

1 large onion, chopped

3 celery stalks, chopped

½ pound fresh mushrooms, sliced (optional)

10 cups dried, unseasoned bread cubes,
preferably whole wheat

2 cups chicken broth, preferably homemade
(page 240)

1¼ teaspoons ground sage or to taste

½ teaspoon coarse salt or to taste

¼ teaspoon freshly ground black pepper or
to taste

In a nonstick skillet, heat olive oil. Add onion and celery; sauté over medium heat until tender. Add mushrooms; sauté 2 to 3 minutes longer. Remove from heat. Add bread cubes. In a small saucepan, heat broth. Moisten bread gradually with broth (don't saturate). Add seasonings. Transfer to baking dish. Bake, uncovered, at 350°F for 30 to 40 minutes, or until piping hot. Serve alongside turkey.

PER ½ CUP STUFFING
Calories - 43
Protein - 2 g
Sodium - 176 mg
Carbohydrates - 6 g
Cholesterol - 0 mg
Total Fat - 1 g
Saturated Fat - 0 g
Dietary Fiber - 0 g

Beef and Other Meats

Classic Grilled Burgers 8 servings

2 pounds extra-lean ground beef*
pinch coarse salt
pinch freshly ground pepper
8 large sesame hamburger buns
2 large firm ripe tomatoes, sliced
8 thin slices white onion
1 head Bibb lettuce, washed and crisped

Shape ground beef into 8 patties. Grill over hot coals, 3 inches from heat, 6 to 7 minutes per side for medium rare or 10 to 11 minutes for well-done, turning meat when juices begin to form on top. Season with salt and pepper. Serve immediately on warm buns with tomato slices, onion slices and lettuce.

PER SERVING
Calories - 318
Protein - 18 g
Sodium - 365 mg
Carbohydrates - 17 g
Cholesterol - 61 mg
Total Fat - 17 g
Saturated Fat - 1 g
Dietary Fiber - 1 g

*An occasional burger can fit nicely into your eating plan. Fifteen percent extra-lean ground beef is considered the best-tasting ground beef for burgers. Nine percent leanest ground beef, while leaner, tends to dry out.

A NOTE ABOUT RED MEAT

Always trim all visible fat from meat before cooking. The difference between a 3-ounce T-bone steak trimmed and untrimmed is about 20 grams of fat. Cook meat to medium or well-done to allow fat to drip off. If you grill regular hamburger meat until it's well-done, you'll end up with as little fat as you'd have if you used lean ground beef.

See page 151 for tips on choosing the leanest cuts.

Sunday Beef Roast 12 servings

A perfect example of weekend cooking/weekday eating. Save the leftovers for French Dip Sandwiches (page 453) later in the week.

> *1 3-pound beef tenderloin roast*
> *4 cloves garlic, minced*
> *pinch coarse salt*
> *pinch freshly ground pepper*
> *Creamy Horseradish Sauce (page 308)*

Place tenderloin on a wire rack in a roasting pan; rub on all sides with garlic, salt and pepper. Insert meat thermometer into center of roast. Roast at 425°F for 45 to 65 minutes, or to desired doneness. Thermometer should register 140°F for rare, 160°F for medium, 170°F for well-done.

Place roast on a warm large platter and let stand at room temperature 10 to 15 minutes before carving. Serve with horseradish sauce.

PER SERVING
Calories - 182
Protein - 24 g
Sodium - 61 mg
Carbohydrates - 0 g
Cholesterol - 70 mg
Total Fat - 9 g
Saturated Fat - 3 g
Dietary Fiber - 0 g

Old-Fashioned Meat Loaf   8 servings

This is a double recipe, so there should be plenty of leftover slices for sandwiches made with light mayonnaise and lettuce.

1 teaspoon extra-virgin olive oil
1 large yellow onion, finely chopped
2 pounds leanest ground beef
1½ cups bread crumbs
2 eggs, lightly beaten
1 teaspoon coarse salt
½ teaspoon freshly ground black pepper
1 teaspoon dry mustard
¼ teaspoon ground thyme
¼ cup finely chopped fresh parsley
½ cup evaporated skim milk

In a nonstick skillet, heat olive oil over medium-high heat; add onion and sauté 4 to 5 minutes. In a large bowl, combine beef, bread crumbs and sautéed onion. In a medium bowl, whisk together eggs, salt, pepper, mustard, thyme, parsley and milk. Pour egg mixture over beef. Using your hands, lightly mix ingredients.

PER SERVING
Calories - 317
Protein - 28 g
Sodium - 556 mg
Carbohydrates - 19 g
Cholesterol - 123 mg
Total Fat - 14 g
Saturated Fat - 5 g
Dietary Fiber - 1 g

Pat meat into a loaf pan. Bake at 350°F for 1½ hours; cover pan with foil for the first half-hour. Meat loaf is done when it begins to shrink from sides of pan.

Remove loaf from oven and let cool 5 to 10 minutes; cut into thick slices.

Nutrition Note: Finding 90% leanest ground beef is worth the search! For an even leaner meat loaf, use a draining meat loaf pan available at most specialty kitchen stores.

Grilled Teriyaki Steak 6 servings

MARINADE
1/2 cup reduced-sodium soy sauce*
1/2 cup dry vermouth
1 tablespoon brown sugar
1 tablespoon Worcestershire sauce
2 garlic cloves, minced
1 1-inch piece fresh ginger, peeled and minced

1 1/2 pounds flank steak, all visible fat removed

Combine soy sauce, vermouth, brown sugar, Worcestershire sauce, garlic and ginger.

Arrange flank steak in a shallow casserole suitable for marinating; pour marinade over top. Cover. Marinate in refrigerator 1 to 24 hours. Drain marinade.

Grill steak over hot coals 6 to 8 minutes on each side, or to desired doneness; remove to a cutting board and cut across grain at a diagonal angle into thin slices.

PER SERVING
Calories - 194
Protein - 23 g
Sodium - 244 mg
Carbohydrates - 1 g
Cholesterol - 57 mg
Total Fat - 9 g
Saturated Fat - 4 g
Dietary Fiber - 0 g

*Reduced-sodium soy sauce contains 46% less sodium than regular soy sauce, with little or no difference in flavor.

Note: You can make leaner cuts of meat more tender by marinating them first in a low-fat marinade.

Italian Steaks 8 servings

> 1½ pounds flank steak
> 1 28-ounce can plum tomatoes, including liquid,
>   diced
> 4 cloves garlic, minced
> ½ teaspoon oregano
> 1 tablespoon chopped fresh basil
> 2 teaspoons olive oil

Arrange steak on a rack in a broiler pan. Broil 3 inches from heat 5 minutes on each side. Remove to a baking pan.

    Combine tomatoes, garlic, oregano, basil and olive oil; pour over meat. Bake at 350°F for 45 minutes, or until sauce is bubbling and meat is cooked. Stir juices to blend. Use sauce for the meat, for pasta or as a dip for bread.

PER 3.5-OZ. SERVING
Calories - 164
Protein - 18 g
Sodium - 221 mg
Carbohydrates - 5 g
Cholesterol - 43 mg
Total Fat - 8 g
Saturated Fat - 3 g
Dietary Fiber - 1 g

Cook's Suggestion: Serve with bow-tie pasta and a Christmas Salad (page 269).

■

Stir-Fried Beef 6 servings

> *SAUCE*
> 2 tablespoons unseasoned rice vinegar
> 2 tablespoons oyster-flavored sauce*
> ¼ cup reduced-sodium soy sauce
> 1 tablespoon olive oil
> ¼ teaspoon Asian hot chili oil or sauce
>   (optional)

2 cups beef broth

2 cups water

1 8-ounce package soba noodles

4 teaspoons olive oil

1 teaspoon finely minced garlic

1 teaspoon peeled and minced fresh ginger

¾ pound boneless beefsteak (top round, flank or sirloin),
*   cut into 1-inch stir-fry strips*

¾ pound snow peas, ends and strings removed

1 red pepper, seeded and cut into ½-inch-wide strips

⅛ teaspoon crushed red pepper (optional)

In a small bowl, combine the rice vinegar, oyster-flavored sauce, soy sauce, olive oil and, if using, chili oil. Set aside.

PER SERVING
Calories - 304
Protein - 24 g
Sodium - 812 mg
Carbohydrates - 36 g
Cholesterol - 37 mg
Total Fat - 9 g
Saturated Fat - 2 g
Dietary Fiber - 2 g

In a medium saucepan, bring broth and water to a boil. Add noodles and cook 5 to 6 minutes, or until noodles are tender. Drain, rinse and set aside.

Preheat a nonstick wok or skillet over medium-high heat and add 2 teaspoons of the olive oil. When oil is hot, add garlic and ginger and cook 2 to 3 minutes; add beef and stir-fry 2 to 3 minutes, or until browned. Remove from wok and set aside. Heat remaining 2 teaspoons of oil. Add snow peas, red pepper and crushed red pepper, if desired. Stir-fry 2 to 3 minutes, or just until crisp-tender. Arrange beef, noodles and vegetables on individual plates. Accompany with sauce.

*Oyster-flavored sauce is available in the Asian section of most supermarkets.

Sodium Alert: Choose low-sodium foods at other meals throughout the day to balance the higher sodium in this recipe.

Grilled Round Steak   8 servings

The acidic nature of lemon juice and wine vinegar tenderizes this lean steak. Keep it in mind for steak sandwiches.

2 teaspoons olive oil
3 tablespoons lemon juice
1 tablespoon red wine vinegar
2 garlic cloves, sliced
pinch fresh or dried thyme
$\frac{1}{2}$ teaspoon chili powder
2 pounds extra-lean round steak
1 large onion, sliced
pinch coarse salt
pinch freshly ground black pepper

Combine olive oil, lemon juice, vinegar, garlic, thyme and chili powder. Pour over steak and top with onion. Cover. Marinate in refrigerator for 2 hours, turning several times to coat. Drain.

Grill steak over hot coals 7 to 8 minutes on each side, or to desired doneness. Sprinkle lightly with salt and pepper.

PER SERVING
Calories - 180
Protein - 26 g
Sodium - 127 mg
Carbohydrates - 3 g
Cholesterol - 74 mg
Total Fat - 7 g
Saturated Fat - 2 g
Dietary Fiber - 0 g

Beef Stroganoff 8 servings

Try this leaner version of an old favorite for an ultimate comfort food.

¾ pound leanest ground beef
¾ cup finely chopped onion
1 garlic clove, minced
½ pound fresh mushrooms, sliced
¼ teaspoon salt
⅛ teaspoon pepper
⅛ teaspoon dried rosemary
1½ cups low-fat (1%) cream of
  chicken soup
1 cup nonfat sour cream
1 pound cooked bow-tie pasta
  (al dente)
2 teaspoons poppy seeds
fresh parsley for garnish

Sauté beef, onion and garlic in a nonstick skillet until beef is browned; drain off excess fat. Add mushrooms; cook 3 to 5 minutes. Stir in salt, pepper and rosemary; simmer, uncovered, 10 minutes. Add chicken soup and heat. Stir in sour cream; heat but do not boil.

Arrange pasta around the edges of a large platter; spoon sauce into center. Sprinkle with poppy seeds. Garnish with parsley.

PER SERVING
Calories - 331
Protein - 18 g
Sodium - 288 mg
Carbohydrates - 51 g
Cholesterol - 30 mg
Total Fat - 6 g
Saturated Fat - 2 g
Dietary Fiber - 2 g

Veal, Mozzarella and Tomatoes

4 servings

Veal is one of the leanest red meats, so you can treat yourself to a mozzarella topping without breaking your fat budget.

3 ripe tomatoes
2 small garlic cloves, minced
3 teaspoons olive oil
¼ teaspoon coarse salt
⅛ teaspoon coarsely ground black pepper
1 tablespoon chopped fresh basil
¼ teaspoon dried oregano
1 pound very thinly sliced veal round steaks
1 cup grated reduced-fat mozzarella cheese

PER SERVING
Calories - 215
Protein - 26 g
Sodium - 298 mg
Carbohydrates - 5 g
Cholesterol - 97 mg
Total Fat - 9 g
Saturated Fat - 4 g
Dietary Fiber - 1 g

Plunge tomatoes into a pot of boiling water and let cook 30 seconds, or until skins crack and loosen. Plunge immediately into cold water. (The skins will fall right off.) Coarsely chop tomatoes and place in a medium saucepan over medium-high heat. Add garlic, one teaspoon of the olive oil, salt, pepper, basil and oregano. Bring just to boiling. Reduce heat and allow to simmer at least 30 minutes.

Preheat a nonstick skillet over medium-high heat. Add remaining 2 teaspoons olive oil; when hot, add veal and sauté 1 to 2 minutes. Turn meat and cook 2 minutes. Sprinkle with cheese. Cover pan with a lid and cook 1 to 2 minutes longer, until cheese is melted.

Serve onto dinner plates. Cover with sauce.

Lemon-Garlic Veal Roast   8 servings

1 2-pound veal loin roast
1 teaspoon olive oil
juice of ½ lemon
pinch fresh or dried thyme
pinch coarse salt
pinch coarsely ground pepper
1 head garlic, separated into cloves
  and peeled
1 recipe Creamy Horseradish Sauce
  (page 308)

Rub veal with olive oil and sprinkle with
lemon juice; season with thyme, salt and
pepper. Place veal fat side up on a rack in
a roasting pan. Stick garlic cloves into meat
by making incisions all over roast with tip
of paring knife. Insert a meat thermometer
through outside fat into thickest part of meat.
Roast, uncovered, at 325°F for 15 to 30
minutes per pound; meat thermometer should
register 170°.

PER 3.5-OZ. VEAL
Calories - 116
Protein - 20 g
Sodium - 91 mg
Carbohydrates - 0 g
Cholesterol - 80 mg
Total Fat - 3 g
Saturated Fat - 1 g
Dietary Fiber - 0 g

Cook's Suggestion: Serve leftover roast on crusty whole-grain bread
or rolls with lettuce, tomato, onion and mustard or horseradish sauce.

Veal, Mushrooms and Artichokes

4 servings

½ cup dry white wine

2 tablespoons fresh lemon juice

2 tablespoons olive oil

1 pound fresh mushrooms, thinly sliced

1 14-ounce can water-packed quartered
artichoke hearts, drained

1 pound very thinly sliced veal round steaks

juice of ½ lemon

½ teaspoon coarse salt

In a nonstick skillet, heat 1 tablespoon of the olive oil over medium heat. Add mushrooms and sauté 8 to 10 minutes, or until mushrooms are tender. Stir in artichoke hearts and heat to serving temperature.

Combine wine and lemon juice in a medium saucepan. Heat just to boiling; immediately reduce heat and allow to simmer.

Meanwhile, heat the remaining tablespoon of olive oil in a nonstick skillet over medium-high heat. Add veal and sauté 3 to 4 minutes. Turn and cook 2 to 3 minutes longer, or until veal is cooked. Transfer veal to heated serving platter. Squeeze lemon juice over veal. Top with mushrooms and artichokes.

Season wine sauce with salt and pour over mushrooms, artichokes and veal.

PER SERVING

Calories - 273

Protein - 29 g

Sodium - 93 mg

Carbohydrates - 16 g

Cholesterol - 88 mg

Total Fat - 11 g

Saturated Fat - 1 g

Dietary Fiber - 2 g

Grilled Rosemary Veal Chops

4 servings

> *1 pound extra-lean veal loin chops*
> *(4 chops)*
> *1 teaspoon extra-virgin olive oil*
> *2 teaspoons fresh lemon juice*
> *3 garlic cloves, minced*
> *1 tablespoon minced fresh thyme*
> *or 1 teaspoon dried*
> *1 tablespoon minced fresh rosemary*
> *or 1 teaspoon powdered*
> *pinch salt*
> *pinch freshly ground pepper*

Rub veal chops with olive oil and lemon juice; season with garlic, thyme, rosemary, salt and pepper. Grill over hot coals or broil on a rack 3 inches from heat. Turn when juices begin to form on top of meat; cook 3 to 4 minutes longer, or to desired doneness.

PER SERVING
Calories - 146
Protein - 23 g
Sodium - 104 mg
Carbohydrates - 1 g
Cholesterol - 90 mg
Total Fat - 5 g
Saturated Fat - 1 g
Dietary Fiber - 0 g

Grilled Lamb in Pita Pockets   10 servings

1 3-pound leg of lamb, boned and butterflied
pinch powdered rosemary
pinch dried thyme
pinch coarse salt
pinch freshly ground black pepper
2 ripe tomatoes, coarsely chopped
2 English cucumbers, peeled and coarsely chopped
2 white onions, peeled and coarsely chopped
4 cups mixed salad greens, rolled like a cigar
* and sliced into ribbons*
¼ cup baba ghanoush* or 1 avocado, peeled,
* seeded and diced*
8 rounds warm pita bread with pockets

Rub lamb all over with rosemary, thyme, salt and pepper. Allow to stand at room temperature for about 1 hour before grilling.

Build a medium-hot fire in grill. Grill lamb 4 inches from heat, turning every 10 minutes, 30 to 40 minutes for rare, 40 to 50 minutes for medium or 50 to 60 minutes for well-done. Place on carving platter and let sit 10 minutes. Carve into diagonal slices. Arrange on serving platter.

Arrange tomatoes, cucumbers, onions, greens and baba ghanoush or avocado in separate bowls. Arrange pita pockets in napkin-lined serving basket. Pass with lamb. Each person makes own lamb pita.

PER 3.5-OZ. SERVING
Calories - 409
Protein - 26 g
Sodium - 386 mg
Carbohydrates - 40 g
Cholesterol - 69 mg
Total Fat - 16 g
Saturated Fat - 6 g
Dietary Fiber - 3 g

*Baba ghanoush, a Middle Eastern puree of charbroiled eggplant, tahini, olive oil, lemon juice and garlic, is available in the deli cases of most supermarkets.

Roast Leg of Lamb   10 servings

1 3-pound boneless lean leg of lamb
juice of 1 lemon
1 tablespoon olive oil
6 cloves garlic, minced
1 teaspoon powdered rosemary
¼ teaspoon coarse salt
¼ teaspoon coarsely ground black pepper

Preheat oven to 425°F. Place lamb in a shallow baking dish. Combine remaining ingredients and pour over roast; turn to coat. Allow to sit at room temperature for 30 minutes to an hour.

Place lamb on a wire rack in a roasting pan. Pour remaining marinade back over meat and into bottom of pan. Roast 20 minutes; reduce heat to 350°F, and roast approximately 1¼ hours, or until desired doneness.

Save leftovers to serve on pita bread.

PER SERVING
Calories - 180
Protein - 25 g
Sodium - 127 mg
Carbohydrates - 1 g
Cholesterol - 81 mg
Total Fat - 8 g
Saturated Fat - 2 g
Dietary Fiber - 0 g

Grilled Lamb Skewers 4 servings

MARINADE
juice of ½ lemon
1½ tablespoons olive oil
6 cloves garlic, crushed
1 tablespoon chopped fresh rosemary
1 tablespoon chopped fresh thyme

1 pound boneless lean leg of lamb,
  cut into 1-inch cubes

Place lamb in a shallow baking dish. Combine lemon juice, olive oil, garlic, rosemary and thyme; pour over lamb. Marinate 30 minutes. Drain.

Arrange lamb on skewers. Grill skewers over hot coals 4 inches from heat for 12 to 15 minutes, turning often and basting frequently with marinade.

PER 3.5-OZ. SERVING
Calories - 170
Protein - 24 g
Sodium - 73 mg
Carbohydrates - 2 g
Cholesterol - 75 mg
Total Fat - 7 g
Saturated Fat - 3 g
Dietary Fiber - 0 g

Cook's Suggestion: Serve with Couscous Salad (page 266).

Roast Pork Tenderloin with Sauerkraut   4 servings

1 pork tenderloin (about 1 pound)
3 cloves garlic, minced
1 teaspoon extra-virgin olive oil
1 tablespoon minced fresh rosemary
  or 1 teaspoon powdered
1 tablespoon freshly ground pepper
8 ounces sauerkraut

Place tenderloin fat side up on a wire rack in a shallow roasting pan. Mix garlic with olive oil; rub on roast. Combine rosemary and pepper; rub on roast. Insert meat thermometer horizontally so tip is in center of thickest part of pork. Roast, uncovered, at 325°F for about 1 hour, or until thermometer registers 150°F for rare, 160°F for medium or 170°F for well-done. Serve with heated sauerkraut.

PER SERVING
Calories - 164
Protein - 25 g
Sodium - 751 mg
Carbohydrates - 3 g
Cholesterol - 79 mg
Total Fat - 5 g
Saturated Fat - 2 g
Dietary Fiber - 0 g

Cook's Suggestions: Serve with Roast Red Potatoes (page 333) or Roast Fingerling Potatoes (page 338), Stir-Fried Peppers and Onions (page 328) and Homemade Applesauce (page 494). Save leftover pork to serve as an appetizer with hot mustard sauce, or warm the pork in BBQ sauce and serve on a crusty roll.

Sandwiches and Wraps

■ Grilled Turkey Sandwiches   Makes 6 sandwiches

LEMON MAYONNAISE
¼ cup light mayonnaise
1½ teaspoons fresh lemon juice
1 teaspoon grated zest of lemon

1 tablespoon extra-virgin olive oil
2 tablespoons fresh lemon juice
1 pound very thin turkey breast fillets
6 sesame hamburger buns or sandwich buns, split
12 large butter lettuce leaves, washed and crisped
1 large firm tomato, sliced
6 thin slices white onion
coarse salt to taste
freshly ground pepper to taste

Combine lemon mayonnaise ingredients and stir to blend. In a separate bowl, combine olive oil and lemon juice. Add turkey fillets and coat on both sides with lemon oil.

Place fillets on a hot grill 4 to 6 inches above coals. Cook 10 to 15 minutes, turning only once, until fillets are white in center. Just before removing fillets from grill, arrange buns on top to warm.

To assemble, place turkey fillets, lettuce, tomato and onion on bottom half of bun. Season. Spread lemon mayonnaise on top half.

PER SANDWICH
Calories - 252
Protein - 21 g
Sodium - 350 mg
Carbohydrates - 25 g
Cholesterol - 50 mg
Total Fat - 7 g
Saturated Fat - 1 g
Dietary Fiber - 1 g

444

Turkey, Cranberry and Cream Cheese Sandwich Makes 1 sandwich

You'll like this sandwich even better once you see how easy it is to make your own cranberry sauce.

CRANBERRY SAUCE IN MINUTES
1 12-ounce bag fresh or frozen cranberries,
*   rinsed and sorted*
1 cup water
1 cup superfine sugar

2 tablespoons fat-free cream cheese or
*   light whipped cream cheese*
2 slices whole-grain bread
2 ounces Roast Breast of Turkey
*   (page 425)*
red or other dark leafy lettuce

To make cranberry sauce, mix sugar and water in a medium saucepan; stir to dissolve sugar. Bring to a boil; add cranberries. Return to a boil; reduce heat and simmer 10 minutes, stirring occasionally. Remove from heat. Cool at room temperature and refrigerate.

    Spread cream cheese onto one slice of the bread. Top with turkey, lettuce and 2 tablespoons of cranberry sauce. Cover with second slice of bread.

PER SANDWICH
WITH 2 TBSP. SAUCE
Calories - 297
Protein - 27 g
Sodium - 491 mg
Carbohydrates - 41 g
Cholesterol - 51 mg
Total Fat - 3 g
Saturated Fat - 1 g
Dietary Fiber - 4 g

Roast Turkey Sandwich   Makes 1 sandwich

It's not just another turkey sandwich once you add the chutney and sliced fruit.

2 slices whole wheat or multigrain bread
1 tablespoon Major Grey's Chutney
2 ounces Roast Breast of Turkey (page 425)
2 thin slices pear (Anjou or Comice) or apple
2 thin slices red or yellow onion
1 romaine lettuce leaf

Spread one slice of bread with chutney; top with remaining ingredients and other slice of bread. Cut sandwich in half or diagonally into quarters and serve.

PER SANDWICH
Calories - 268
Protein - 19 g
Sodium - 430 mg
Carbohydrates - 42 g
Cholesterol - 37 mg
Total Fat - 3 g
Saturated Fat - 1 g
Dietary Fiber - 5 g

Quick Chicken Sandwich   Makes 1 sandwich

2 slices whole wheat or multigrain bread
2 teaspoons light mayonnaise
2 ounces Quick Chicken (page 413)
2 Bibb lettuce leaves
2 tomato slices

Spread one slice of bread with mayonnaise; top with remaining ingredients and other bread slice. Cut sandwich in half or diagonally into quarters and serve.

Variation: Instead of mayo, use Major Grey's Chutney.

PER SANDWICH
Calories - 282
Protein - 24 g
Sodium - 423 mg
Carbohydrates - 31 g
Cholesterol - 52 mg
Total Fat - 8 g
Saturated Fat - 2 g
Dietary Fiber - 5 g

Pesto Chicken on Olive Bread

Makes 1 sandwich

Pull out your bite-size frozen pesto the night before so it's ready to use in this nutritious sandwich recipe.

> *1 tablespoon Pesto (page 309)*
> *1 white onion, sliced*
> *1 tomato, sliced*
> *2 ounces Roast Chicken (page 424),*
> > *Grilled Herbed Chicken Breast (page 420)*
> > *or Quick Chicken (page 413)*
> *2 slices rustic olive bread*

Spread one slice of bread with pesto; top with remaining ingredients and other bread slice. Cut sandwich in half or diagonally into quarters and serve.

PER SANDWICH
Calories - 275
Protein - 21 g
Sodium - 355 mg
Carbohydrates - 29 g
Cholesterol - 43 mg
Total Fat - 8 g
Saturated Fat - 1 g
Dietary Fiber - 2

Pesto Chicken on a Roll Makes 1 sandwich

1 crusty French roll
1 tablespoon Pesto (page 309)
2 tablespoons dried cranberries
2 ounces Quick Chicken (page 413)
2 green lettuce leaves

Slice roll in half. Spread each half with pesto.
Layer cranberries, then chicken and lettuce.

PER SANDWICH
Calories - 367
Protein - 32 g
Sodium - 384 mg
Carbohydrates - 41 g
Cholesterol - 73 mg
Total Fat - 9 g
Saturated Fat - 2 g
Dietary Fiber - 2 g

Chicken and Shrimp Club Makes 1 sandwich

3 slices whole wheat toast
1½ teaspoons light mayonnaise
1 ounce cooked chicken breast, sliced
6 red lettuce leaves, rolled like a cigar
and cut into ribbons
3 tomato slices
1 ounce small cooked shrimp

Top one slice of toast with mayonnaise,
chicken and lettuce. Cover top with second
slice of toast; add tomato slices and shrimp.
Cover with third slice of toast. Slice diagonally
into quarters.

PER SANDWICH
Calories - 319
Protein - 23 g
Sodium - 590 mg
Carbohydrates - 43 g
Cholesterol - 77 mg
Total Fat - 8 g
Saturated Fat - 2 g
Dietary Fiber - 6 g

Shrimp Sandwiches Makes 3 sandwiches

2 tablespoons light mayonnaise

1 tablespoon lemon juice

2 teaspoons grated white onion

½ pound cooked shrimp

6 slices 9-grain bread

3 slices ripe tomato

1½ cups mixed salad greens

In a small bowl, combine mayonnaise, lemon juice and onion. Add shrimp and mix gently. Spread mixture over 3 slices of bread. Top with tomato, salad greens and remaining bread slices. Cut into halves.

PER SERVING

Calories - 279

Protein - 23 g

Sodium - 566 mg

Carbohydrates - 33 g

Cholesterol - 153 mg

Total Fat - 7 g

Saturated Fat - 1 g

Dietary Fiber - 5 g

Cucumber Shrimp Baguette 6 servings

1 12-inch multigrain baguette

1 tablespoon safflower mayonnaise

6 tomato slices

12 English cucumber slices

2 cups shredded lettuce

½ pound cooked shrimp

Cut the baguette in half lengthwise. Spread mayonnaise over each half. Layer bottom half with remaining ingredients and cover with top half. Cut diagonally into 6 servings.

PER SERVING

Calories - 257

Protein - 15 g

Sodium - 486 mg

Carbohydrates - 37 g

Cholesterol - 75 mg

Total Fat - 5 g

Saturated Fat - 1 g

Dietary Fiber - 2 g

The Big Tuna Makes 3 sandwiches

½ teaspoon fresh lemon juice
1 6-ounce can water-packed tuna, drained
3 tablespoons minced onion
2 tablespoons minced celery
2 tablespoons finely chopped water chestnuts
⅓ cup light mayonnaise
dash prepared mustard
6 slices whole-grain or rye bread
6 ripe tomato slices
6 large dark lettuce leaves

Sprinkle lemon juice over tuna; mix in onion, celery and water chestnuts. Moisten with mayonnaise and mustard. Spread 3 slices of bread with filling; top each with tomato and lettuce and second slice of bread. Cut each sandwich in half.

PER SANDWICH
Calories - 291
Protein - 18 g
Sodium - 628 mg
Carbohydrates - 33 g
Cholesterol - 18 mg
Total Fat - 10 g
Saturated Fat - 2 g
Dietary Fiber - 4 g

Variations: 1) Omit the celery, water chestnuts and mustard. Add roasted red pepper and red tomato salsa. 2) Omit the water chestnuts and mustard. Add apples and sunflower seeds.

■

Monte Cristo Makes 3 sandwiches

1 6-ounce can water-packed tuna, drained
¼ cup light mayonnaise
6 slices whole wheat bread
2 eggs, lightly beaten

Moisten tuna with mayonnaise. Dip one slice of bread into beaten egg; place on a preheated nonstick griddle. Spread with tuna. Dip second slice of bread into beaten egg; place over tuna. Brown sandwiches in a skillet on both sides, turning only once. Repeat. Cut each sandwich in half and serve.

Variation: Add slices of tomato or white onion.

PER SANDWICH
Calories - 315
Protein - 24 g
Sodium - 687 mg
Carbohydrates - 28 g
Cholesterol - 149 mg
Total Fat - 12 g
Saturated Fat - 3 g
Dietary Fiber - 4 g

■

The Big Crab   Makes 4 sandwiches

½ pound crabmeat
2 tablespoons minced celery
2 tablespoons minced white onion
3 tablespoons light mayonnaise
½ teaspoon lemon juice
8 slices rustic sourdough bread
8 tomato slices
8 red-leaf lettuce leaves, rolled like a cigar
    and cut into ribbons

Combine crabmeat, celery, onion, mayonnaise and lemon juice in a medium bowl. Toss. Divide filling over 4 slices of bread. Layer each with 2 tomato slices and lettuce. Cover with remaining slices. Cut sandwiches in half.

Cook's Suggestion: Try these sandwiches with our Artichoke and Tomato Soup (page 258).

PER SANDWICH
Calories - 269
Protein - 17 g
Sodium - 600 mg
Carbohydrates - 34 g
Cholesterol - 30 mg
Total Fat - 7 g
Saturated Fat - 1 g
Dietary Fiber - 3 g

Lox and Bagels 4 servings

2 fresh whole wheat bagels
3 tablespoons nonfat cream cheese
4 thin slices white onion (optional)
¼ pound thinly sliced lox or smoked salmon
1 tomato, thinly sliced
lettuce leaves or young baby spinach leaves

Slice bagels in half. Spread each half with cream cheese. Top with onion and lox or smoked salmon. Garnish with tomato slices and lettuce or spinach leaves.

PER ½ BAGEL
Calories - 147
Protein - 11 g
Sodium - 513 mg
Carbohydrates - 22 g
Cholesterol - 8 mg
Total Fat - 2 g
Saturated Fat - 0 g
Dietary Fiber - 1 g

Just Egg Salad Makes 2 sandwiches

I always loved the egg salad sandwiches they made at our local deli. One day, I asked for their secret. Was it a special mustard? No, they just used the regular old ballpark kind, along with mayo, salt and pepper. I went straight home and made it their way. Here it is.

2 hard-boiled eggs, diced
1 tablespoon light mayonnaise
dash coarse salt
dash freshly ground pepper
4 slices whole wheat or 9-grain bread
yellow mustard

Combine egg with mayonnaise. Season with salt and pepper. Spread one slice of bread with mustard. Top with egg filling and second slice of bread. Repeat.

PER SANDWICH
Calories - 229
Protein - 11 g
Sodium - 530 mg
Carbohydrates - 27 g
Cholesterol - 190 mg
Total Fat - 9 g
Saturated Fat - 2 g
Dietary Fiber - 4 g

PBG Sandwich Makes 1 sandwich

Wish you were a kid again? Try this updated version.

> *2 tablespoons peanut butter**
> *1 tablespoon granola*
> *½ teaspoon honey*
> *2 slices raisin or whole-grain bread*

Spread peanut butter, granola and honey
on one slice of bread. Top with second slice.
Cut in half and serve.

**Be sure to select a peanut butter made with
nonhydrogenated rather than partially
hydrogenated oil.*

PER SANDWICH
Calories - 361
Protein - 12 g
Sodium - 378 mg
Carbohydrates - 41 g
Cholesterol - 0 mg
Total Fat - 18 g
Saturated Fat - 7 g
Dietary Fiber - 5 g

■

French Dip Sandwich Makes 1 sandwich

An easy makeover for a Sunday roast.

> *1 6-inch crusty baguette*
> *2 teaspoons Creamy Horseradish Sauce (page 308)*
> *2 ounces cooked Sunday Beef Roast (page 429)*
> *½ cup beef broth*

Cut the baguette lengthwise. Spread sauce
lightly over bottom half; top with beef.

Heat broth to boiling; ladle into shallow
bowl. Serve with sandwich as dipping sauce.

PER SANDWICH
Calories - 277
Protein - 24 g
Sodium - 441 mg
Carbohydrates - 31 g
Cholesterol - 40 mg
Total Fat - 6 g
Saturated Fat - 1 g
Dietary Fiber - 2 g

453

Vegetarian Wraps 4 servings

> 4 whole wheat or flour tortillas
> 8 teaspoons light mayonnaise
> 4 ounces sharp cheddar or Monterey Jack cheese
> 1 tomato, sliced
> ½ onion, diced
> ½ cucumber, sliced
> 2 cups shredded lettuce
> 4 peperoncini, sliced

Lay each tortilla flat. Spread with mayonnaise. Top with remaining ingredients. Roll tightly. Slice into rounds.

PER WRAP
Calories - 229
Protein - 10 g
Sodium - 592 mg
Carbohydrates - 17 g
Cholesterol - 33 mg
Total Fat - 13 g
Saturated Fat - 7 g
Dietary Fiber - 10 g

Roast Beef, Roasted Red Pepper and Onion Wraps 4 servings

> 4 whole wheat or flour tortillas
> ½ cup Creamy Horseradish Sauce (page 308)
> 8 ounces roast beef tenderloin, cut into strips
> 1 roasted red pepper, sliced
> ¼ sweet onion, sliced
> 8 dark lettuce leaves

Lay each tortilla flat. Spread with horseradish sauce. Top with remaining ingredients. Roll tightly. Slice into rounds.

PER WRAP
Calories - 219
Protein - 15 g
Sodium - 287 mg
Carbohydrates - 15 g
Cholesterol - 39 mg
Total Fat - 11 g
Saturated Fat - 2 g
Dietary Fiber - 10 g

Herbed Turkey Wraps 4 wraps

Whole wheat tortillas help to ease the transition to whole grains.
It's worth the search to find your favorite brand.

4 whole wheat or flour tortillas
8 tablespoons Avocado Spread (page 313)
8 ounces Roast Breast of Turkey (page 425),
        cut into strips
¼ red onion, sliced
1 ripe tomato, sliced
8 romaine lettuce leaves, rolled like a cigar
        and sliced into ribbons

Lay each tortilla flat. Smooth avocado spread
over tortilla. Top with remaining ingredients.
Roll tightly. Slice into rounds.

PER WRAP
Calories - 194
Protein - 17 g
Sodium - 246 mg
Carbohydrates - 17 g
Cholesterol - 37 mg
Total Fat - 6 g
Saturated Fat - 1 g
Dietary Fiber - 11 g

Chicken in Lettuce Wraps 6 servings

SAUCE

1 tablespoon hoisin sauce

2 tablespoons oyster sauce

1 tablespoon reduced-sodium soy sauce

1 tablespoon rice wine vinegar

1 teaspoon sesame oil

1 tablespoon olive oil

2 cups chicken broth, preferably homemade (page 240)

2 cups water

1 6-ounce package somen noodles

1 pound boned and skinned chicken breasts, diced

2 teaspoons potato starch

1 tablespoon olive oil

2 teaspoons peeled and minced fresh ginger

2 cloves garlic, minced

1 hot jalapeño pepper, minced

2 green onions, minced

1 5-ounce can water chestnuts, drained and minced

1/2 pound shiitake mushrooms, minced

1 8-ounce can bamboo shoots, drained and minced

1 head red-leaf lettuce

In a small saucepan, combine ingredients for sauce. Keep warm over low heat.

Bring broth and water to a boil in a medium saucepan. Add noodles; cook until tender. Drain, rinse and chop. Set aside.

Place chicken in a shallow bowl; toss with potato starch. Heat 1½ teaspoons of the olive oil in a nonstick skillet. Add chicken; stir-fry

PER SERVING
Calories - 292
Protein - 25 g
Sodium - 908 mg
Carbohydrates - 31 g
Cholesterol - 45 mg
Total Fat - 7 g
Saturated Fat - 1 g
Dietary Fiber - 3 g

2 to 3 minutes, or until done. Remove from pan; set aside. Heat remaining 1½ teaspoons olive oil in the skillet. Add ginger, garlic, jalapeño pepper and onions; stir-fry 1 to 2 minutes. Add water chestnuts, mushrooms and bamboo shoots; stir-fry 2 minutes. Return chicken to pan. Add sauce.

Arrange noodles in a shallow serving bowl. Pour chicken mixture over noodles; toss. Spoon about ¼ cup of mixture into each lettuce leaf and roll. Or serve a bowl of leaf each lettuce alongside chicken and noodle filling for each person to make wraps.

For a delicious soup, heat leftover filling in chicken broth. See the recipe for Monday Soup (page 252).

Sodium Alert: Choose low-sodium foods at other meals throughout the day to offset the higher sodium in this recipe.

■

Chicken and Black Bean Wraps 4 wraps

4 whole wheat or flour tortillas
4 tablespoons Black Bean Dip (page 310)
8 ounces Quick Chicken (page 413)
1 large tomato, diced
1 roasted red pepper, sliced
8 dark green lettuce leaves, rolled like a cigar
*   and sliced into ribbons*
¼ cup chopped onion
4 tablespoons grated sharp cheddar
*   cheese*

Lay each tortilla flat. Spread with black bean dip. Layer with remaining ingredients. Roll tightly. Slice into rounds.

PER WRAP
Calories - 266
Protein - 21 g
Sodium - 503 mg
Carbohydrates - 19 g
Cholesterol - 50 mg
Total Fat - 11 g
Saturated Fat - 2 g
Dietary Fiber - 12 g

Finger Sandwiches Makes 4 sandwiches

8 slices 7-grain bread, crusts removed
whipped light cream cheese

Choose a Filling*
8 ounces thinly sliced Black Forest ham**
½ large cucumber, thinly sliced
8 ounces crab or shrimp meat

Select a filling. Spread bread with cream cheese and selected filling. Top with second slice of bread. Cut into squares or triangles. Keep sandwiches under a damp kitchen towel until ready to serve.

*Round out filling with 8 ounces of egg salad and/or 8 ounces of lox or smoked salmon. (Watch the sodium content in the latter.)

**Be sure to check labels. Some brands of Black Forest ham are high in sodium.

PER HAM SANDWICH
Calories - 226
Protein - 19 g
Sodium - 480 mg
Carbohydrates - 26 g
Cholesterol - 31 mg
Total Fat - 5 g
Saturated Fat - 2 g
Dietary Fiber - 3 g

PER CUCUMBER SANDWICH
Calories - 148
Protein - 7 g
Sodium - 331 mg
Carbohydrates - 26 g
Cholesterol - 1 mg
Total Fat - 2 g
Saturated Fat - 1 g
Dietary Fiber - 4 g

PER CRAB OR SHRIMP SANDWICH
Calories - 204
Protein - 19 g
Sodium - 414 mg
Carbohydrates - 25 g
Cholesterol - 87 mg
Total Fat - 3 g
Saturated Fat - 1 g
Dietary Fiber - 3 g

Pita Pockets

The sky's the limit when it comes to filling a pita pocket.

> *1 whole-grain pita pocket*
>
> STUFFING*
> *Grilled Chicken Salad (page 293)*
> *Grilled Steak and Onion Salad (page 296)*
> *tuna salad*
> *egg salad*
> *shrimp salad*
>
> ADD-ONS**
> *sliced tomatoes*
> *sliced roasted red peppers*
> *sun-dried tomatoes*
> *romaine or other dark green leafy lettuces*
> *baby spinach leaves*
> *shredded cabbage*
> *broccoli slaw (found in refrigerated deli case)*
> *sliced onions*
> *olives*
> *peperoncini*
> *apple slices*
> *pear slices*

Stuff pita with your choice of stuffing. Tuck in your choice of add-ons.

See nutritional information for individual recipes.

**All add-ons will add a few more calories, sodium and, in some cases, healthy monounsaturated fat.*

Pizza and Breads

Pizza Crust Makes 2 9-inch crusts

Although preparing a homemade crust takes time, it's something the whole family can do together. Hand-kneading the dough in this recipe creates a delicious crust that rewards the extra effort.

> *1 package active dry yeast*
> *¾ cup warm water*
> *4 cups all-purpose flour*
> *½ teaspoon sugar*
> *½ teaspoon salt*
> *2 tablespoons olive oil*
> *1 egg, beaten*
> *dab of tub-type safflower margarine*

Dissolve yeast in warm water. Mix flour with sugar and salt; add to yeast along with olive oil and egg, and stir until mixed. Knead on a heavily floured board until smooth and elastic. (Add water if needed for moisture.)

Place the dough in a bowl greased with margarine; cover and let rise in a warm place for 1 hour. Punch down. Knead slightly. Let rise 1 hour longer. Punch down. Knead slightly. Let rise one more hour.

Divide dough in half. Roll into two 9-inch crusts.

Variation: If you have a bread machine, follow the manufacturer's suggested recipe for pizza crust.

PER SERVING
(⅙ OF 1 CRUST)
Calories - 182
Protein - 5 g
Sodium - 107 mg
Carbohydrates - 32 g
Cholesterol - 16 mg
Total Fat - 3 g
Saturated Fat - 1 g
Dietary Fiber - 1 g

A NOTE ABOUT PIZZA CRUSTS

When selecting a commercially prepared pizza crust, be sure to read labels. Whole wheat crusts are more nutritious than those made with white flour, and some crusts have little or no total fat or saturated fat. Once you get the toppings on, you won't notice the difference.

You can buy delicious crusts from your local pizza parlor. Buy two at a time and keep one in your freezer. This way, you can have your pizza on the table in less time than it takes to have one delivered.

Neapolitan Pizza Sauce Makes 1½ cups

When you find a spare five minutes, make a batch of this homemade pizza sauce to have on hand.

> *1 14½-ounce can Italian-style plum tomatoes,*
>   *including liquid, diced*
> *1 tablespoon tomato paste*
> *1 tablespoon olive oil*
> *¼ teaspoon coarse salt*

Mix tomatoes and ½ cup of the liquid with tomato paste and olive oil. Season with salt.

PER 1½ CUPS
Calories - 240
Protein - 4 g
Sodium - 1,501 mg
Carbohydrates - 29 g
Cholesterol - 0 mg
Total Fat - 14 g
Saturated Fat - 2 g
Dietary Fiber - 1 g

Tomato, Basil and Olive Pizza

Makes 8 slices

1 pound ripe plum tomatoes, chopped
3 garlic cloves, finely chopped
1½ tablespoons olive oil
¼ cup chopped fresh basil
½ cup chopped kalamata olives
1 9-inch pizza crust
1 cup grated part-skim mozzarella cheese

Combine tomatoes, garlic and 1 tablespoon of the olive oil. Let stand 1 hour at room temperature. Add basil and olives.

Preheat oven to 450°F. Move oven rack to highest position. If using a baking stone, place stone on rack and heat at least 30 minutes.

Rub pizza crust with remaining olive oil. Sprinkle with cheese. Place on pizza baking pan or directly on baking stone. Bake 10 to 15 minutes, or until crust is golden (time will vary depending on type of crust). Remove from oven onto serving round.

Top crust with tomato mixture. Use a pizza wheel to slice.

PER SLICE
Calories - 226
Protein - 8 g
Sodium - 448 mg
Carbohydrates - 29 g
Cholesterol - 19 mg
Total Fat - 9 g
Saturated Fat - 2 g
Dietary Fiber - 2 g

Pizza Marinara   Makes 8 slices

1 9-inch pizza crust
¾ cup Neapolitan Pizza Sauce (page 461)
3 tablespoons chopped fresh basil
⅓ cup pitted and sliced kalamata olives
½ cup grated part-skim mozzarella cheese

Preheat oven to 450°F. Move oven rack to highest position. If using a baking stone, place stone on rack and heat at least 30 minutes.

Lay pizza crust flat. Remove diced tomatoes from pizza sauce with slotted spoon and spread over crust. Sprinkle with basil and olives. Top with cheese. Bake 20 minutes, or until crust is cooked.

PER SLICE
Calories - 207
Protein - 7 g
Sodium - 557 mg
Carbohydrates - 29 g
Cholesterol - 17 mg
Total Fat - 7 g
Saturated Fat - 2 g
Dietary Fiber - 1 g

Variation: Add other toppings, such as quartered artichoke hearts, anchovies, roasted red peppers, sun-dried tomatoes, sliced mushrooms, peperoncini, crumbled meatless soy burger or leanest ground round.

Veggie Pizza Makes 8 slices

1 9-inch pizza crust
1 teaspoon olive oil
1 cup grated part-skim mozzarella cheese

¼ cup olive oil
2 tablespoons balsamic vinegar
¼ teaspoon coarse salt
dash freshly ground pepper
4 cups shredded hearts of romaine
½ cup diced red onion
1 tomato, diced
¼ cup pitted and halved kalamata olives
1 ripe Hass avocado, diced

Preheat oven to 450°F. Move oven rack to highest position. If using a baking stone, place stone on rack and heat at least 30 minutes.

Rub pizza crust with 1 teaspoon olive oil. Sprinkle with cheese. Place on pizza baking pan or directly on baking stone. Bake 10 to 15 minutes, or until crust is cooked (time will vary depending on type of crust).

Combine remaining olive oil, vinegar, salt and pepper in a jar with lid. Shake. Combine romaine, red onion, tomato and olives in a medium salad bowl. Pour dressing over salad and toss.

Remove pizza from oven onto serving round. Use a pizza wheel to slice. Place slices onto individual dinner or salad plates. Top with salad. Garnish with avocado.

PER SLICE
Calories - 299
Protein - 9 g
Sodium - 336 mg
Carbohydrates - 29 g
Cholesterol - 19 g
Total Fat - 16 g
Saturated Fat - 3 g
Dietary Fiber - 3 g

Pesto, Onion and Sun-Dried Tomato Pizza   Makes 6 slices

Out of energy? Keep some pesto in your freezer and a pizza crust in your pantry. You'll have dinner on the table in a matter of minutes.

1/2 cup dry-packed sun-dried tomatoes

2 cups water

1 9-inch pizza crust

1/3 cup Pesto (page 309)

3/4 cup medium-diced red pepper

3/4 cup red onion, quartered and thinly sliced

1 cup grated part-skim mozzarella cheese

Slice each tomato in half lengthwise and then into strips (approximately 6 strips per half). Place strips in a bowl. Bring 2 cups water just to boiling. Pour over tomatoes. Let tomatoes sit 5 minutes to plump. Drain and pat dry with paper towels.

Lay pizza crust flat. Spread pesto over crust. Top with tomatoes, red pepper and onion. Sprinkle with cheese. Bake 8 to 10 minutes, or until crust is golden.

PER SLICE

Calories - 299

Protein - 12 g

Sodium - 344 mg

Carbohydrates - 38 g

Cholesterol - 26 mg

Total Fat - 11 g

Saturated Fat - 3 g

Dietary Fiber - 3 g

Combination Pizza   Makes 6 slices

Topping the grated fat-free mozzarella with part-skim mozzarella slices seems to be what makes this pizza work. As long as the cheeses are layered in the order given, any other toppings may be substituted.

¼ pound leanest Italian sausage
1 9-inch pizza crust
1 teaspoon extra-virgin olive oil
10 fresh basil leaves, chopped
⅓ to ½ cup Neapolitan Pizza Sauce (page 461)
1 7-ounce can mushroom stems and pieces, drained
1 4-ounce can sliced black olives, drained
½ cup shredded fat-free mozzarella cheese
3-ounces very thinly sliced part-skim mozzarella cheese
    or ⅔ cup shredded

Preheat oven to 450°F or 500°F (the highest setting, but not broil). Move oven rack to highest position. If using a baking stone, place stone on rack and heat at least 30 minutes.

PER 1½ SLICE
Calories - 274
Protein - 16 g
Sodium - 771 mg
Carbohydrates - 31 g
Cholesterol - 23 mg
Total Fat - 10 g
Saturated Fat - 2 g
Dietary Fiber - 1 g

Preheat a nonstick skillet over medium-high heat. Slit sausage open; remove and discard casing. Add sausage to skillet and cook 6 to 8 minutes, breaking it apart as it browns. Drain on paper towels and pat dry with additional toweling to remove all excess fat. Set aside.

Slide crust onto a nonstick pizza pan; rub with olive oil, but do not dampen the edges. Combine basil and pizza sauce; spread ⅓ to ½ cup of the sauce over crust, again taking care not to dampen edges.

Sprinkle pizza evenly with sausage, mushrooms and olives. Top with shredded fat-free mozzarella, then part-skim mozzarella slices. Bake 12 to 15 minutes, or until crust is golden brown.

Tex-Mex Pizza Makes 6 slices

1 15-ounce can black beans, drained and rinsed

1 teaspoon olive oil

1 tablespoon plus ¼ teaspoon chili powder

1 8-ounce can tomato sauce

½ teaspoon ground cumin

¼ teaspoon coarse salt

¼ teaspoon coarsely ground black pepper

1 9-inch pizza crust

1 cup quartered cherry or grape tomatoes

⅓ cup chopped yellow onion

½ cup chopped kalamata olives

½ pound fresh mozzarella cheese, sliced

Preheat oven to 450°F or 500°F (the highest setting, but not broil). Move oven rack to highest position. If using a baking stone, place stone on rack and heat at least 30 minutes.

In a small bowl, combine black beans, olive oil and 1 tablespoon chili powder; set aside. In a separate bowl, combine tomato sauce, cumin, ¼ teaspoon chili powder, salt and pepper.

Lay pizza crust flat. Roll edges up slightly and spread a layer of sauce over crust. (Freeze remaining sauce for another pizza.) Sprinkle black beans over sauce; add tomatoes, onions and olives. Layer cheese over top. Bake 8 to 10 minutes, or until crust is golden.

Cook's Suggestion: Serve with our Save-the-Day Fresh Fruit Salad (page 299).

PER SLICE
Calories - 401
Protein - 21 g
Sodium - 910 mg
Carbohydrates - 53 g
Cholesterol - 36 mg
Total Fat - 12 g
Saturated Fat - 5 g
Dietary Fiber - 6 g

Bruschetta   8 servings

2 tablespoons extra-virgin olive oil
1 large ripe tomato, seeded and diced
1 tablespoon finely chopped fresh basil
2 teaspoons minced garlic
¼ to ½ teaspoon coarse salt
¼ teaspoon freshly ground black pepper
8 ½-inch-thick slices rustic bread
extra-virgin olive oil cooking spray

In a small bowl, combine olive oil, tomatoes, basil, garlic, salt and pepper. Set aside.

Spray each bread slice lightly on both sides with olive oil, about 5 seconds or until coated. In a preheated broiler, toast bread until lightly browned, turning once. Serve onto individual bread plates. Pass tomato topping.

PER SLICE
Calories - 144
Protein - 4 g
Sodium - 441 mg
Carbohydrates - 23 g
Cholesterol - 0 mg
Total Fat - 4 g
Saturated Fat - 1 g
Dietary Fiber - 0 g

Roasted Garlic Bread   12 1-inch slices

No regrets for the missing butter. Roasted garlic wins hands down!

4 tiny (3-inch) loaves rustic bread
olive oil cooking spray
Roasted Garlic (page 327)

Cut each loaf of bread into 3 slices. Lightly spray top of each slice with olive oil. Place under broiler 2 to 3 minutes, or until lightly toasted. Pass toasted bread with warm garlic spread.

PER SLICE
Calories - 41
Protein - 1 g
Sodium - 72 mg
Carbohydrates - 6 g
Cholesterol - 0 mg
Total Fat - 1 g
Saturated Fat - 0 g
Dietary Fiber - 0 g

Tuscan Bread with Olives and Tomatoes   Makes 16 ½-inch slices

Good with soups and pasta. Even better on a picnic with roasted
or grilled chicken.

1 pound fresh ripe plum tomatoes, chopped
3 garlic cloves, finely chopped
2 tablespoons olive oil
1 loaf Italian, Tuscan or peasant bread
16 kalamata olives, pitted and chopped
¼ cup chopped fresh basil

Combine tomatoes, garlic and olive oil;
let stand at room temperature for 1 hour.

Meanwhile, slice a loaf of bread into
approximately 16 half-inch slices. Toast
under a preheated broiler or in a toaster
oven for 2 to 3 minutes, until bread browns
on both sides.

Just before serving, add olives and basil
to tomato mixture. Spoon mixture into a medium bowl and place
in center of a basket or serving tray. Ring with toasted bread.

PER SERVING
Calories - 95
Protein - 3 g
Sodium - 239 mg
Carbohydrates - 15 g
Cholesterol - 0 mg
Total Fat - 3 g
Saturated Fat - 0 g
Dietary Fiber - 0 g

Breakfasts

■ Old-Fashioned Oatmeal 2 servings

On oatmeal mornings, start the oatmeal as soon as you get up.
By the time you're dressed, the cereal will be ready.

> *1 cup water*
> *½ cup steel-cut rolled oats*
> *¼ cup raisins**

Bring water to a boil in a medium saucepan.
Stir in rolled oats. Reduce heat to medium.
Cook uncovered for 2 to 3 minutes. Turn off
heat. Stir in raisins. Cover and let oatmeal
sit 10 to 12 minutes, or until moisture is
absorbed.

**No measuring is necessary if you use the
1½-ounce snack-size box of raisins.*

PER SERVING
Calories - 174
Protein - 5 g
Sodium - 4 mg
Carbohydrates - 36 g
Cholesterol - 0 mg
Total Fat - 2 g
Saturated Fat - 0 g
Dietary Fiber - 4 g

Breakfast in a Bowl 1 serving

> 1 cup mixed berries
> 4 to 6 ounces nonfat fruit-sweetened yogurt
> ½ cup breakfast cereal (Cheerios, Kashi GOLEAN,
>   Flax Plus, Fiber One, All-Bran)
> ½ banana, sliced
> 1 tablespoon walnuts, chopped almonds or ground flaxseed

Layer ingredients in a bowl in the order given.

PER SERVING
Calories - 335
Protein - 11 g
Sodium - 236 mg
Carbohydrates - 63 g
Cholesterol - 0 mg
Total Fat - 7 g
Saturated Fat - 1 g
Dietary Fiber - 8 g

Breakfast on the Run 1 serving

> 1 cup fresh or unsweetened frozen berries
> 1 6-ounce carton nonfat fruit-sweetened yogurt
> 2 tablespoons nonfat milk or enriched soy milk
> ⅔ cup crushed ice
> ½ banana
> 1 tablespoon wheat germ, sliced almonds or ground flaxseed

Combine ingredients in a blender until frothy.

PER SERVING
Calories - 287
Protein - 12 g
Sodium - 113 mg
Carbohydrates - 60 g
Cholesterol - 1 mg
Total Fat - 2 g
Saturated Fat - 0 g
Dietary Fiber - 9 g

◼ Artichoke Frittata   6 servings

If someone in the family doesn't like artichokes, you can leave them out and still have a great breakfast. You can also use another type of vegetable or even some diced lean ham.

> *10 eggs*
> *½ teaspoon salt*
> *½ teaspoon pepper*
> *1 15-ounce can water-packed artichoke hearts,*
> *   drained and quartered*
> *extra-virgin olive oil cooking spray*
> *2 tablespoons freshly grated Parmesan cheese*

In a large bowl, beat eggs with salt and pepper. Stir artichoke hearts into egg mixture.

Preheat a 10-inch nonstick skillet over medium-high heat. When skillet is hot, spray lightly with olive oil. Pour in egg mixture. Cover and cook until eggs are set and starting to brown on bottom. Off the heat, place a 12-inch plate over skillet. Invert frittata onto plate. Return pan to heat. Spray lightly with olive oil. Slide frittata off plate and back into skillet, topside down. Cook 1 to 2 minutes, or until lightly brown. Sprinkle with cheese.

Invert pan and turn frittata onto serving platter. Cut into wedges and serve.

PER SERVING
Calories - 151
Protein - 12 g
Sodium - 569 mg
Carbohydrates - 4 g
Cholesterol - 356 mg
Total Fat - 9 g
Saturated Fat - 3 g
Dietary Fiber - 2 g

Huevos Rancheros 4 servings

1 4-ounce can whole green chilies, drained

3 tablespoons grated reduced-fat Monterey Jack cheese

1½ cups egg substitute, beaten

2 tablespoons grated reduced-fat cheddar cheese

4 6-inch whole wheat flour or corn tortillas

2 cups Pico de Gallo (page 315)

Carefully slit each chili lengthwise and remove seeds. Stuff with Monterey Jack. Press slit edges together to hold cheese in. Cut stuffed chilies into bite-size pieces.

Preheat a nonstick skillet over medium-high heat. Add stuffed chilies and cook until cheese begins to melt; pour in beaten egg substitute. When eggs start to firm, lift chilies slightly to allow uncooked eggs to run underneath. When almost fully cooked, sprinkle cheddar cheese on top. When cheese melts, remove skillet from heat.

Serve with tortillas and pico de gallo.

PER SERVING
Calories - 224
Protein - 17 g
Sodium - 821 mg
Carbohydrates - 20 g
Cholesterol - 3 mg
Total Fat - 9 g
Saturated Fat - 2 g
Dietary Fiber - 10 g

Variation: If you haven't had eggs this week, you can use 6 whole eggs or 6 egg whites plus 2 egg yolks in place of the egg substitute.

Egg on a Muffin 1 serving

1 whole wheat English muffin
1 raw egg
1 ounce Canadian bacon, sliced
1 ounce sliced reduced-fat cheese

Toast muffin in a toaster. Place egg in a custard cup sprayed with nonstick spray coating. Prick egg with a fork and place in microwave with a plate or saucer on top. Microwave for 1 minute, or until cooked through. Assemble egg, bacon and cheese on muffin. Microwave 30 seconds.

PER SERVING
Calories - 283
Protein - 23 g
Sodium - 937 mg
Carbohydrates 28 g
Cholesterol - 207 mg
Total Fat - 9 g
Saturated Fat - 3 g
Dietary Fiber - 4 g

Omelet for Two 2 servings

To treat yourself especially well, buy eggs from your local farmer's market that have been laid by free-range chickens.

2 large whole eggs
1 large egg white
2 tablespoons nonfat milk
olive oil cooking spray
¼ cup chopped green onion
¼ cup diced small red pepper
¼ cup grated reduced-fat sharp
*   cheddar cheese*

Break 2 eggs into a small bowl with egg white and beat with a fork until frothy. Stir in milk.

Preheat a nonstick skillet over medium-high heat. When pan is hot, spray with olive oil cooking spray. Pour in egg mixture. Cover pan and cook 2 minutes to allow eggs to set. Add vegetables and cheese. Cover and cook 1 to 2 minutes, or until eggs look cooked (they stay set when you tilt the pan). Fold omelet and cut in half. Cook 1 minute longer to seal cut edges.

PER SERVING
Calories - 122
Protein - 12 mg
Sodium - 187 mg
Carbohydrates - 4 g
Cholesterol - 216 mg
Total Fat - 6 g
Saturated Fat - 2 g
Dietary Fiber - 1 g

■

Egg Beater Scramble   2 servings

Doctor up your scrambled eggs with your favorite fresh veggies.

1 teaspoon olive oil
2 teaspoons chopped onion
1 teaspoon finely chopped red pepper
¼ cup sliced fresh mushrooms
1 cup egg substitute

Heat olive oil in a nonstick skillet over medium-high heat. Sauté onion 4 to 5 minutes. Add red pepper and mushrooms, and sauté 3 to 4 minutes. Remove from skillet and set aside.

PER SERVING
Calories - 129
Protein - 15 g
Sodium - 223 mg
Carbohydrates - 2 g
Cholesterol - 1 mg
Total Fat - 6 g
Saturated Fat - 1 g
Dietary Fiber - 0 g

Beat egg substitute lightly with a fork. Pour into skillet and stir rapidly. When eggs begin to set, add sautéed onions, peppers and mushrooms. Continue to stir until egg is cooked throughout but still glossy and moist.

Variation: Use 4 egg whites in place of egg substitute.

French Omelet Makes 2 omelets

Omelets aren't just for breakfast. You can make a nice light dinner by serving an omelet with a salad.

FILLING OPTIONS
1 tablespoon chopped onion
¼ cup sliced mushrooms
1 teaspoon minced red pepper
2 tablespoons grated reduced-fat cheddar cheese
1 teaspoon minced fresh chives
2 teaspoons chopped fresh flat-leaf parsley
2 teaspoons diced green chilies
2 tablespoons chopped tomato
2 tablespoons crabmeat

OMELET
1 cup egg substitute
2 tablespoons water
dash salt
dash pepper
4 slices tomato for garnish
fresh flat-leaf parsley for garnish

Select your filling. For onion, mushrooms and red pepper, heat 2 teaspoons olive oil in a nonstick skillet over medium-high heat, add vegetables and sauté until tender.

Beat egg substitute, water, salt and pepper with a fork until mixture is well blended but not frothy. Preheat an 8-inch nonstick skillet over medium heat until a drop of water sizzles when sprinkled on the pan. Pour in egg mixture; tilt pan to spread evenly throughout and at an even depth.

PER OMELET
WITH CHEESE
AND VEGETABLES
Calories - 79
Protein - 13 g
Sodium - 484 mg
Carbohydrates - 4 g
Cholesterol - 5 mg
Total Fat - 1 g
Saturated Fat - 1 g
Dietary Fiber - 0 g

Using a fork, stir rapidly through top of uncooked eggs. Shake pan frequently to keep eggs moving. When eggs are set but still shiny, remove pan from heat. Spoon filling across center. Flip sides of omelet over, envelope style, to hold in filling. Tilt pan and roll omelet onto plate. Garnish with tomato and parsley.

PER OMELET WITH CHEESE, CRAB AND VEGETABLES
Calories - 93
Protein - 15 g
Sodium - 523 mg
Carbohydrates - 4 g
Cholesterol - 10 mg
Total Fat - 2 g
Saturated Fat - 1 g
Dietary Fiber - 0 g

■

Vegetables Benedict   2 servings

2 eggplant slices, each ⅛ inch thick
2 yellow squash slices, each ⅛ inch thick
2 tomato slices, each ⅛ inch thick
1 tablespoon olive oil
1 whole wheat English muffin, split and
*   toasted*
2 eggs, sunny-side up

Brush eggplant, squash and tomatoes on both sides with olive oil. Arrange slices on a rack in a broiler pan and broil 2 minutes on each side. On each muffin half, layer one slice eggplant, squash and tomato. Top with egg. Serve at once.

PER SERVING
Calories - 218
Protein - 9 g
Sodium - 270 mg
Carbohydrates - 20 g
Cholesterol - 187 mg
Total Fat - 12 g
Saturated Fat - 2 g
Dietary Fiber - 4 g

Prosciutto with Melon 12 servings

I put this traditional appetizer in the breakfast section because it's a delicious accompaniment to omelets and scrambled eggs.

1 small cantaloupe
¼ pound thinly sliced prosciutto

Cut cantaloupe into 12 thin wedges and remove rind. Wrap each wedge with a slice of prosciutto.

PER SERVING
Calories - 32
Protein - 3 g
Sodium - 192 mg
Carbohydrates - 3 g
Cholesterol - 2 mg
Total Fat - 1 g
Saturated Fat - 0 g
Dietary Fiber - 0 g

Breakfast Burrito 1 serving

1 6-inch whole wheat tortilla
¼ cup nonfat refried beans
1 egg, scrambled
chopped tomato
shredded lettuce
1 tablespoon shredded reduced-fat cheddar cheese
6 olives or ⅛ avocado (optional)

Top tortilla with refried beans, scrambled egg, tomato, lettuce, cheese and olives or avocado, if desired.

PER SERVING
Calories - 269
Protein - 14 g
Sodium - 487 mg
Carbohydrates - 33 g
Cholesterol - 195 mg
Total Fat - 9 g
Saturated Fat - 3 g
Dietary Fiber - 5 g

Cook's Suggestion: Serve with half a grapefruit or Citrus Salad (page 276).

Nutrition Note: Adding olives increases the calories to 291 and the fat to 11 grams. Adding avocado increases the calories to 309 and the fat to 13 grams.

A NOTE ABOUT YOGURT

Yogurt comes in low-fat and fat-free versions, but be sure to read the labels. Many low- and nonfat types have traded fat for high-fructose corn syrup. Your best bet is to buy organic fruit-sweetened or plain yogurt with whole fruit added, or add your own fruit, nuts, seeds and cinnamon.

Breakfast Smoothies   Makes 4 cups (2 servings)

1 papaya, peeled, seeded and chopped
1 mango, peeled, seeded and chopped
1 banana
¾ cup freshly squeezed orange juice
¾ cup nonfat milk or 6 ounces nonfat
*   vanilla or fruited yogurt*
2 cups ice

Combine fruit, orange juice and milk in a blender. Process until smooth. Add ice and process 1 to 2 minutes longer.

PER SERVING
Calories - 126
Protein - 3 g
Sodium - 26 mg
Carbohydrates - 30 g
Cholesterol - 1 mg
Total Fat - 1 g
Saturated Fat - 0 g
Dietary Fiber - 3 g

■

Berry Smoothies   2 servings

1 6-ounce container nonfat
*   fruit-sweetened yogurt*
½ cup nonfat milk
¼ cup fresh blueberries
1 medium banana
1½ cups chopped ice

Combine all ingredients in a blender and process until smooth.

PER SERVING
Calories - 88
Protein - 4 g
Sodium - 48 mg
Carbohydrates - 19 g
Cholesterol - 4 mg
Total Fat - 0 g
Saturated Fat - 0 g
Dietary Fiber - 1 g

Silver Dollar Pancakes Makes 18 pancakes

2 eggs
½ cup egg substitute
½ cup whole wheat flour, sifted
¼ teaspoon salt
1 teaspoon baking soda
2 cups nonfat sour cream
3 tablespoons water

Combine eggs and egg substitute; beat lightly. Combine flour, salt and baking soda; using a wire whisk, blend with eggs and sour cream. Stir in water. (If batter is too thick, add up to 2 tablespoons of additional water.)

Pour enough batter for each pancake onto a preheated nonstick griddle. Cook until top side is bubbly and a few bubbles have broken. Turn and brown other side.

PER PANCAKE
Calories - 50
Protein - 3 g
Sodium - 141 mg
Carbohydrates - 7 g
Cholesterol - 23 mg
Total Fat - 1 g
Saturated Fat - 0 g
Dietary Fiber - 0 g

Variation: Substitute all-purpose flour for whole wheat; add water to blended batter ingredients only if necessary.

Cook's Suggestion: Consider topping your pancakes with warmed applesauce, berries, 100% fruit spread or, if desired and calories permit, a tablespoon of maple syrup.

■ Rustic French Toast Makes 6 slices

Serve this toast on Sunday morning for a special treat.

> *2 eggs**
> *⅓ cup nonfat milk*
> *¼ teaspoon sugar*
> *½ teaspoon cinnamon*
> *6 slices day-old crusty rustic bread*
> *2 tablespoons tub-style safflower margarine*
> *½ cup light maple syrup or strawberry or*
>   *raspberry syrup or preserves*

Beat eggs. Add milk, sugar and cinnamon.
Blend.

Preheat a nonstick griddle over medium-
high heat. Dip bread one slice at a time into
egg mixture, coating both sides evenly, and
place on griddle. Brown 2 to 3 minutes. Turn
and brown other side, 2 to 3 minutes longer.
Remove to warm serving platter. Serve with
margarine and syrup on the side.

PER SLICE
Calories - 88
Protein - 3 g
Sodium - 143 mg
Carbohydrates - 6 g
Cholesterol - 63 mg
Total Fat - 5 g
Saturated Fat - 1 g
Dietary Fiber - 1 g

**Using an egg substitute reduces the cholesterol, total fat and
saturated fat to 0 and the calories to 66.*

Bran Muffins Makes 14 muffins

1 cup whole wheat flour
½ cup enriched white flour
½ cup oatmeal
2 teaspoons baking soda
dash salt
½ cup wheat bran
1 cup raisins
1 egg
½ cup canola oil
1 cup skim milk
¼ cup honey

In a large bowl, combine flours, oatmeal, baking soda, salt, wheat bran, raisins and egg. In a separate bowl combine oil, milk and honey; add to flour mixture. Blend with a wooden spoon. Pour ¼ cup batter into each paper-lined muffin cup. Bake at 400°F for 12 to 15 minutes.

PER SERVING
Calories - 190
Protein - 4 g
Sodium - 214 mg
Carbohydrates - 27 g
Cholesterol - 14 mg
Total Fat - 9 g
Saturated Fat - 1 g
Dietary Fiber - 3 g

Note: A single bran muffin is not a nutritional powerhouse. Pair it with ½ cup cottage cheese and ½ cup fresh pineapple or a peach for a healthy breakfast.

Fresh Fruit Endings and Other Desserts

■ Summer Fruit with Lemon Ice 4 servings

½ pint frozen lemon or berry ice
½ cup watermelon, cut into 2-inch cubes
½ cup cantaloupe, cut into 2-inch cubes
½ cup honeydew, cut into 2-inch cubes
½ cup pineapple, cut into 2-inch cubes
1 cup raspberries, strawberries or blueberries
fresh mint

Scoop lemon or berry ice into four 4-ounce custard cups. Center each cup on a salad plate. Ring with fruits and garnish with mint.

Cook's Suggestion: For a nice finish to a company meal, cut tops from whole lemons; squeeze out juice (reserve for lemonade), remove pulp and fill shells with lemon or berry ice. Garnish with violets or with blueberries and a sprig of mint.

PER SERVING
Calories - 80
Protein - 1 g
Sodium - 6 mg
Carbohydrates - 26 g
Cholesterol - 0 mg
Total Fat - 0 g
Saturated Fat - 0 g
Dietary Fiber - 1 g

A NOTE ABOUT DESSERTS

You'll notice that fresh fruit is central to most of our dessert recipes. That's because we know it's the best choice. But we also know we have to be realistic. The new guidelines make room for some discretionary calories if you've taken care of business and eaten all the nutrient-rich foods you need.

Fresh Dipped Strawberries 4 servings

1¹/₂ pints fresh strawberries, hulled
4 sprigs fresh mint (optional)
4 tablespoons brown sugar
¹/₂ cup nonfat sour cream or
  nonfat vanilla yogurt

Arrange fresh strawberries in a pretty serving bowl. Garnish with mint, if desired.

Place brown sugar and sour cream in separate small, custard-size bowls. Dip strawberries first in sour cream, then in brown sugar.

PER SERVING
Calories - 99
Protein - 3 g
Sodium - 27 mg
Carbohydrates - 24 g
Cholesterol - 0 mg
Total Fat - 0 g
Saturated Fat - 0 g
Dietary Fiber - 2 g

Warm Berries and Ice Cream

4 servings

This tastes so good that you'll start looking for things to put it on. Some of our favorites are pancakes, waffles, English muffins, plain nonfat vanilla or fruit-sweetened yogurt, and now and then a dish of nonfat vanilla ice cream. Use frozen berries when fresh ones aren't available.

2 cups raspberries
2 cups blueberries
2 cups blackberries
2 tablespoons superfine sugar
2 cups light vanilla ice cream
4 sprigs fresh mint

Combine 1 cup raspberries, 1 cup blueberries, 1 cup blackberries and sugar in a saucepan; bring to a boil. Reduce heat and simmer, uncovered, about 10 minutes. Stir in remaining berries.

Place a cup of fruit in each of 4 bowls. Add a scoop of ice cream. Garnish with mint.

PER SERVING
Calories - 231
Protein - 4 g
Sodium - 62 mg
Carbohydrates - 45 g
Cholesterol - 11 mg
Total Fat - 5 g
Saturated Fat - 2 g
Dietary Fiber - 10 g

Fresh Strawberries with Strawberry Sorbet

4 servings

If you've used up your fat budget but want something sweet to end your meal, sorbet and fresh fruit may be just what you're looking for.

1 pint strawberry sorbet
4 cups fresh strawberries, washed, hulled and slightly crushed
fresh mint

Scoop sorbet into stemmed glasses. Top with berries. Garnish with mint.

PER SERVING
Calories - 175
Protein - 1 g
Sodium - 2 mg
Carbohydrates - 43 g
Cholesterol - 0 mg
Total Fat - 1 g
Saturated Fat - 0 g
Dietary Fiber - 3 g

Strawberry Shortcake

8 servings

Our goal with this dessert was to give the feel of the real thing while reducing fat and calories. For a fun Valentine's Day dessert, cut the biscuits into heart shapes with a cookie cutter.

4 cups hulled strawberries
8 biscuits made from reduced-fat biscuit mix
2 cups light vanilla ice cream

Set aside a few whole berries for garnish. Place remaining berries in a bowl and crush them slightly.

Split still-hot biscuits and place bottoms on individual dessert plates. Add crushed berries and a dollop of ice cream. Cover with top halves. Add more ice cream and crushed berries. Garnish with reserved whole berries.

PER SERVING
Calories - 180
Protein - 5 g
Sodium - 336 mg
Carbohydrates - 31 g
Cholesterol - 3 mg
Total Fat - 4 g
Saturated Fat - 2 g
Dietary Fiber - 1 g

Strawberry Rhubarb Sauce   6 servings

1 pound rhubarb (about 6 cups)
cut into ½-inch pieces
2 tablespoons freshly squeezed orange juice
1 cup sliced strawberries
¾ cups superfine sugar

Combine rhubarb and orange juice in a medium saucepan. Cover and cook 20 minutes over low heat. Add strawberries and sugar. Cook about 10 minutes, or until rhubarb is tender. Serve warm or refrigerate until well chilled.

PER SERVING
Calories - 92
Protein - 1 g
Sodium - 3 mg
Carbohydrates - 23 g
Cholesterol - 0 mg
Total Fat - 0 g
Saturated Fat - 0 g
Dietary Fiber - 1 g

Variation: Spoon vanilla nonfat yogurt into parfait glasses. Top with warm rhubarb sauce. Sprinkle with chopped walnuts.

Note: When selecting rhubarb, choose the thinnest stalks. They're the most tender and the least bitter. Always discard the leaves before cooking; they contain oxalic acid, which can be quite poisonous.

Fresh Pineapple, Papaya and Berries 8 servings

The papaya puree adds a nice touch to this refreshing dessert.

> *1 ripe pineapple*
> *2 ripe papayas*
> *1½ cups strawberries, raspberries*
>   *or blueberries*

Cut off the top and bottom of the pineapple. Peel off the brown skin, cutting fairly deep. Remove any brown "eyes" that may remain. Cut pineapple into rings, then cut rings into quarters.

Peel papayas; cut in half and remove seeds. Place papaya halves in food processor and puree. Divide puree among individual dessert plates. Arrange pineapple quarters over the top. Garnish with berries.

PER SERVING
Calories - 86
Protein - 1 g
Sodium - 3 mg
Carbohydrates - 21 g
Cholesterol - 0 mg
Total Fat - 1 g
Saturated Fat - 0 g
Dietary Fiber - 4 g

Fresh Fruit in a Pineapple 10 servings

Presentation is an important part of the whole eating experience.
Delight your family and friends by serving this fruit salad in a
pineapple boat.

1 fresh pineapple
1 cup strawberries, stemmed and halved
1 cup blueberries
½ small cantaloupe, peeled and
    cut into 1-inch cubes
1 papaya, peeled, seeded and cut up
1 cup seedless green grapes
fresh mint for garnish

Cut pineapple in half horizontally, leaving the
stem end intact. Using a curved grapefruit
knife, carefully remove the pineapple flesh from
the shell and cut into cubes. Place half of the
cubes in a salad bowl (reserve remaining half
for later use). Add remaining fruit and toss.

Transfer fruit to pineapple shells. Garnish
with mint.

PER SERVING
Calories - 60
Protein - 1 g
Sodium - 5 mg
Carbohydrates - 15 g
Cholesterol - 0 mg
Total Fat - 0 g
Saturated Fat - 0 g
Dietary Fiber - 2 g

Simple Indulgence 1 serving

½ cup orange sherbet
¼ cup freshly squeezed orange juice
fresh mint

Scoop sherbet into a bowl. Pour orange juice over sherbet. Garnish with mint.

Variation: Scoop ½ cup fat-free lemon sorbet into a bowl; pour ¾ cup sugar-free lemonade over sorbet.

PER SERVING
Calories - 185
Protein - 2 g
Sodium - 36 mg
Carbohydrates - 4 g
Cholesterol - 4 mg
Total Fat - 2 g
Saturated Fat - 1 g
Dietary Fiber - 0 g

Fresh Peaches in Warm Raspberry Sauce 4 servings

1 10-ounce package frozen raspberries
¼ cup freshly squeezed orange juice
1½ tablespoons superfine sugar
1 teaspoon cornstarch
2 tablespoons cold water
4 fresh peaches, seeded and thinly sliced

In a 2-quart saucepan, combine raspberries, orange juice and sugar; heat to boiling. In a small bowl, combine cornstarch and water; stir until smooth and gradually add to raspberry sauce. Boil one minute, stirring constantly until sauce thickens. Ladle sauce onto deep dessert plates. Arrange peaches symmetrically over sauce.

PER SERVING
Calories - 95
Protein - 1 g
Sodium - 0 mg
Carbohydrates - 24 g
Cholesterol - 0 mg
Total Fat - 0 g
Saturated Fat - 0 g
Dietary Fiber - 7 g

Cook's Suggestion: Substitute Save-the-Day Fresh Fruit Salad (page 299) for the peaches in this recipe. Arrange the fruit in symmetrical piles on a serving plate with a cup-size bowl of the raspberry sauce in the center. You'll love the presentation, and dipping the fruit in the sauce adds to the fun.

∎

Warm Caramel Pears   4 servings

Here's a dessert that will satisfy the cravings of even the most serious sweet tooth.

> *½ cup water*
> *½ cup brown sugar*
> *½ vanilla bean, 4 inches long*
> *4 ripe but firm Bosc or Anjou pears*
> *¼ cup caramel dessert topping*

In a small saucepan, combine water, brown sugar and vanilla bean. Simmer 5 minutes to dissolve sugar.

PER SERVING
Calories - 243
Protein - 1 g
Sodium - 111 mg
Carbohydrates - 60 g
Cholesterol - 0 g
Total Fat - 1 g
Saturated Fat - 0 g
Dietary Fiber - 4 g

Meanwhile, carefully peel pears and use an apple corer to remove cores. Slice a small piece off the bottom of each pear and stand in a shallow ovenproof casserole. Pour brown sugar mixture over top. Cover casserole with aluminum foil and bake at 425°F for 30 to 40 minutes, occasionally basting pears with syrup in casserole.

Serve pears on deep-lip dessert plates. Ladle sauce over the pears. Warm caramel topping and drizzle 1 tablespoon over each pear.

Poached Pears with Raspberry Sauce

4 servings

Another elegant dessert with only a trace of fat.

4 Bosc or Bartlett pears
2 cups dry white wine
½ vanilla bean, 4 inches long
1 10-ounce box frozen raspberries, thawed
3 to 4 tablespoons cornstarch
½ cup cold water
1 cup sliced fresh strawberries
1 cup fresh blueberries
fresh mint

Carefully peel pears, leaving stems intact; slice a small piece off the bottom of each pear. Pour wine into a deep saucepan; add vanilla bean. Bring to a boil, reduce heat to low and simmer 10 minutes. Stand pears upright in wine. Cover pan with lid; simmer 20 to 30 minutes, or until pears are tender when tested with a fork.

PER SERVING
Calories - 278
Protein - 2 g
Sodium - 13 mg
Carbohydrates - 50 g
Cholesterol - 0 mg
Total Fat - 1 g
Saturated Fat - 0 g
Dietary Fiber - 11 g

Heat raspberries in a saucepan. While berries are warming, use the back of a spoon to smooth them out. In a small bowl, mix cornstarch with cold water to make a smooth paste; gradually add to warm raspberries.

Divide raspberry sauce among 4 dessert plates. Stand pears upright in center of sauce. Drizzle each pear with 1 teaspoon of poaching liquid. Ring with fresh strawberries and blueberries. Garnish with mint. Serve warm.

Pears in Citrus Sauce   2 servings

You can feel good about this dessert. While you're enjoying something really sweet and tasty, you're getting a healthy serving of fiber right along with it.

> *2 firm ripe pears*
> *¼ cup freshly squeezed lemon juice*
> *1 cup white wine*
> *½ vanilla bean, 4 inches long*
> *¼ cup freshly squeezed orange juice*

Peel and quarter pears. Dip in lemon juice (reserve juice).

Bring wine and vanilla bean to a boil in a medium saucepan with a steamer insert. Arrange pears in basket; cover, reduce heat and steam 8 to 10 minutes, or until tender.

Remove pears to individual dessert bowls. Boil poaching liquid 2 to 3 minutes to reduce slightly. Mix 2 tablespoons of liquid with orange juice and reserved lemon juice. Pour sauce over pears. Serve warm.

PER SERVING
Calories - 166
Protein - 1 g
Sodium - 7 mg
Carbohydrates - 33 g
Cholesterol - 0 mg
Total Fat - 1 g
Saturated Fat - 0 g
Dietary Fiber - 6 g

Homemade Applesauce 8 servings

You'll never want to buy another jar of applesauce once you've tried this recipe. Sprinkling red-hot cinnamon candies on top adds a kid-friendly touch.

8 to 10 large tart cooking apples
1/2 cup water
1/2 cup granulated sugar
1 teaspoon ground cinnamon

Wash and peel apples; core and cut into quarters. Place apples in a medium saucepan, add water and bring to a boil. Reduce heat, cover and simmer 8 to 10 minutes, stirring frequently, until apples are barely tender. Add sugar and continue cooking about 10 minutes, or until apples are tender and sugar is dissolved. Remove from heat. Stir in cinnamon. Serve in bowls.

PER 1/2 CUP
Calories - 130
Protein - 0 g
Sodium - 1 mg
Carbohydrates - 34 g
Cholesterol - 0 mg
Total Fat - 0 g
Saturated Fat - 0 g
Dietary Fiber - 3 g

Sautéed Apples with Raisins

4 servings

1 tablespoon butter

3 tablespoons brown sugar

4 Gala, Honey Crisp or Granny Smith apples,
sliced into thin wedges

¼ cup raisins

½ cup apple cider

½ teaspoon ground cinnamon

Melt butter in a nonstick skillet. Stir in sugar. Add apples and top with raisins. Cook over medium-high heat 6 to 8 minutes. Pour in cider and mix in the cinnamon. Bring to a boil and cook 2 to 3 minutes, or until apples are tender. Serve on dessert plates.

PER SERVING
Calories - 170
Protein - 1 g
Sodium - 34 mg
Carbohydrates - 380 g
Cholesterol - 8 g
Total Fat - 3 g
Saturated Fat - 2 g
Dietary Fiber - 4 g

Apple Cranberry Crisp   12 servings

Butter-laden desserts are no longer part of a heart-healthy lifestyle.
Enjoy this updated version of an old favorite.

> *6 tart cooking apples (such as McIntosh, Macoun*
> *or Granny Smith), peeled and sliced*
> *1 tablespoon freshly squeezed lemon juice*
> *1 tablespoon freshly squeezed orange juice*
> *1 teaspoon lemon zest*
> *1 teaspoon orange zest*
> *¼ cup superfine granulated sugar*
> *1 teaspoon cinnamon*
> *⅔ cup dried cranberries*
>
> *TOPPING*
> *½ cup flour*
> *¾ cup steel-cut rolled oats*
> *⅓ cup brown sugar*
> *⅓ cup superfine granulated sugar*
> *½ cup tub-style safflower oil margarine*

In a medium bowl, toss the apples with lemon
juice, orange juice, lemon zest and orange
zest. Sprinkle with ¼ cup sugar and
cinnamon. Toss again. Add cranberries and
toss. Put mixture in a greased ovenproof
baking dish.

   In the bowl of an electric mixer, combine
flour, oats, brown sugar, superfine sugar and
margarine. Using the paddle attachment to the mixer, mix until
mostly smooth but still a little crumbly. Using your hands, crumble
mixture over apples. Bake at 350°F for 1 hour.

PER SERVING
Calories - 240
Protein - 3 g
Sodium - 105 mg
Carbohydrates - 40 g
Cholesterol - 0 mg
Total Fat - 9 g
Saturated Fat - 1 g
Dietary Fiber - 3 g

Baked Apples 4 servings

4 tart cooking apples (such as Granny Smith or McIntosh)
⅓ cup brown sugar
zest of 1 orange
1 tablespoon tub-style margarine
½ cup dried cranberries or raisins*
¾ cup water
2 tablespoons granulated sugar

Wash apples and remove core to ½ inch of the bottom. Arrange apples in an ovenproof baking dish. Using a fork, combine brown sugar, orange zest and margarine; stir in cranberries. Fill each apple center with the mixture.

In a small container, combine water and granulated sugar; pour around apples. Bake at 375°F for about 30 minutes, or until apples are tender but not mushy. Remove from oven and baste apples several times with pan juices. If juices are thin, remove apples to individual serving bowls and reduce pan juices before glazing. Serve warm with ice cream.

*Dried cranberries are plumper and sweeter than raisins. Kids aren't the only ones who love them.

PER SERVING
Calories - 257
Protein - 1 g
Sodium - 48 mg
Carbohydrates - 60 g
Cholesterol - 0 mg
Total Fat - 3 g
Saturated Fat - 1 g
Dietary Fiber - 5 g

Homemade Apple Pie 8 servings

1 9-inch double pie crust
6 cups pared and sliced tart apples
   (such as Granny Smith, McIntosh or Macoun)
2 tablespoons freshly squeezed lemon juice
¼ cup granulated sugar
½ teaspoon cinnamon
1 tablespoon all-purpose flour

Prepare the double pie crust according to package instructions. Line a 9-inch pie plate with bottom crust.

Toss apples with lemon juice. In a bowl, combine sugar, cinnamon and flour; mix with apples. Spoon into pie crust. Add top crust, leaving a 1-inch overhang; seal and flute edges with thumb. Cover edges of crust with a 3-inch strip of aluminum foil to prevent excessive browning. Cut slits in top crust so that steam can escape. Bake at 450°F for 10 minutes. Reduce heat to 375°F and bake 30 to 40 minutes longer, or until crust is brown and juices begin to bubble through slits in crust. Remove foil during last 15 minutes of baking.

PER SERVING
Calories - 296
Protein - 2 g
Sodium - 200 mg
Carbohydrates - 46 g
Cholesterol - 0 mg
Total Fat - 12 g
Saturated Fat - 2 g
Dietary Fiber - 2 g

Cook's Suggestion: If you want to save room for an apple pie dessert, start out with a lean dish like French Lentil Salad (page 291).

Almost Apple Pie Makes 10 cups

One day I bought the apples and made the filling, but then ran out of time and never made the crust. The filling was so delicious, I served it warm with a scoop of light vanilla ice cream. We didn't even miss the pie crust, and we saved a lot of fat and calories.

> *8 to 10 large cooking apples (such as Macoun or*
> *McIntosh, Granny Smith, Gala, or Honey Crisp)*
> *zest of 1 large orange*
> *juice of 2 large oranges*
> *zest of 1/2 lemon*
> *juice of 1 lemon*
> *1/4 cup brown sugar*
> *1/4 cup granulated sugar*
> *1 teaspoon cinnamon*

Put apples, orange zest, orange juice, lemon zest and lemon juice in a large saucepan; cover and simmer, stirring frequently, until apples are barely tender. Add sugars and continue cooking 25 to 30 minutes, or until mostly smooth. Stir in cinnamon.

PER 1/2 CUP
Calories - 54
Protein - 0 g
Sodium - 0 mg
Carbohydrates - 14 g
Cholesterol - 0 mg
Total Fat - 0 g
Saturated Fat - 0 g
Dietary Fiber - 2 g

Seasonal Berry Pie   8 servings

1 9-inch double pastry crust
1 tablespoon all-purpose flour
½ cup granulated sugar
1 teaspoon salt
4 cups fresh blackberries, strawberries
   or raspberries
1 teaspoon freshly squeezed lemon juice

Prepare double pastry crust according to package directions. Line a 9-inch pie plate with bottom crust.

Mix together flour, sugar and salt; sprinkle a quarter of the mixture on bottom crust. Coat berries with lemon juice and toss with remaining sugar mixture; spoon onto crust.

Add top crust, leaving a 1-inch overhang; seal and flute edges with thumb. Cover edges with a 3-inch strip of aluminum foil to prevent excessive browning. Cut slits in top crust so that steam can escape. Bake at 450°F for 15 minutes. Reduce heat to 350°F and continue baking 20 to 25 minutes, or until crust is brown and juices begin to bubble through slits in crust. Remove foil during last 15 minutes of baking.

PER SERVING
Calories - 266
Protein - 3 g
Sodium - 234 mg
Carbohydrates - 41 g
Cholesterol - 0 g
Total Fat - 10 g
Saturated Fat - 1 g
Dietary Fiber - 0 g

Strawberry Rhubarb Pie   8 servings

Pie is a special occasion food, not an everyday choice. I like to serve this one to friends at the end of a light dinner.

1 9-inch double pastry crust
½ cup sugar
¼ cup all-purpose flour
¼ teaspoon salt
¼ teaspoon nutmeg
3 cups sliced rhubarb stalks, all leaves removed
1 cup sliced strawberries

Prepare double pastry crust according to package directions. Line a 9-inch pie plate with bottom crust.

    Combine sugar, flour, salt, and nutmeg. Add rhubarb and strawberries. Toss to coat. Let stand 20 minutes. Spoon into pie crust. Add top crust. Flute edges. Prick. Bake at 400°F for 40 to 45 minutes, or until crust is brown and juices begin to bubble through slits in crust.

PER SERVING
Calories - 258
Protein - 3 g
Sodium - 269 mg
Carbohydrates - 39 g
Cholesterol - 0 mg
Total Fat - 10 g
Saturated Fat - 1 g
Dietary Fiber - 0 g

Cook's Suggestion: When the berries and rhubarb are at their peak, serve this pie with a light dish like Salade Niçoise (page 298).

Pumpkin Pie   8 servings

The key to allowing yourself a slice of pumpkin pie on Thanksgiving is to keep the portions small and replace regular evaporated milk with evaporated skim milk.

> 1 9-inch pie shell
> 1 1-pound can pumpkin
> ¾ cup firmly packed brown sugar
> 3 lightly beaten eggs
> ¼ teaspoon salt
> 1 teaspoon cinnamon
> ½ teaspoon ground ginger
> ½ teaspoon nutmeg
> ¼ teaspoon ground cloves
> 1 12-ounce can evaporated skim milk

Prepare pie shell according to package instructions. Line a 9-inch pie plate with crust. Trim edges, leaving a 1-inch overhang; flute edges with thumb.

Measure remaining ingredients into a medium mixing bowl. Mix with a wire whisk or a spoon until well blended. Pour into pie shell. Cover edges of crust with a 3-inch strip of aluminum foil to prevent excessive browning. Bake at 400°F for 50 minutes, or until knife inserted in center of pie comes out clean.

PER SERVING
Calories - 253
Protein - 8 g
Sodium - 279 mg
Carbohydrates - 35 g
Cholesterol - 72 mg
Total Fat - 11 g
Saturated Fat - 3 g
Dietary Fiber - 2 g

Angel Food Cake with Strawberries

12 servings

It's not strawberry "shortcake" without a dollop of whipped cream. We suggest *only* a dollop to keep this dessert almost fat-free.

1 box angel food cake mix
3 cups crushed fresh strawberries
3 cups sliced fresh strawberries
12 tablespoons whipped cream
12 whole berries for garnish

Prepare angel food cake according to package instructions. Cool thoroughly and cut into 12 slices. Top each slice with ¼ cup crushed berries, ¼ cup sliced berries, 1 tablespoon of whipped cream and one whole berry for garnish.

PER SERVING
Calories - 168
Protein - 4 g
Sodium - 257 mg
Carbohydrates - 37 g
Cholesterol - 2 mg
Total Fat - 1 g
Saturated Fat - 0 g
Dietary Fiber - 3 g

Variation: Use mini angel food cake pans, available at kitchen stores. Each muffin-type pan makes 6 mini angel food cakes.

Angel Food Cake with
Seven-Minute Icing 12 servings

This is the birthday cake of choice at our house because it's so
low in fat.

1 box angel food cake mix

FROSTING
2 egg whites
1¼ cups granulated sugar
dash salt
½ cup water
¼ teaspoon cream of tartar
1 teaspoon vanilla extract

Prepare angel food cake according to package
instructions. Let cake cool.

In the bottom of a double boiler, bring
2 cups water to a boil. In the top of the
double boiler, combine egg whites, sugar,
salt, ½ cup water and cream of tartar; beat
1 minute. Place over boiling water. Using
highest speed of electric mixer, beat
constantly for 5 to 7 minutes, or until frosting stands in stiff peaks.
Remove from heat. Stir in vanilla. Spread frosting over top and sides
of cake.

PER SERVING
Calories - 214
Protein - 4 g
Sodium - 224 mg
Carbohydrates - 51 g
Cholesterol - 0 mg
Total Fat - 0 g
Saturated Fat - 0 g
Dietary Fiber - 0 g

CHOCOLATE GLAZE. In a small bowl, combine 1 cup confectioners'
sugar, sifted, and 2 tablespoons cold nonfat milk; stir until smooth.
Add 1 teaspoon unsweetened cocoa powder; stir until smooth.
Spread glaze over top of cake and allow to drizzle down sides.
(Each serving has approximately 170 calories and 172 milligrams
sodium; other amounts remain the same.)

ORANGE GLAZE. In a small bowl, combine 1 cup confectioners' sugar, 2 tablespoons chilled fresh orange juice and 1 tablespoon orange zest; stir until smooth. Spread glaze over top of cake and allow to drizzle down sides. (Each serving has approximately 170 calories and 170 milligrams sodium; other amounts remain the same.)

■

Granita de Caffé con Pane   <small>6 servings</small>

The next best thing to sitting in an Italian espresso bar on a hot summer day . . .

> *½ cup water*
> *½ cup superfine sugar*
> *2 cups brewed espresso*
> *½ teaspoon vanilla*
> *¼ cup whipped cream (optional)*

Combine water and sugar in a medium saucepan. Bring to a boil over medium heat, stirring frequently. Boil 5 minutes without stirring; remove from heat and stir again. Cool completely. Add espresso and vanilla; stir thoroughly.

PER SERVING
Calories - 76
Protein - 0 g
Sodium - 10 mg
Carbohydrates - 18 g
Cholesterol - 2 mg
Total Fat - 1 g
Saturated Fat - 0 g
Dietary Fiber - 0 g

Pour mixture into a glass casserole and place in freezer for 30 minutes. Remove from freezer and stir with a fork to break up crystals. Return to freezer for 30 minutes. Remove from freezer and again break up crystals by stirring with a fork. Repeat three or four times. Cover with plastic wrap and store in freezer for up to 48 hours.

When ready to serve, break up crystals with a fork. Spoon ½ cup of the mixture into each of 6 champagne glasses. Top with a dollop of whipped cream.

Cobbler Dough 8 servings

1 cup all-purpose flour, sifted
1/2 teaspoon salt
1 1/2 teaspoons baking powder
1/3 cup nonfat milk
3 tablespoons safflower oil

Combine flour, salt and baking powder.
Mix milk with oil; add to flour mixture.
Using a fork or pastry blender, work dough
into a ball.

PER SERVING
Calories - 106
Protein - 2 g
Sodium - 139 mg
Carbohydrates - 13 g
Cholesterol - 0 mg
Total Fat - 5 g
Saturated Fat - 0 g
Dietary Fiber - 1 g

Very Berry Cobbler 8 servings

Keep some berries in the freezer, and this delicious cobbler can come
together in minutes—all year round.

1/2 cup cold water
2 tablespoons cornstarch
1/2 cup granulated sugar
6 cups strawberries, raspberries, blueberries or blackberries
1 recipe Cobbler Dough (above)

In a medium saucepan, combine water,
cornstarch and sugar; bring to a boil over
high heat. Cook 1 minute, stirring constantly.
Remove from heat and gently stir in berries.
Pour into a 9-inch pie plate and drop
spoonfuls of dough onto fruit. Bake at 425°F
for 20 to 25 minutes, or until topping is lightly
browned.

PER SERVING
Calories - 179
Protein - 2 g
Sodium - 141 mg
Carbohydrates - 31 g
Cholesterol - 0 mg
Total Fat - 5 g
Saturated Fat - 0 g
Dietary Fiber - 2 g

Rhubarb Cobbler   8 servings

There's no "top" to a cobbler, the way there is to a pie, so the fat is cut in half.

6 cups sliced rhubarb stalks,
*   all leaves removed*
½ cup sugar
2 to 3 tablespoons water
2 tablespoons cornstarch
1 recipe Cobbler Dough (page 506)

In a medium saucepan, combine rhubarb, sugar, water and cornstarch. Bring to a boil; cook 1 minute, stirring constantly. Pour into a 9-inch pie plate and drop spoonfuls of dough onto fruit. Bake at 425°F for 25 to 30 minutes, or until topping is lightly browned. Serve warm from the oven.

PER SERVING
Calories - 170
Protein - 2 g
Sodium - 140 mg
Carbohydrates - 29 g
Cholesterol - 0 mg
Total Fat - 5 g
Saturated Fat - 0 g
Dietary Fiber - 2 g

Variation: To make a strawberry rhubarb cobbler, use 3 cups of rhubarb and 1 cup of sliced strawberries.

Cookbook

Menus

Planning Ahead

The key to success is planning ahead. Eating healthfully requires a change in habits as well as menus, so it's vitally important to spend a few minutes each week making a meal plan. Take into account the menu, the beverages, the company, preparation time and the schedules of family members.

It also helps to keep a list of meals that can be prepared quickly. Working late on a deadline, driving kids in a soccer carpool, running out of time to shop and cook . . . these realities of life can undo the best intentions. If it's six P.M. and you're just arriving at the food store, your planned dinner may no longer be feasible. You need a fallback. Find three favorite dinners that you know you can get on the table quickly and keep the ingredients on hand. Tape a copy of the recipes and menus on the inside of your cupboard door and put another in your car, purse or briefcase, so you can make the right shopping choices. You'll be able to stick to a plan rather than buy on a whim, as often happens when you're hungry as you shop. It's a simple alternative and is much more healthful than picking up fast food or cooking hot dogs. My six favorite fallback menus are Pasta with 20-Minute Marinara Sauce; Chicken Cutlets and Mac and Peas; Stir-Fried Scallops and Prawns; Three-Bean Chili; Grilled Steak and Onion Salad; and Linguine with Shrimp. The last two suggestions even work for company.

In the menus that follow, dishes preceded by asterisks are included in the recipe section.

Down-Home Cooking

Pasta with *20-Minute Marinara Sauce or
*Five-Star Marinara Sauce
*Field Greens with Chickpeas and Tomatoes
*Sautéed Spinach with Pine Nuts

Both pasta sauces are delicious, but the 20-Minute Marinara Sauce takes a third of the time to prepare.

*French Lentil Soup
*Watercress and Radicchio Salad
Seasonal Fruit

*Grilled Salmon and Shiitake Mushrooms
*Wild Rice, Brown Rice and Barley
*Grilled Parmesan Tomatoes
*Spinach, Strawberry and Walnut Salad

Miso Soup
*Asian Stir-Fry with Noodles
*Fresh Fruit in a Pineapple

*Tortilla Soup
Tricolored Melon Ball Salad:
Watermelon, Cantaloupe, Honeydew

*SEA BASS WITH SUN-DRIED TOMATO CRUST
*ROAST FINGERLING POTATOES
*ROASTED BABY VEGETABLES
*FRESH PEACHES IN WARM RASPBERRY SAUCE

*ROAST CHICKEN
*RICE AND BEANS
*SPINACH, STRAWBERRY AND WALNUT SALAD

*VEGGIE CHILI
*HOMEMADE TORTILLA CHIPS
*PICO DE GALLO
*SPINACH AND TANGERINE SALAD

*SPLIT-PEA SOUP
*ROASTED GARLIC BREAD
*WARM PEAR SALAD WITH BLUE CHEESE AND PECANS

*BAKED SALMON
*ROASTED ROOT VEGETABLES
*NEW YEAR'S EVE SALAD

*40 CLOVES OF GARLIC CHICKEN
*TUSCAN BEAN SALAD
RUSTIC BREAD
WATERMELON, GRAPES AND CHERRIES

Quick-Fix Dinners

ROASTED TOMATO SOUP
*GRILLED STEAK AND ONION SALAD
CRUSTY WHOLE-GRAIN BREAD
SLICED FRESH PEARS OR MELON

*CITRUS MARINATED CHICKEN
*COUSCOUS SALAD
*ROASTED CARROTS OR *ROASTED ASPARAGUS WITH PARMESAN
SEASONAL FRUIT

*GRILLED FISH TACOS
REFRIED NONFAT BEANS OR STEAMED BLACK OR PINTO BEANS
FRUIT SALAD OF ORANGES, BANANAS, PINEAPPLE AND KIWI

*Luckily, stores now carry refried beans made without lard or animal fats.
Read labels to make the healthiest choices.*

*LINGUINE WITH SHRIMP
*CHRISTMAS SALAD
*GRILLED PARMESAN ZUCCHINI

---

*ASIAN GRILLED FISH
STIR-FRIED VEGETABLES
SLICED ASIAN PEAR

---

*SNAPPER AND CAPERS
*POLENTA WITH PARMESAN
*SAUTÉED SPINACH WITH GARLIC
*FIELD GREENS WITH BALSAMIC DRESSING

---

*ARTICHOKE FRITTATA
SLICED HEIRLOOM TOMATOES
*COUNTRY FRIED POTATOES WITH GARLIC
CITRUS SALAD

---

*GRILLED CHICKEN BURGERS
*JUMBO OVEN FRIES
DARK GREEN LETTUCE, TOMATO, ONION, DILL PICKLE, CUCUMBER, MUSTARD
WATERMELON WEDGES

---

*SAUTÉED SHRIMP
*WILD RICE WITH MUSHROOMS
*TOMATO, FRESH MOZZARELLA AND BASIL SALAD
SEASONAL FRUIT

Dinner with Friends

---

*STIR-FRIED SCALLOPS AND PRAWNS

*PASTA WITH PESTO AND TOMATOES

*PAN-STEAMED ASPARAGUS

*VERY BERRY COBBLER

MELON AND PROSCIUTTO

*JUST GRILLED SALMON

*PASTA AND SUN-DRIED TOMATOES

BROCCOLINI

*ANGEL FOOD CAKE WITH STRAWBERRIES

---

*ROAST LEG OF LAMB

*OLIVE BREAD SALAD

*GREEN BEANS WITH ARTICHOKES AND RED PEPPERS

*SUMMER FRUIT WITH LEMON ICE

The combined fat content for this meal is higher than most. Make lower-fat choices throughout the day.

---

*ANTIPASTO

SOUTH OF THE BORDER STEW

CRUSTY BREAD FOR DIPPING

SEASONAL FRUIT

---

*Tortilla Soup
*Pan-Seared Tuna
Mexicali Corn Salad
*Fresh Dipped Strawberries

*Grilled Swordfish with Olives and Capers
*Grilled Vegetables
*Just Long-Grain Rice
Seasonal Fruit

*Rotelle with Prawns, Tomatoes and Olives
Fresh Asparagus
Rustic Bread
Seasonal Fruit or *Seasonal Berry Pie or
*Very Berry Cobbler

Corn Chowder
Caesar Salad
Cracked Crab with Spicy Sauce
*Seasonal Berry Pie

*Grilled Rosemary Veal Chops or
Lemon-Garlic Veal Roast
*Mostaccioli with Fresh Tomatoes and Basil
Prawns on Endive with Avocado
Seasonal Fruit

Comfort Foods

---

*Southern Fried Chicken

*Yukon Gold Smashed Potatoes

*Green Beans with Shallots

*Baked Apples

---

*Chicken Cutlets

*Mac and Peas

*Four-Bean Salad

---

*Mac and Cheese

*Raw Veggies in a Basket

*Save-the-Day Fresh Fruit Salad

---

*Old-Fashioned Meat Loaf

Corn on the Cob

Sugar Snap Peas

*Jalapeño-Stuffed Potatoes

Sliced Fresh Peaches with Blueberries

---

*Tuna Casserole

Broccolini

Baby Carrots

Apples, Pears, Red Grapes

Weekend Cooking, Weekday Eating

---

*SPAGHETTI WITH MEATBALLS

MIXED GREEN SALAD WITH CUCUMBERS AND TOMATOES

*ITALIAN VINAIGRETTE

Slice leftover meatballs for meatball sandwiches made with rustic bread. Serve leftover sauce without the meatballs over penne on another pasta night; accompany with a big mixed green salad.

---

*ROAST PORK TENDERLOIN WITH SAUERKRAUT

*ROAST RED POTATOES

*GREEN BEANS WITH ARTICHOKES AND RED PEPPERS

*HOMEMADE APPLESAUCE

---

*COUNTRY-STYLE CHICKEN NOODLE SOUP

*ROMAINE, EDAMAME AND FETA CHEESE

*SAUTÉED APPLES WITH RAISINS

It's worth the effort. A soup is only as good as its broth. Make Homemade Chicken Broth on a Saturday. Skim the fat from the refrigerated broth and make Country Style Soup on a Sunday.

Freeze any remaining broth for Get-Well Soup for a rainy day.

---

*Roast Breast of Turkey

*Couscous with Cranberries and Almonds

*Spinach with Tomatoes, Blue Cheese and Pecans

---

*Minestrone

*Caprese Salad on Rustic Bread

*Apple Cranberry Crisp

Leftover minestrone gets a whole new look when served alongside our All-in-One Pasta Salad and some sliced seasonal fruit.

General Index

G

Recipe Index

Acknowledgments

It takes a team of dedicated people to put a book together. In particular, we are grateful to the numerous medical professionals who gave of their time and expertise, providing information, insight and valuable suggestions.

We especially want to thank Bev Utt, M.S., M.P.H., C.D., and Deborah Robinette, M.A., R.D., C.D., whose expertise and personal commitment to healthy eating were invaluable. Both made important contributions to the text as well as the recipes. Bev analyzed each recipe for the nutritional data, and her personal motto—"where healthy meals meet good taste"—kept us focused on our approach. Each of our menus was analyzed by Deborah to ensure that foods were paired and partnered for maximum nutritional content. Her insight into making sure our recipes and menus were not only heart-healthy but in keeping with today's busy lifestyles reinforced our belief that the road to a healthy heart does indeed run through the kitchen.

We are forever grateful to Lita Dawn Stanton for her expertise in the design of the nutritional charts, the initial layout and recipe design, as well as her tireless inputting of recipes into the computer. Most important, we are grateful for her friendship and belief in our work throughout the writing process.

Our heartfelt thanks to our family and friends, who tirelessly support us on the road to heart health. Deepest thanks to our mothers, Mary Petri and Mary Piscatella, who taught us from childhood about the importance of good nutrition and balanced meals. They passed down much more than favorite recipes; they taught us to find the positive even in adversity.

And finally, our thanks to our Workman family, with whom we have worked for 23 years. Their belief in our work and constant support transcend a business relationship. Our most sincere thanks to Susan Bolotin, Lynn Strong, Megan Nicolay and Mary Ann McLaughlin for their fine editorial hands, and most especially their patience; to Kim Hicks and Sarah O'Leary for their undying dedication in publicizing the book; to Paul Gamarello for his skillful use of graphics; to Katie Workman, Jenny Mandel and Lily Tilton for their creative approach to sales and for listening to our unending thoughts on marketing; and most especially to Peter Workman, for his wisdom, clear vision, enduring faith in our work and our long years of friendship.